COTTON RESEARCH

Edited by **Ibrokhim Y. Abdurakhmonov**

Cotton Research
http://dx.doi.org/10.5772/61914
Edited by Ibrokhim Y. Abdurakhmonov

Contributors

Ademar Pereira Serra, Yali Zhang, Xiaoping Yi, Wangfeng Zhang, Wah Soon Chow, Yuanyuan Hu, Chao Zhang, Dongxia Zhan, Yuksel Bolek, Adem Bardak, Khezir Hayat, Muhammad Tehseen Azhar, Franco Ferrero, Gianluca Migliavacca, Monica Periolatto, Marina Sanamyan, Makamov Abdusalom, Bobokhucshaev Shuhrat, Buriev Zabardasdt, Sukumar Saha, Guoqiang Yin, Hangbo Yue, Yingde Cui, Seloame Tatu Nyaku, Yonathan Tilahun, Kathy Lawrence, Abreotta Williams, Govind Sharma, Venkateswara Sripathi, Issa Mousa El Nahhal, Abdelraouf Elmanama, Nadia Amara, Andrew Price, Mv Venugopalan, Abdul Qayyum Rao, Muhammad Azmat Ullah Khan, Kamran Shehzad Bajwa, Tahir Iqbal, Muhammad Azam, Adnan Iqbal, Ahmad Ali Shahid, Tayyab Husnain, Hezhong Dong, Jianlong Dai, Ibrokhim Abdurakhmonov

Published by InTech

Janeza Trdine 9, 51000 Rijeka, Croatia

Publishing Process Manager Romina Rovan

Technical Editor SPi Global

Cover InTech Design team

First published November, 2016

Printed in Croatia

Additional hard copies can be obtained from orders@intechopen.com

Cotton Research, Edited by Ibrokhim Y. Abdurakhmonov

p. cm.

Print ISBN 978-953-51-2736-9
Online ISBN 978-953-51-2737-6

For EU product safety concerns:
IN TECH d.o.o., Prolaz Marije Krucifikse Kozulić 3, 51000 Rijeka, Croatia,
info@intechopen.com or visit our website at intechopen.com.

Meet the editor

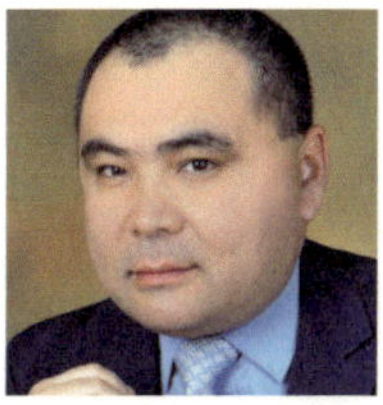

Ibrokhim Y. Abdurakhmonov received his BS degree (1997) in *biotechnology* from the National University of Uzbekistan, MS degree in *plant breeding* (2001) from Texas A&M University of the USA, PhD degree (2002) in *molecular genetics*, Doctor of Science degree (2009) in *genetics*, and full professorship (2011) in *molecular genetics and molecular biotechnology* from the Institute of Genetics and Plant Experimental Biology, Academy of Sciences of Uzbekistan. He founded (2012) and is currently leading the Center of Genomics and Bioinformatics of Uzbekistan. He serves as an associate editor/editorial board member of several international and national journals in plant sciences. He received government awards—2010 chest badge "Sign of Uzbekistan," 2010 TWAS prize, and "ICAC Cotton Researcher of the Year 2013" for his outstanding contribution to cotton genomics and biotechnology. He was elected as The World Academy of Sciences (TWAS) fellow (2014) on *agricultural science* and as a cochair/chair of "Comparative Genomics and Bioinformatics" workgroup (2015) of the International Cotton Genome Initiative (ICGI).

Contents

Foreword

Cotton Research is edited by Dr. Ibrokhim Y. Abdurakhmonov, a young scientist who has gained an excellent international research reputation. He has received many awards for his innovative research in cotton breeding. The book describes the status of the current research in cotton from a worldwide perspective. The authors for the individual chapters are primarily from outside the United States. Individual chapter authors are from Australia, Brazil, China, Ghana, India, Iran, Italy, Pakistan, Palestine, Tunisia, Turkey, the United States, and Uzbekistan. Collectively, they present a picture of cotton research around the world. Not all topics of interest to cotton scientists are included in the book chapters, but they do represent some current highlights of research that has been conducted in cotton. What the book does accomplish is to provide the reader with a current view of research scientists primarily working in major cotton-producing countries. This is an important perspective, as cotton is a world commodity and these international authors collectively describe the current status of cotton research in their countries as well as including relevant references from elsewhere. The book is not intended to be a comprehensive review of all cotton research but is composed of selected topics across the broad areas of production and utilization of cotton. It will be useful to practicing researchers, academics, PhD students, and those who want to understand the breadth of the cotton research community on a worldwide basis. It emphasizes some of the latest technologies and potential research approaches in cotton. It serves a worthwhile objective, by providing selected views of research in major cotton laboratories around the world.

Johnie N. Jenkins
Research Leader
Genetics and Sustainable Agriculture Research Unit
ARS, USDA
Mississippi State, MS

Preface

Scientific research on *Gossypium* genus and its products is important because cotton is a unique natural fiber producing cash crop. It brings significant worldwide economic impact with a large clothing and household usage, followed by production of industrial items that account for many thousands of bales. Besides its fiber, cotton is valued for its cotton seed products (meal and hulls), which are used for livestock feed; people use cotton seed oil as an ingredient in food products as well as a premium cooking oil and salad dressing. Furthermore, the cotton stalks and leaves are used as an organic matter to enrich soil as well as to obtain biogas and/or biofertilizers and firewood for primary energy in cooking process in rural areas.

Cotton fiber has been utilized by humans for more than seven thousand years, and cotton started to be grown for its fiber around three thousand years ago. Over this long historic period, up to date, cotton investigations have been timely developed and advanced from simple utilization of its fiber/products from naturally grown perennial shrubs to unintentional collection of seeds and plant selection, leading to domesticated, annually propagated primitive genotypes. These historic advances, efforts, and demand for cotton products resulted in worldwide cultivation of cotton in 32–36 million-hectare area in over 80 countries of the world, spreading cotton to virtually all tropical and northernmost agricultural latitudes as Uzbekistan.

Cotton research is progressively advanced over the past 100 years with the increased demand for cotton products, introduction and replacement of diploid cultivars with more productive allotetraploid varieties, development of germplasm resources, and understanding and advances on technologies in breeding/genetics, agronomy and crop management, and fiber and textile processing. This progress resulted in the development of novel cotton cultivars with high yield, early maturity, and superior fiber quality. For the past 30 years, scientific advances on genetics, breeding, agronomy, molecular biology and genetic engineering, and decoding of cotton genomes, as well as developments made in ginning, fiber processing, fiber dyeing, and textile technologies, have greatly accelerated cotton research. These advances have helped to address key issues of cotton production and farming although negative genetic correlations between the key fiber and agronomic traits, as well as a low genetic diversity among cultivars, continue to be a major limiting factor of cotton improvement. There is an increasing need for more feed and food products and demand for better-quality natural fiber production to make cotton completive over the man-made synthetic fibers.

Therefore, the objective of this *Cotton Research* book, written by the international team of cotton researchers, is to provide the latest updates on cotton research. This book is compiled into 13 chapters including an introductory chapter that describe and discuss cotton research structures; advances on cotton genetics, variety development, and molecular breeding; and latest developments on cotton transformation, agronomy, physiology, and crop management technologies, covering key traits for sustainable cotton production. The chapters also cover cotton fiber processing, textile, and other by-product research updates. I hope all chapter materials of this book should be useful for university students, life science researchers, and interested readers.

I am thankful for the InTech book department and its publication manager Ms. Romina Rovan for the opportunity to work on this book project and help with my editorial duties. All authors of the book chapters are gratefully acknowledged for their valuable chapter contributions and cooperations.

Ibrokhim Y. Abdurakhmonov
Center of Genomics and Bioinformatics
Academy of Sciences of Uzbekistan
Tashkent, Uzbekistan

Section 1

Introductory

Chapter 1

Introductory Chapter: Cotton Research Highlights

Ibrokhim Y. Abdurakhmonov

Additional information is available at the end of the chapter

http://dx.doi.org/10.5772/65456

1. Introduction

Cotton, derived from the Arabic word 'quotn' [1], belongs to *Gossypium* genus, which was also derived from the Arabic word 'goz', meaning a soft substance [2]. Cotton is a unique natural fiber producing most common fiber crop of the world, which provides humanity with cloth and vegetable oil, medicinal compounds, meal and hull for livestock feed, energy sources, organic matter to enrich soil, and industrial lubricants [3]. The genus *Gossypium* includes five 52-chromosome species (2n=4x=52) that arose some 1–2 million years ago [4–6] through allotetraploidization between the extinct representatives of A and D cotton genomes. Current representatives of putative ancestor-like A-genome species (2n=2x=26) are *G. herbaceum* (A_1) and *G. arboretum* (A_2), referred as the Old World cottons, whereas a putative ancestor like 'D-genome' species is *G. raimondii* (D_5) Ulbrich (2n=2x=26), referred as the New World cottons. There are five allotetraploids and 45 extant diploid cotton species that are classified into eight genomic groups (A to G, and K) [4]. The two allotetraploid cultivated species include the *G. hirsutum* $[AD]_1$ and *G. barbadense* $[AD]_2$. The remaining three wild tetraploids, *G. tomentosum* $[AD]_3$, *G. mustelinum* $[AD]_4$, and *G. darwinii* $[AD]_5$, are endemic to the Hawaii, Brazil, and Galapagos Islands, respectively.

Based on archeological evidence, humans utilized cotton fiber from at least more than four to seven thousand years ago, and cotton started to be grown as a fiber crop around three thousand years ago [1, 7]. Demands for natural fiber and cotton products had historically developed that advanced cotton research for the past century. Progressive scientific advances on cotton biotechnology and decoding of cotton genomes have resulted in the development of novel cotton cultivars with high yield, early maturity, improved resistance to pests, and superior fiber quality; however, a negative correlation between fiber traits and yield components/ maturity as well as genetic "bottlenecks" in cultivar germplasm still hinders to overcome conventionally longstanding problems of simultaneous yield and quality improvements in cotton [3, 8].

Cotton is grown on around 32–36 million-hectares area of tropical and northernmost agricultural latitudes in over 80 countries of the world [8, 9] to fulfill the current global needs of humanity for the natural fiber. For the past decade, however, global cotton production, demand, and market significantly fluctuated that caused a pressure on farmers, consumers, and traders. Area for cotton farming decreased by 9% to 31.1 million hectares leading to a total annual production of 21.74 million metric tons (MMTs) in 2015/16 [10]. The world average yield was 699 kg per hectare in 2015/16 and also decreased by 9% compared to previous season although the average yield is expected to increase to 735 kg/ha that would lead to increase a total world production by ~5% to 22.7 million tons in 2016/17 [10]. Similarly, world cotton consumption saw its 'ups' and 'downs' from 2007 and has been on decline since 2011 (~23 MMT) [11]; it has been 23.7 million tons in 2015/16 [12] with a similar expected consumption of 23.7 million tons in 2016/17 [10]. In other words, for the past two years world cotton production did not match world consumption of cotton, making the deficit to be covered from cotton stocks [13].

The significant fluctuations in world cotton production and consumption and decreasing yields require world cotton science to pursue new research directions and develop innovations to substantially increase and stabilize cotton production worldwide [14, 15]. In that, innovations on increasing yield with the improvements of fiber quality without affecting the maturity and other key agronomic traits are the key challenges faced by the cotton research community. In parallel, due to global climate change, increased heat and drought stress and biosecurity issues, it is demanded to improve drought, salt and heat tolerance traits as well as to increase the resistance characteristics of cotton cultivars to better respond to existing and emerging bacterial, fungal, and insect pest infestations [15, 16]. At the same time, increasing human population highlights an urgent need for investigations on cottonseed feed and food product qualities as well as cottonseed marketing, which moved cotton research and its increased financing in this direction for the past decade period [17]. Moreover, a continuous lower price of synthetic fibers compared to cotton prompts researchers to make cotton competitive with manmade fibers through improvements in quality, while being friendly to the environment [3, 15, 16].

2. Cotton research updates and advances

Cotton research has witnessed many progressive developments over the past half a century to address the above-mentioned challenges and limitations, and cotton researchers worldwide have initiated and performed largely coordinated research projects in every aspects of cotton sciences. These efforts have greatly accelerated cotton research worldwide and helped to address the key issues of cotton production and farming [7, 14].

Some of the best examples of these progressive developments of cotton research can be the worldwide collection, maintenance, and inventory efforts of 53,000 [18] to 63,946 [14, 19] world cotton germplasm resources preserved in major cotton-growing countries. Cotton research community has extensively developed cotton genetic mapping population resources, and characterized large sets of DNA-based molecular markers such as simple sequence repeats (SSRs) and other restriction site-derived polymorphisms [20]. Researchers have widely and successfully applied molecular marker technology [21] to create densely covered genetic linkage maps of cotton genome(s) using various mapping populations. Scientists also succeeded to characterize cotton germplasm resources using both traditional quantitative trait loci (QTL) and modern linkage disequilibrium (LD)-based association mapping strategies [20–23]. Furthermore, cotton researchers have successfully developed a SNP marker system, and with the emergence and application of high-throughput next generation sequencing (NGS) technologies, a large number of SNPs were developed and made available for cotton research and breeding [24–27]. These advances provided an opportunity of shifting molecular marker applications from restriction enzyme or SSR-based characterizations toward SNP-based analyses and high-throughput genotyping by sequencing (GBS)-based mapping methods [14, 24].

As a result of advances on molecular markers and genetic mapping of important cotton traits, cotton breeding research has enriched with molecular breeding techniques and "breeding by design" approaches such as modern marker assisted-selection and genomic selection. This has not only accelerated the development of superior cotton cultivars with reduced cost and time, but it also helped in widening the "conventionally-narrow" genetic base of novel cultivars via introducing 'yet-unexploited' genetic diversities from cotton germplasm resources [8, 14, 20–23, 28]. Further, molecular marker technology has helped to establish and genetically differentiate 13 homeologous chromosome pairs accelerating cotton cytogenetics and genetics studies [29]. Detailed cytogenetic studies and the characterization of aneuploidy and translocation lines identified almost all 26 chromosomes of allotetraploid cottons and provided an innovative way of replacing the *G. hirsutum* (referred to as Upland cotton [8]) chromosome pairs with corresponding chromosome pairs of other cultivated and wild allotetraploids such as *G. barbadense, G. mustelinum,* and *G. tomentosum*. This effort created unique sets of chromosome substitution backcross (CS-B) cotton germplasm resources of Upland cottons that are widely used as a novel direction in cotton improvement, supplementing and enhancing conventional cotton breeding programs worldwide [30, 31].

Development of cotton genetic engineering (GE) and somatic embryogenesis research have further revolutionized cotton science and production for the past 30-year period, resulting in the development and commercialization of "biotech" cotton varieties of insect-pest and herbicide tolerance traits [7]. GE research with transgenic, cisgenic, and intergenic approaches and its integration with traditional and modern breeding methods such as backcross, gene staking, and forward breeding [32] have helped and carry a great promise to boost the yield and quality of cotton, which undoubtedly opened a new era for cotton production worldwide [3, 7].

Most revolutionizing efforts and achievements of cotton research for the past 10 years, however, were the successful completion and assembly of whole genomes of the two diploids (D_5 and A_2 genomes) [33–35] and two widely cultivated Upland (*G. hirsutum)* [36, 37] and Sea Island allotetraploid cotton genomes (*G. barbadense*) [38]. These achievements have greatly accelerated current cotton research programs and undoubtedly will foster the exploitation of genetic signatures behind the key cotton traits, helping to overcome the above-mentioned negative correlation and narrow diversity obstacles through a 'skilled' utilization and introduction of the complex effect genetic signatures. For example, due to understanding cotton genomes and genetic signatures, cotton researchers have discovered the key genes conditioning major fiber quality traits of cotton, where the improvement of key characteristics of fiber quality is the most priority task of cotton biotechnology worldwide [15, 20]. As an example, these findings include but not limited to the characterization and biotechnological utilization of (1) *GhMYB2A* and *GhMYB2D* genes and its trans-acting regulatory miR828 and miR858 signatures in trichome and fiber development [39]; (2) cotton phytochrome gene family and its RNA interference (RNAi) in simultaneous improvement of major fiber characteristics and several important agronomic traits of Upland cotton [40]; and (3) phytosulfokine-α (PSK-α) signaling genes, affecting cotton fiber development through the regulation of the respiratory electron-transport chain and reactive oxygen species [41]. These advances, with many other seminal discoveries [7] that could not be covered in this short introduction chapter, provided novel biotechnological strategies to improve complex cotton fiber quality traits and paved the ways and opportunities to compete with man-made fibers.

The characterization of small RNA and microRNA world of cotton, including long noncoding natural antisense transcript (lncNAT) and long noncoding RNA (lncRNA) loci in *Gossypium* spp [15] and their functional associations with the genetic and epigenetic regulation of many complex traits of cotton were the other seminal achievements of cotton research in the past decade. "All of these natural miRNAs, lncRNA, and lncNAT are the key candidate loci to elucidate many challenging functional questions in cotton that will serve as a base for designing novel RNAi approaches and studies in the near future" [15]. These innovative developments in cotton research have provided "golden" opportunities for improving fiber quality parameters, oil and seed quality traits, cotton fertility and embryogenesis, pests, viral, bacterial, and fungal disease, and abiotic stresses through application of novel transgenomics (e.g., antisense and RNAi) [9, 15, 42] and genome editing tools (e.g., CRISPR/Cas) for cotton [43].

Cotton research advances for the past decade period include also the development of cotton bioinformatics research and resources to analyze and utilize a large volume of "gossypomics" data [44, 45] in the plant genomics and postgenomics era. This opened a new paradigm for the development of fine-tuned innovations for cotton breeding and farming with the integration of knowledge gained from "omics" sciences, system biology, and chemical genomics as well as from the translation of the concept of "personalized agriculture" [28], which should increase cotton production worldwide [14].

Similarly, progressive advances were made to understand cotton crop physiology in a complex view from seed germination to maturation stages under different temperatures, water, light, and nutrient applications, as well as in the event of global climate change scenarios [46, 47], which affects cotton yield and quality [16]. Cotton farming and management practices, the utilization of new generation of chemical and biological fertilizers and their assessment tools, including modern conservation tillage, winter cover cropping, site-specific nutrient applications [48], and remote sensing technologies [49], as well as integrated pest and disease management programs [50] have greatly accelerated and improved cotton production worldwide.

Cotton research community has also witnessed the advancements of cotton harvesting mechanizations and machinery [51], modifications in cotton ginning equipment and approaches [52], improvements in cotton fiber quality testing methodology and instrumentation such as high volume instrumentations (HVIs) and advanced fiber information system (AFIS) and cotton classification. All these along with developments in cotton combing, spinning, fabric manufacturing as well as fiber and yarn finishing technologies [53] have not only helped to grow the cotton industry, and increase the satisfaction and demand of consumers for natural fiber but also equipped cotton genetics/breeding programs with in-depth-trait-analysis tools to breed superior quality varieties of cotton and consumers demand.

At the same time, the above-highlighted past-decade scientific and technological advances; current challenges and demand of cotton production, market fluctuations; global climate change and increased biosecurity issues due to adapted and emerging pests and diseases; and global food security policies, as mentioned above, emphasize an urgent need to determine future new research directions, priority tasks and updated approaches and view for cotton research, which recently is well highlighted by world cotton research community under the leadership of International Cotton Advisory Committee (ICAC) [54]. This document highlights many new cotton research directions and grand tasks ahead requiring global collaborations, preparation of new generation of cotton scientists, large investments, and funding. In this context, to timely update, enhance, coordinate, and initiate largely integrated collaborative research and educational programs, discussions, and conferences on global cotton science, cotton researchers have recently established a new international organization, International Cotton Researchers Association (ICRA) [55], that together with ICAC and its member governments, International Cotton Genome Initiative (ICGI), universities and research institutions, is trusted to be a key player for the development and address new directions of cotton research in future.

3. Highlights of chapters

The book aimed to collect the latest research results of to cover some of the past decade achievements and updates on cotton research. Topics are generally divided in five sections including (1) cotton research structure and institutions, cotton agronomy, physiology and crop management, (2) cotton genetics, breeding and biotechnology, and (3) cotton-based products and textile research.

In particular, among many other proposed chapters from Iran and Uzbekistan, the first section incorporated a chapter from Venugopalan and his colleagues of the Central Institute for Cotton Research, India on cotton research structure and institutions in India, the largest cotton growing country in the world with about 12 million-hectares production area in 2016/17 [10]. Venugopalan and his colleagues successfully traced historical evolution of cotton research of the country with current research directions, developments, achievements, and "institutional mechanism responsible for varietal release, seed production and transfer of technology". The chapter has also discussed future challenges and solutions of the cotton sector in the country and beyond.

In the cotton agronomy, physiology and crop management topic, Yali Zhang and his colleagues from the Shihezi University of China and Australian National University of Australia reviewed the mechanisms of cotton photoprotection during the leaf movement and drought conditions in nonfoliar organs, its impact on photosynthetic capacity and enzymes influencing the cotton yield. A multi-institutional joint chapter authored by Ademar Pereira Serra and his colleagues from Brazil and Tunisia presented a methodology chapter on the use of compositional nutrient diagnosis (CND) to better and efficiently assess the status, dynamics, interactions, and demand of nutrients in cotton that have advantages over the traditional methods of fertilizer management. Cotton research advances in farming and cultivation of cotton are well discussed by Jianlong Dai and Hezhong Dong from Shandong Academy of Agricultural Science, China. In a Chinese example, authors reviewed "the achievements, challenges, countermeasures and prospects for intensive cotton cultivation" highlighting a need to apply the light and simplified farming and cultural system for future sustainable cotton production in China. Further, Price and his colleagues from USDA-ARS, USA have presented a research study on the use of winter cover crops in a corn and cotton plantings. Results have shown an importance of early cover plant planting and its late termination that leaded to increased biomass accumulation, helping to suppress early-season weeds in cotton and corn plantations. Researchers have suggested optimal schemes for winter cover crops using crimson clover or rye crops.

The cotton genetics, breeding and biotechnology section has included four chapters. The first chapter of Yuksel Bolek and his collegues from Kahramanmaras Sutcu Imam University and Agriculture University Faisalabad of Pakistan has been devoted to review the achievements and perspectives of molecular breeding of cotton. The chapter has described the development and types of DNA markers, genetic mapping approaches and mapping population resources, breeding challenges for polygenic traits and schemes for molecular breeding, including marker-assisted backcrossing, pedigree selection, gene pyramiding, and marker-assisted recurrent selection as well as database resources in cotton. Authors also reviewed the efforts on some advanced approaches and technologies such as NGS, GBS, association mapping, and 'targeting induced local lesions in genomes (TILLING)'. The review demonstrated significant advances made on molecular breeding and genomics of cotton for the past decade and highlighted future perspectives. Multi-institutional collaborative chapter of Marina Sanamyan and her colleagues from Uzbekistan and the USA has described advances made on the molecular and cytogenetic characterization of "yet-unexplored" cotton cytogenetic collection of Uzbekistan. Using microsatellite markers and a well-defined tester set of translocation lines, authors succeeded to detect the chromosome identity of "unknown" monosomic lines from the collection, which will be useful for cotton genetics and improvement programs. In a continuation of highlighting the cotton genetics and breeding advances of cotton research community, Seloame Nyaku and his colleagues from research institutes of Ghana and the USA reviewed the achievements of world laboratories on the identification of tolerance and resistance mechanisms, and evaluation, introgression and functional analysis of reniform nematode resistance genes in cotton. It is noteworthy to mention that reniform nematode is one of the most devastating diseases causing approximately $130 million loss every year in the U.S. cotton belt [56]. Authors provided a positive conclusion on great perspectives of current omics-derived results to solve reniform resistance problems in cotton.

A book chapter on cotton biotechnology has incorporated the chapter by Abdul Qayyum Rao and his colleagues from the University of the Punjab and the University of Central Punjab, which reviewed the advances made on plant transformation techniques, and its application and suitability for tissue culture of cotton. Authors have described plant regeneration, embryo formation, and genetic vector constructions used in cotton transformation, largely concentrating on all major transformation techniques and methods used in plant transformation, their advantages and disadvantages, and suitability for cotton transformation.

The last section of the book consists of three chapters on cotton-based products and textile research efforts. Multi-institutional group of H.-B. Yue and his colleagues presented their research results on the utilization of glandless cotton seed flour to produce environmentally nonhazardous bioplastic films. Authors have investigated optimum synthesis conditions and various chemical modifications with the analysis and characterization of structure, stability, and biodegradability of obtained bioplastics in different thermal and water treatment conditions. This chapter concluded the usefulness of these cottonseed-derived bioplastics, and among other important points in this direction, highlighted that the cotton seed-derived bioplastics can be significantly improved through the genetic modifications of amino acid compositions of specific cotton seed proteins. The two other chapters are related to modern approaches for textile finishing of cotton fibers. In particular, Franco Ferro and his colleagues from Italy have presented a chapter on UV-assisted differential cotton fiber dyeing using direct and reactive dyes that yields various chromatic effects. This chapter highlighted UV-aided surface modifications of cotton fabrics to improve oil and water repellency, and the use of UV grafting based chitosan finishing to obtain washing resistant antimicrobial cotton fabrics. Similarly, Issa M. El Nahal and his colleagues from Al-Azhar and Islamic Universities of Gaza, Palestine, investigated different methods of synthesis of metal oxide nanoparticles and their deposition onto cotton fibers that resulted in enhancement of antimicrobial activity of cotton fabrics. Authors' contributions exemplified the advances made on application of modern nanotechnologies for cotton textile research.

4. Conclusions

The cotton research has significantly progressed in the last 30 years that resulted in many seminal and historic discoveries in many aspects of cotton science. Cotton research community decoded whole genome of important cotton species, and thus opened a new era for more "targeted" research than ever. Highlighting some updates, all 12 chapters compiled in this book cover a wide range of cotton research topics and describe the latest developments in cotton science and research from both developed and developing country perspectives. The editor of this book is sure that the chapter materials will enrich data, results, and opinions on the progress of worldwide cotton research that should be useful for readers interested with this unique and the most important fiber crop of our planet.

Acknowledgements

I am thankful to the Cabinet of Ministries of Uzbekistan, Academy of Sciences of Uzbekistan, Committee for Coordination of Science and Technology Development, Ministry of Agriculture and Water Resources, "Uzpakhtasanoatexport" holding company, Center "SIFAT", and the Ministry of Foreign Economic Relations, Investments and Trades of Uzbekistan for continual in-house capacity building and scientific research grants for conducting modern cotton "omics" research in Uzbekistan. I gratefully acknowledge the Office of International Research Programs (OIRP) of the United States Department of Agriculture (USDA) – Agricultural Research Service (ARS), Texas A&M University and U.S. Civilian Research & Development Foundation (CRDF) for collaborative programs and continual financial support of cotton genomics and bioinformatics research in Uzbekistan. I thank Dr. M. Rafiq Chaudhry, Head Technical Information Section of the International Cotton Advisory Committee, Washington D.C., USA, for his detailed review and suggestions on this chapter material.

Author details

Ibrokhim Y. Abdurakhmonov

*Address all correspondence to: ibrokhim.abdurakhmonov@genomics.uz; genomics@uzsci.net

Center of Genomics and Bioinformatics, Academy of Science of the Republic of Uzbekistan, Tashkent, Uzbekistan

References

[1] Lee JA, Fang DD. Cotton as a world crop: origin, history, and current status. In: Fang D, Percy R, editors. Cotton. 2nd ed. Madison: American Society of Agronomy; 2015. p. 1–24. doi: 10.2134/agronmonogr57.2013.0019.

[2] Gledhill D. The Names of Plants. 4th ed. Cambridge: Cambridge University Press; 2008. 426 p.

[3] Abdurakhmonov IY. Role of genomic studies in boosting yield. In: Proceedings of International Cotton Advisory Board (ICAC); 20 September – 4 October 2013; Cartagena. 2013. p. 7–22.

[4] Cronn RC, Small RL, Haselkorn T, Wendel JF. Rapid diversification of the cotton genus (*Gossypium*: Malvaceae) revealed by analysis of sixteen nuclear and chloroplast genes. Am J Bot 2002;89:707–725.

[5] Adams KL, Cronn R, Percifield R, Wendel JF. Genes duplicated by polyploidy show unequal contributions to the transcriptome and organ-specific reciprocal silencing. Proc Natl Acad Sci U S A 2003;100:4649–4654. DOI: 10.1073/pnas.0630618100.

[6] Adams KL, Wendel JF. Allele-specific, bidirectional silencing of an alcohol dehydrogenase gene in different organs of interspecific diploid cotton hybrids. Genetics 2005;171:2139–2142. DOI: 10.1534/genetics.105.047357.

[7] Fang D, Percy R, editors. Cotton. 2nd ed. Madison: American Society of Agronomy; 2015. 796 p. DOI: 10.2134/agronmonogr57.

[8] Abdurakhmonov IY, Buriev ZT, Shermatov SS, Abdullaev AA, Urmonov K, Kushanov F, Egamberdiev S, Shapulatov U, Abdukarimov A, Saha S, Jenkins J, Kohel RJ, Yu JZ, Pepper AP, Kumpatla SP, Ulloa U. Genetic diversity in *Gossypium* genus. In: Caliskan M, editor. Genetic Diversity in Plants. Rijeka: InTech; p. 331–338. DOI: 10.5772/35384.

[9] Sunilkumar G, Campbell LM, Puckhaber L, Stipanovic RD, Rathore KS. Engineering cottonseed for use in human nutrition by tissue-specific reduction of toxic gossypol. Proc Natl Acad Sci U S A 2006;103:18054–18059. DOI: 10.1073/pnas.0605389103.

[10] Better yields to boost cotton production in 2016/17. International Cotton Advisory Committee (ICAC) press release [Internet]. 2016. Available at: https://www.icac.org/Press-Release/2016/PR-14-Better-Yields-to-Boost-Cotton-Production-in [accessed: 2016-08-18].

[11] United States Department of Agriculture (USDA) report: Cotton and wool outlook, released on May 14, 2013 [Internet]. 2013. Available at: http://www.ers.usda.gov/publications/cws-cotton-and-wool-outlook/cws-13e.aspx#.UjhSRRzCBmg [accessed: 2016-08-18].

[12] Stable World Cotton Trade Expected in 2015/16. International Cotton Advisory Committee (ICAC) press release [Internet]. 2015. Available at: https://www.icac.org/Press-Release/2015/PR-22-Stable-World-Cotton-Trade-Expected-in-2015-1 [accessed: 2016-08-18].

[13] Powell M. World cotton outlook. Origin Africa Magazine [Internet]. 2016. Available at: http://actifafrica.1kcloud.com/edlv_Vi3SA/#24 [accessed: 2016-08-18].

[14] Abdurakhmonov IY. Focus on some new directions and priority tasks for worldwide cotton genetics, breeding, genomics, and biotechnology research. ICAC Rec 2016;34:10–12.

[15] Abdurakhmonov IY, Ayubov MS, Ubaydullaeva KA, Buriev ZT, Shermatov SE, Ruziboev HS, et al. RNA interference for functional genomics and improvement of cotton (*Gossypium* spp.). Front Plant Sci 2016;7:202. DOI: 10.3389/fpls.2016.00202.

[16] Hake K. Climate disruptions to fiber yield growth [Internet]. 2012. Available at: http://www.cicr.org.in/isci-image/3.pdf [accessed: 2016-08-18].

[17] Hake K, Nichols RL, Barnes EM, Wedegaertner T, Jones D, Kurtz RW. 40 years of Ag research funding at cotton incorporated – an update. In: Proceedings of Cotton Beltwide Conference; 5–7 January 2016; New Orleans: National Cotton Council; 2016. p. 17099.

[18] Campbell BT, Saha S, Percy R, Frelichowski J, Jenkins JN, Park W, et al. Status of global cotton germplasm resources. Crop Sci 2010;50:1161–1179. DOI: 10.2135/cropsci2009.09.0551.

[19] Abdurakhmonov IY, editor. World Cotton Germplasm Resources. Rijeka, Croatia: InTech Press; 2014. 320 p. DOI: 10.5772/56978.

[20] Zhang HB, Li Y, Wang B, Chee PW. Recent advances in cotton genomics. Int J Plant Genomics 2008;2008:742304. doi: 10.1155/2008/742304.

[21] Abdurakhmonov IY. Exploiting genetic diversity. In: Proceedings of 4th World Cotton Research Conference; 10–14 September 2007; Lubbock: ICAC; 2007. P2153. Available at: https://www.icac.org/meetings/wcrc/wcrc4/presentations/data/papers/Paper2153.pdf [accessed: 2016-08-18].

[22] Abdurakhmonov IY, Saha S, Jenkins JN, Buriev ZT, Shermatov SE, Scheffler BE, Pepper AE, Yu JZ, Kohel RJ, Abdukarimov A. Linkage disequilibrium based association mapping of fiber quality traits in *G. hirsutum* L. variety germplasm. Genetic. 2009;136:401–417. DOI: 10.1007/s10709-008-9337-8.

[23] Abdurakhmonov IY, Kohel RJ, Yu JZ, Pepper AE, Abdullaev AA, Kushanov FN, Salakhutdinov IB, Buriev ZT, Saha S, Scheffler BE, Jenkins JN, Abdukarimov A. Molecular diversity and association mapping of fiber quality traits in exotic *G. hirsutum* L. germplasm. Genomics. 2008;92:478–487. DOI: 10.1016/j.ygeno.208.07.013.

[24] Logan-Young CJ, Yu JZ, Verma SK, Percy RG, Pepper AE. SNP discovery in complex allotetraploid genomes (*Gossypium* spp., Malvaceae) using genotyping by sequencing. Appl Plant Sci 2015;3:1400077. DOI: 10.3732/apps.1400077.

[25] Hulse-Kemp AM, Lemm J, Plieske J, Ashrafi H, Buyyarapu R, Fang DD, et al. Development of a 63K SNP array for cotton and high-density mapping of intra- and interspecific populations of *Gossypium* spp. G3. 2015;5:1187–1209. DOI: 10.1534/g3.115.018416.

[26] Wang S, Chen J, Zhang W, Hu Y, Chang L, Fang L, Wang Q, Lv F, Wu H, Si Z, Chen S, Cai C, Zhu X, Zhou B, Guo W, Zhang T. Sequence-based ultra-dense genetic and physical maps reveal structural variations of allopolyploid cotton genomes. Genome Biol 2015;16:108. DOI: 10.1186/s13059-015-0678-1.

[27] Van Deynze A, Stoffel K, Lee M, Wilkins TA, Kozik A, Cantrell RG, Yu JZ, Kohel RJ, Stelly DM. Sampling nucleotide diversity in cotton. BMC Plant Biol 2009;9:125. DOI: 10.1186/1471-2229-9-125.

[28] Abdurakhmonov IY. Genomics era for plants and crop species: advances made and needed tasks ahead. In: Abdurakhmonov IY, editor. Rijeka, Croatia: InTech Press; 2016. p. 3–26. DOI: 10.5772/62083.

[29] Zhang T, Endrizzi JE. Cytology and cytogenetics. In: Fang D, Percy R, editors. Cotton. 2nd ed. Madison: American Society of Agronomy; 2015. p. 129–154. DOI: 10.2134/agronmonogr57.2013.0023.

[30] Saha S, Stelly DM, Raska DA, Wu J, Jenkins JN, McCarty JC, Makamov A, Gotmare V, Abdurakhmonov IY, Campbell BT. Chromosome substitution lines: concept, development and utilization in the genetic improvement of Upland cotton. In: Abdurakhmonov IY, editor. Plant Breeding. Rijeka: InTech; 2012. p. 107–128. DOI: 10.5772/35585.

[31] Stelly D, Saha S, Raska D, Jenkins J, McCarty J, Gutierrez O. Registration of 17 Upland (*Gossypium hirsutum*) germplasm lines disomic for different *G. barbadense* chromosome or arm substitutions. Crop Sci. 2005;45:2663–2665. DOI: 10.2135/cropsci2004.0642.

[32] Zhang J. Transgenic cotton breeding. In: Fang D, Percy R, editors. Cotton. 2nd ed. Madison: American Society of Agronomy; 2015. p. 229–254. DOI: 10.2134/agronmonogr57.2013.0026.

[33] Wang K, Wang Z, Li F, Ye W, Wang J, Song G, Yue Z, Cong L, Shang H, Zhu S, Zou C, Li Q, Yuan Y, Lu C, Wei H, Gou C, Zheng Z, Yin Y, Zhang X, Liu K, Wang B, Song C, Shi N, Kohel RJ, Percy RG, Yu JZ, Zhu YX, Wang J, Yu S. The draft genome of a diploid cotton *Gossypium raimondii*. Nat Genet 2012;44:1098–1103. DOI: 10.1038/ng.2371.

[34] Paterson AH, Wendel JF, Gundlach H, Guo H, Jenkins J, Jin D, et al. Repeated polyploidization of *Gossypium* genomes and the evolution of spinnable cotton fibres. Nature 2012;492:423–427. DOI: 10.1038/nature11798.

[35] Li F, Fan G, Wang K, Sun F, Yuan Y, Song G, et al. Genome sequence of the cultivated cotton *Gossypium arboreum*. Nat Genet 2014;46:567–572. DOI: 10.1038/ng.2987.

[36] Zhang T, Hu Y, Jiang W, Fang L, Guan X, Chen J, et al. Sequencing of allotetraploid cotton (*Gossypium hirsutum* L. acc. TM-1) provides a resource for fiber improvement. Nat Biotechnol. 2015;33:531–537. DOI: 10.1038/nbt.3207.

[37] Li F, Fan G, Lu C, Xiao G, Zou C, Kohel RJ, et al. Genome sequence of cultivated Upland cotton (*Gossypium hirsutum* TM-1) provides insights into genome evolution. Nat Biotechnol 2015;33:524–530. DOI: 10.1038/nbt.3208.

[38] Liu X, Zhao B, Zheng HJ, Hu Y, Lu G, Yang CQ, et al. *Gossypium barbadense* genome sequence provides insight into the evolution of extra-long staple fiber and specialized metabolites. Sci Rep 2015;5:14139. DOI: 10.1038/srep14139.

[39] Guan X, Pang M, Nah G, Shi X, Ye W, Stelly DM, Chen ZJ. miR828 and miR858 regulate homoeologous MYB2 gene functions in Arabidopsis trichome and cotton fibre development. Nat Commun. 2014;5:3050. DOI: 10.1038/ncomms4050.

[40] Abdurakhmonov IY, Buriev ZT, Saha S, Jenkins JN, Abdukarimov A, Pepper AE. Phytochrome RNAi enhances major fibre quality and agronomic traits of the cotton *Gossypium hirsutum* L. Nat Commun 2014;5:3062. DOI: 10.1038/ncomms4062.

[41] Han J, Tan J, Tu L, Zhang X. A peptide hormone gene, GhPSK promotes fibre elongation and contributes to longer and finer cotton fibre. Plant Biotechnol J 2014;12:861–871. DOI: 10.1111/pbi.12187.

[42] Mao YB, Cai WJ, Wang JW, Hong GJ, Tao XY, Wang LJ, Huang YP, Chen XY. Silencing a cotton bollworm P450 monooxygenase gene by plant-mediated RNAi impairs larval tolerance of gossypol. Nat Biotechnol 2007;25:1307–1313. DOI: 10.1038/nbt1352.

[43] Iqbal Z, Sattar MN, Shafiq M. CRISPR/Cas9: a tool to circumscribe cotton leaf curl disease. Front Plant Sci 2016;7:475. DOI: 10.3389/fpls.2016.00475.

[44] Sripathi VR, Buyyarapu R, Kumpatla SP, Williams AJ, Nyaku ST, Tilahun Y, Kalavacharla VC, Sharma GC. Bioinformatics tools and genomic resources available in understanding the structure and function of *Gossypium*. In: Abdurakhmonov IY, editor. Rijeka, Croatia: InTech Press; 2016. p. 231–258. DOI: 10.5772/64325.

[45] Yu J, Main D. Role of bioinformatic tools and databases in cotton research. In: Fang D, Percy R, editors. Cotton. 2nd ed. Madison: American Society of Agronomy; 2015. p. 303–338. DOI: 10.2134/agronmonogr57.2013.0043.

[46] Snider JL, Oosterhuis DM. Physiology. In: Fang D, Percy R, editors. Cotton. 2nd ed. Madison: American Society of Agronomy; 2015. p. 339–400. DOI: 10.2134/agronmonogr57.2013.0044.

[47] Conaty W, Brodrick R, Mahan J, Payton P. Climate and its interaction with cotton morphology. In: Fang D, Percy R, editors. Cotton. 2nd ed. Madison: American Society of Agronomy; 2015. p. 401–418. DOI: 10.2134/agronmonogr57.2013.0021.

[48] Bauer PJ. Crop growing practices. In: Fang D, Percy R, editors. Cotton. 2nd ed. Madison: American Society of Agronomy; 2015. p. 419–438. DOI: 10.2134/agronmonogr57.2013.0029.

[49] Huang Y, Thomson SJ. Remote sensing for cotton farming. In: Fang D, Percy R, editors. Cotton. 2nd ed. Madison: American Society of Agronomy; 2015. p. 439–464. DOI: 10.2134/agronmonogr57.2013.0030.

[50] Luttrell RG, Teague TG, Brewer MJ. Cotton insect pest management. In: Fang D, Percy R, editors. Cotton. 2nd ed. Madison: American Society of Agronomy; 2015. p. 509–546. DOI: 10.2134/agronmonogr57.2014.0072.

[51] Wanjura JD, Barnes EM, Kelley MS, Boman RK. Harvesting. In: Fang D, Percy R, editors. Cotton. 2nd ed. Madison: American Society of Agronomy; 2015. p. 571–608. DOI: 10.2134/agronmonogr57.2013.0047.

[52] Hughs E, Holt G. Ginning. In: Fang D, Percy R, editors. Cotton. 2nd ed. Madison: American Society of Agronomy; 2015. p. 609–664. DOI: 10.2134/agronmonogr57.2013.0048.

[53] Kelly B, Abidi N, Ethridge D, Hequet EF. Fiber to fabric. In: Fang D, Percy R, editors. Cotton. 2nd ed. Madison: American Society of Agronomy; 2015. p. 665–744. DOI: 10.2134/agronmonogr57.2013.0031.

[54] New directions in cotton research. The ICAC Recorder. 2016;34:3–14.

[55] International Cotton Researchers Association (ICRA) [Internet]. 2016. Available at: http://www.icracotton.org [accessed: 2016-08-20].

[56] The search for nematode-resistant cotton [Internet]. 2016. Available at: https://agresearchmag.ars.usda.gov/2012/jul/cotton [accessed: 2016-08-18].

Section 2

Cotton Research Structure and Institutions, Cotton Agronomy, Physiology and Crop Management

Chapter 2

Institutional Structure of Cotton Research in India

Mangat V. Venugopalan,

Mahendra Singh Yadav and Vandana Satish

Additional information is available at the end of the chapter

http://dx.doi.org/10.5772/63798

Abstract

The chapter traces the landmark events in the contemporary history of cotton in India. The achievements in research and development that transformed India from a chronic importer of cotton to the largest producer and a net exporter of cotton are highlighted. The structure of cotton research undertaken by the institutes under the National Agricultural Research and Education System (NARES) are also elaborated. The institutional mechanism responsible for varietal release, seed production and transfer of technology are briefly described. The immediate challenges facing the cotton sector and approaches to tackle them are also discussed.

Keywords: ICAR-CICR, ICAR-CIRCOT, AICRP on Cotton, cotton research, transfer of technology

1. Introduction

India is the country with primarily an agrarian economy. Despite massive industrialization and rapid growth of tertiary sector following the economic liberations in 1990s, agriculture sector still contributes about 14% to the national gross domestic product (GDP). Agriculture supports the livelihood of about 50% of its population. In the post-independence era, huge investments were made in agricultural research for the expansion of irrigation and soil water conservation and to increase the adoption of new agricultural technologies.

The Indian Council of Agricultural Research (ICAR) is the apex agriculture research organization under the Department of Agricultural Research and Education (DARE), Ministry of Agriculture, Government of India. It coordinates, guides, and manages research, education and extension services in the agriculture sector comprising field crops, horticultural crops, agro-forestry, animal sciences and fisheries. These functions are discharged through the NARES comprising 96 ICAR research institutes, 77 'All India Coordinated Research Projects/ Networks', 4 deemed to be Universities [Indian Agricultural Research Institute (IARI), Indian Veterinary Research Institute (IVRI), National Dairy Research Institute (NDRI) and Central Institute of Fisheries Education (CIFE)], 62 State Agricultural/Veterinary/Horticulture/Fishery Universities and 641 Krishi Vigyan Kendra [1]. The ICAR played a key role in ushering the green revolution and subsequent sector-wise development that transformed in India from a chronic importer to an era of self-sufficiency in food grains and allied agricultural products. The technologies developed through the NARES system helped farmers to increase the production of food grains from 50 million metric tonnes (MMTs) in 1950 to 264 MMTs in 2013. During the same period, there was a 6-fold increase in horticultural crops, 12-fold increase in fish production, 8-fold increase in milk production, 27-fold increase in egg production [1] and an 11-fold increase in cotton production from 0.58 MMT in 1950/1951 to 6.7 MMT in 2013/2014.

2. Role of cotton in the Indian economy

The textile and clothing industry has a long history in India. Today, this sector contributes 6% of the GDP and 14% of India's exports [2]. Around 65% of textile production and over 75% of textile exports are based on cotton. During 2014/2015, India produced 6.5 MMT of cotton fibres from 11.96 million hectares (m ha) area. The cotton cultivation sector engages around 10 million farmers and involves another about 30 million people operations related to cotton cultivation, cotton trade and its processing such as ginning, spinning, weaving and garmenting. Out of the total cotton consumed, 94% is spun into yarn and the rest used in the production of surgical cotton and other applications [3].

Cotton is a multi-component crop, and apart from lint, it provides valuable by-products such as cotton seed, linter, oil, meal and biomass (cotton stalk). Considering the importance of cotton to India's economy, the ICAR supports research on cotton production through the ICAR—Central Institute for Cotton Research (CICR) and All India Coordinated Research Project on Cotton (AICRP on Cotton). Research on post-harvest technology and value addition is led by ICAR—Central Institute for Research on Cotton Technology (CIRCOT).

3. Issues and challenges in cotton production research

During the post-independence period, the cotton sector faced several challenges at different periods and the cotton R&D continuously changed its priorities to address these challenges. The first task of independent India was to ensure sufficient cotton to its domestic mills. During partition, 21% of the prime cotton area that provided 40% of the total production became a part of Pakistan, but 409 out of the 423 cotton mills remained in the Indian Union. This caused a huge shortage of domestic cotton. To tide over this crisis and reduce imports, the 'GROW MORE COTTON' programme was implemented between 1951/1952 and 1960/1961. Special schemes were initiated to increase in area under cotton, increase in area under irrigation, supply improved seeds and fertilizers at subsidized rates and raise the basic ruling price [4]. The net result was an increase in area from 4.3 m ha in 1947/1948 to 7.61 m ha in 1960/1961.

During 1950s, India was producing more of short staple cotton and a huge quantity of long and extra-long staple was imported. Focus of research hence shifted to replace indigenous *Gossypium arboreum* and *Gossypium herbaceum* cotton by Indian *Gossypium hirsutum* varieties. The resulting 'Madras Combodia' series and 'Laxmi' in south India, inter-specific Indo-American varieties 'Deviraj' and 'Devitej' in Gujarat and Maharashtra and the Punjab-American cottons 'P 216F' and '320F' brought about substantial quality improvement [5]. Agronomic field trials to optimize yields from these varieties were initiated. Because of these efforts, the area under *G. hirsutum* cotton increased from 3% in 1947/1948 to 29% in 1960/1961 and 50% in 1970/1971 [6]. Basu [7] has reviewed the cotton genetics and breeding work carried out during the 1970s and 1980s. To further increase the productivity of cotton and widen the quality spectrum, hybrids *viz.* 'Hybrid 4' (intra- *hirsutum*) and 'DCH 32' (*hirsutum* × *barbadense*) were released. These became popular and heralded in the hybrid cotton era in India. Extra-long staple 'Suvin' was introduced in the 1970s.

A large-scale replacement of indigenous cotton with G. *hirsutum* varieties and increase in the application rates of fertilizers changed the pest complex. Whitefly (*Bemisia tabaci*) and American bollworm (*Helicoverpa armigera*) replaced the conventional insect pest-spotted bollworm (*Erias vitella*), spiny bollworm (*Erias insulana*) and pink bollworm (*Pectinophora gossypiella*) and emerged as major pests of cotton [8]. Insecticides were introduced in the 1960s. The availability of carbamates and organophosphates shifted research focus on chemical-based pest control in cotton. Pyrethroids were introduced in 1985. Elimination of natural enemies and subsequent outbreaks of whitefly and bollworms promoted research and development of integrated pest management (IPM) systems [9] in the 1990s. The phase between 1992 and 2002 saw the emergence of private sector as a major contributor to seed and pesticide research. To modernize the entire cotton scenario, the government initiated the 'Technology Mission on Cotton' in 2000. Repeated crop failure and rising pesticide resistance to bollworms led to the promotion of insecticide resistance management (IRM) strategies and subsequently the introduction of *Bacillus thuringiensis* toxin containing (Bt) cotton in 2002.

3.1. Current challenges facing cotton in the post-Bt era

A critical note on the contemporary challenges being confronted by the cotton farmer is available in [10]. Here, we highlight some key challenges:

Declining the total factor productivity and soil health and fertility. A widespread adoption of Bt hybrids converted traditional multi-cropping systems (i.e. inter cropping, crop rotations, mixed cropping, etc.) to mono-cropping systems. An imbalanced application of fertilizers in favour of N and progressive depletion of macro and micro-nutrients has deteriorated soil heath and fertility. From 2002 to 2012, the fertilizer use for cotton cultivation increased about 8.1% per annum [11], but the partial factor productivity (expressed as kg of lint/kg of fertilizer applied) for fertilizers declined. Research is, therefore, necessary to rationalize fertilizer use through soil enriching cropping systems.

Resurgence of leaf hoppers and whitefly, and emergence of minor pests. Minor pests, such as thrips, mirid bugs, mealy bugs, stem weevil, etc., have emerged as serious pests. Bt-cotton seeds are treated with imidacloprid to protect the crop from sucking pests. Repeated over the top application of the same molecule made jassids resistant to this chemical. The resurgence of whitefly caused huge economic loss to farmers in the North India. Alternate pest management strategies are needed.

Pink bollworm resistance to Bt toxin. Transgenic Bt-cotton conferring resistance to bollworms was introduced to provide protection against bollworms. Poor stewardship, such as extending the crop duration from 180 days to 220 or even 250 days by providing additional irrigation and fertilizers, non-compliance of refugia put Indian cotton at the doorstep of an era of resistance to Bt toxins. The damage in Bollgard II® (BG II) and Bt-hybrid in parts of Gujarat and Andhra Pradesh by pink bollworms is compelling researchers to reformulate the pest management strategies.

Increasing the production cost and declining the profitability. During the last decade, there has been a tremendous increase in the input usage particularly fertilizers. There has been a reduction in partial factor productivity of fertilizers (kg yield/kg of fertilizer) and increase in the cost of production [11].

Lack of synchrony between input requirement by crop and input availability/supply in rainfed cotton. About 60% of the cotton is cultivated under rainfed conditions, mostly in the Central and South India. Sowing commences with the onset of the monsoon in June and the monsoon recedes by mid September. The present-day hybrids are of long duration with a long fruiting window beginning from the end of September during the post-monsoon phase. The peak water requirement during early boll development phase coincides with the receding soil moisture phase. This induces moisture stress and reduces yield. Similarly, the peak nutrient requirement is when the crop is 90–120 days old. Lack of nutrient in soil (due to lopsided application schedule) or inadequate soil moisture to solubilize nutrients causes nutrient deficiency adversely affecting yield. Early maturing genotypes and revised nutrient scheduling based on demand/supply synchrony is another challenge.

Labour shortage, delays in sowing and cropping operations that lead to reducing yields. The entire cotton produced in India is handpicked. Non-availability of low-cost machines adoptable by small farmers is another major challenge and will remain the focus of research.

4. Brief history of cotton research and development in India

Indian sub-continent is recognized as the home of diploid cotton and the cotton-based clothing, and textile industry flourished even during the pre-Christian era. India is globally recognized as a traditional home of cotton and cotton textile. The domestication of diploid Asiatic cotton (*G. arboreum* and *G. herbaceum*) for commercial cultivation to meet the clothing needs is considered to have begun from Harappan civilization [12]. Only *G. arboreum* and *G. herbaceum* cotton were grown until the middle of eighteenth century.

The East India Company in 1790 first attempted to grow 'Bourbon' (*G. hirsutum* race punctatum) in Bombay and Madras Provinces, but the efforts were not successful. In 1840, trials with *G. hirsutum* cotton was carried out in Gujarat, the Deccan and Konkan regions and the introduction of New Orleans (*G. hirsutum* race latifolium) proved partly successful in Hubli (Karnataka). Attempts to introduce American, Peruvian, Egyptian and Sea Island varieties of *Gossypium barbadense* cotton in 1905 in Coimbatore were also not successful [13].

The first significant research achievement was the successful introduction of *G. hirsutum* (Cambodian cotton) during 1904/1905 in the Madras State [14]. Agriculture Departments in various provinces of India were established in 1904. Staff posted in the Department of Agriculture in Bombay, Punjab, Madras, Central Provinces and Berar and United Provinces initiated cotton improvement work through the selection of superior lines for yield and fibre quality from the existing mixtures. The efforts resulted in the development of 'Co 1', 'Co 2', 'Cawnpore American No. 9', '4 F' in *G. hirsutum*, 'V 262', 'V 434', 'N 14', 'C 520' in *G. arboreum* and 'H 1' in *G. herbaceum* suitable for various cotton growing tracts [15].

The establishment of the Indian Central Cotton Committee (ICCC) in Bombay as a Technical Advisory body to the Government in 1921 is considered as a major landmark in the history of cotton research in India. The Indian Cotton Cess Act was enacted in 1923 to levy a cess on cotton consumed by the domestic textile mills or exported to generate funds to promote systematic research on cotton. The ICCC became a statutory body with funds at its disposal for promoting research in cotton. It established the Cotton Technological Research Laboratory (CTRL) [later rechristened as Central Institute for Research on Cotton Technology (CIRCOT)] at Bombay in 1924 with Dr. A. J. Turner as its founder Director [16]. It undertook two main activities: (1) conducting spinning tests on various strains of cotton received from Agricultural Departments situated in various locations of the country and (2) conducting tests on fibre properties to relate fibre properties with the spinning value of cotton. Emphasis was also given to the development and standardization of testing procedures for fibre evaluation and spinning performance [16].

From 1924 to 1937, the ICCC funded the Department of Agriculture of the Provincial Governments for the improvement of cotton cultivation in the country. Systematic research on cotton breeding, varietal improvement, seed production, agronomy, entomology and physiology were initiated. ICCC organized the first conference of cotton workers in Bombay in 1937 during which a historic decision to intensively pursue cotton breeding and varietal improvement work in *G. hirsutum* cotton for increasing the yield and fibre quality was adopted. This chartered the future of cotton research in India, and it received further impetus after the partition and independence of India in 1947.

The concerted, research and development efforts under the aegis of ICCC helped independent India to increase the cotton area to 7.8 m ha and the production to 5.3 million bales (a bale is equal to 170 kg) by 1966/1967. The ICCC was abolished in 1966, and CTRL was placed under the administrative control of ICAR. The ICAR reorganized its research set-up in 'Crop Sciences' and the 'All India Coordinated Cotton Improvement project' (AICCIP) [now rechristened as All India Coordinated Research Project on Cotton (AICRP on Cotton)] was launched in 1967 with its headquarters in Coimbatore (Tamil Nadu) with a network of cotton research centres. This set-up, along with basic and strategic research on cotton production conducted at the ICAR-Central Institute for Cotton Research (Nagpur) and that on fibre quality testing and post-harvest value chain at ICAR-CIRCOT, forms the present structure of cotton research.

The Ministry of Agriculture, Government of India set up the Directorate of Cotton Development (DOCD) in Bombay in 1966 for implementing developmental schemes on cotton. To cater to the marketing of cotton and to provide remunerative prices to farmers, the Ministry of Textiles, Government of India, established the Cotton Corporation India, in 1970 with its headquarters in Bombay. The launching of Technology Mission on Cotton (TMC) in 2000 to boost research and extension capabilities as well as modernize the marketing and processing sectors was another landmark by the Government of India [12].

5. Present structure of cotton research in India

The ICAR-CICR (Nagpur), ICAR-CIRCOT (Mumbai) along with the AICRP on Cotton together conducts/coordinates the research work on cotton (**Figure 1**). The CICR, a premier national institute under the ICAR, is the nodal agency for cotton production research. With its headquarters in Nagpur and regional stations at Sirsa (north India) and Coimbatore (south India), CICR conducts basic and strategic research on all aspects of cotton production. From 2000, it is also coordinating the TMC (Mini Mission I) being carried out in a networking mode with Agricultural Universities located in the cotton growing regions and sister ICAR institutes. The AICRP on Cotton with headquarters at Coimbatore has a network of 22 cotton research centres located in 11 cotton-growing states. AICRP on Cotton conducts multi-location and multi-disciplinary research on applied aspects of cotton including varietal development and evaluation/site-specific modifications of agro-technologies. Research on post-harvest processing of seed cotton and value addition of cotton is carried out at the ICAR-CIRCOT (Mumbai). Its regional centres assist the AICRP on Cotton for fibre quality analysis of cultures and spinning test of varieties developed.

The Government of India approved the commercial cultivations of Bt transgenic cotton in 2002. Currently, Bt hybrids are developed by private seed companies under license from Monsanto. For their release, one year of field trial in State Agricultural Universities is mandatory. These hybrids are then released by event-based approval mechanism (EBAM) committee under Review Committee on Genetic Manipulation (RCGM)/Genetic Engineering Approval Committee (GEAC) based on criteria laid out by GEAC.

http://dx.doi.org/10.5772/63798

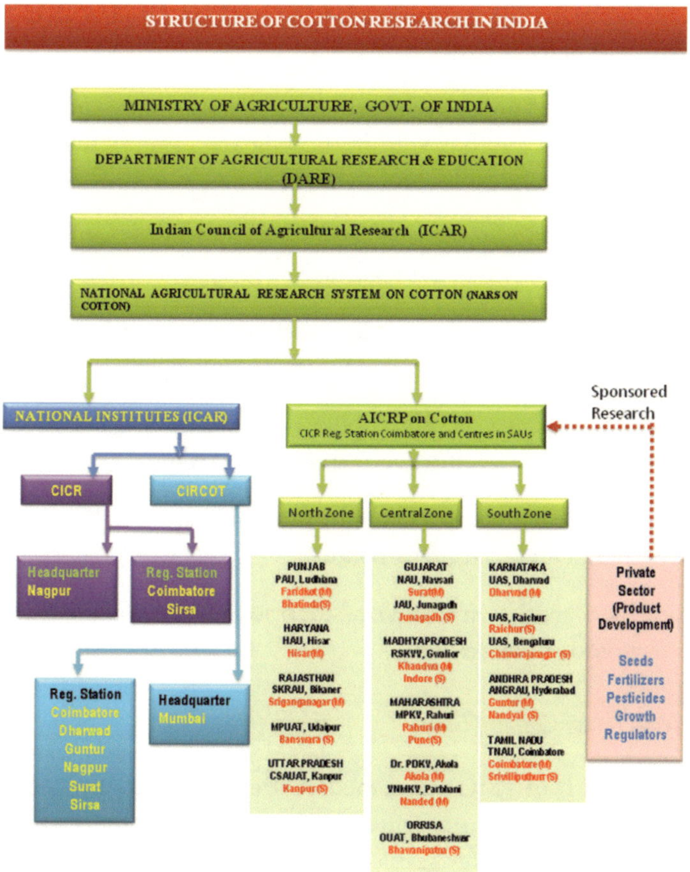

Figure 1. Structure of cotton research in India.

6. Cotton research institutes

6.1. ICAR-Central Institute for Cotton Research (CICR)

The ICAR-CICR was established at Nagpur, Maharashtra (central India), in 1976. ICAR-CICR is **mandated** to conduct basic and strategic research to improve yield and quality of cotton and to create new genetic variability in cotton to facilitate location/cropping system-based adoption. It also facilitates technology transfer to different user agencies and extends consultancy and linkage with national and international agencies.

6.1.1. Research projects/programmes under plan scheme

Details regarding the research programmes undertaken in the past have been made available by International Cotton Advisory Committee (ICAC) [17], and hence it is not presented here.

The programmes being undertaken during XII five year Plan (2012/2013 to 2016/2017) under plan scheme are enlisted here:

1. Genetic improvement and precision breeding of different cotton varieties for specific agro-eco sub-regions with an emphasis on improving the crop architecture, harvest index, ginning outturn, fibre quality, resistant to biotic and abiotic stresses;

2. Documentation of genetic diversity of cotton germplasm through DNA barcoding and utilization of molecular markers in breeding;

3. Discovery of novel genes for resistance to insect pests, leaf-curl virus, water logging and drought for transgenic development;

4. Development of sustainable precision input management systems through consolidation of integrated weed, water and nutrient management strategies;

5. Consolidating ecologically compatible and profitable sustainable crop health management for conventional and transgenic cotton;

6. Priority setting and market intelligence to prioritize 'demand driven research' and appropriate 'technology placement'.

6.1.2. Technology Mission on Cotton (TMC)

The Mini Mission-I (MM-I) of TMC was aimed at strengthening strategic cotton research to provide critical interventions to improve the production, productivity and quality of cotton. ICAR-CICR is the nodal agency for implementing these research programmes through a network of partners under the NARES selected based on human resource/infrastructure present at different centres. The programmes undertaken under TMC MM-I during XII five-year plan period are summarized below:

1. Development of indigenous multi-gene constructs and Bt transgenic varieties:

2. Development of varieties resistant to cotton leaf curl disease (CLCuD), bacterial leaf blight (BLB) and nematodes through marker-assisted breeding;

3. Consolidation of repository of high-strength cotton genotypes. Evaluation of genotypes and standardization of agro-techniques for high-density planting and surgical cotton production;

4. Simulation models/electronic gadgets to predict insect infestation, bollworm resistance to Bt cotton, area, production and price of cotton;

5. Voice call-based e-Kapas network and technology documentation for effective dissemination;

6. Development of cotton picker for small scale cotton production systems.

http://dx.doi.org/10.5772/63798

6.1.3. Structure

ICAR-CICR has its headquarters at Nagpur (Maharashtra) and regional stations at Sirsa (Haryana) and Coimbatore (Tamil Nadu). Presently, there are 65 scientists belonging to 16 disciplines. **Figure 2** describes the organizational structure of ICAR-CICR with details of scientists working in different disciplines.

6.1.4. Research achievements

ICAR- CICR is globally acclaimed for its basic and strategic research outputs that led to the development of several products, processes and technologies. A detailed account of the research achievements is available in ICAR-CICR Vision 2030 and Vision 2050 document and in the Annual Reports uploaded in [18]. A summary is presented here.

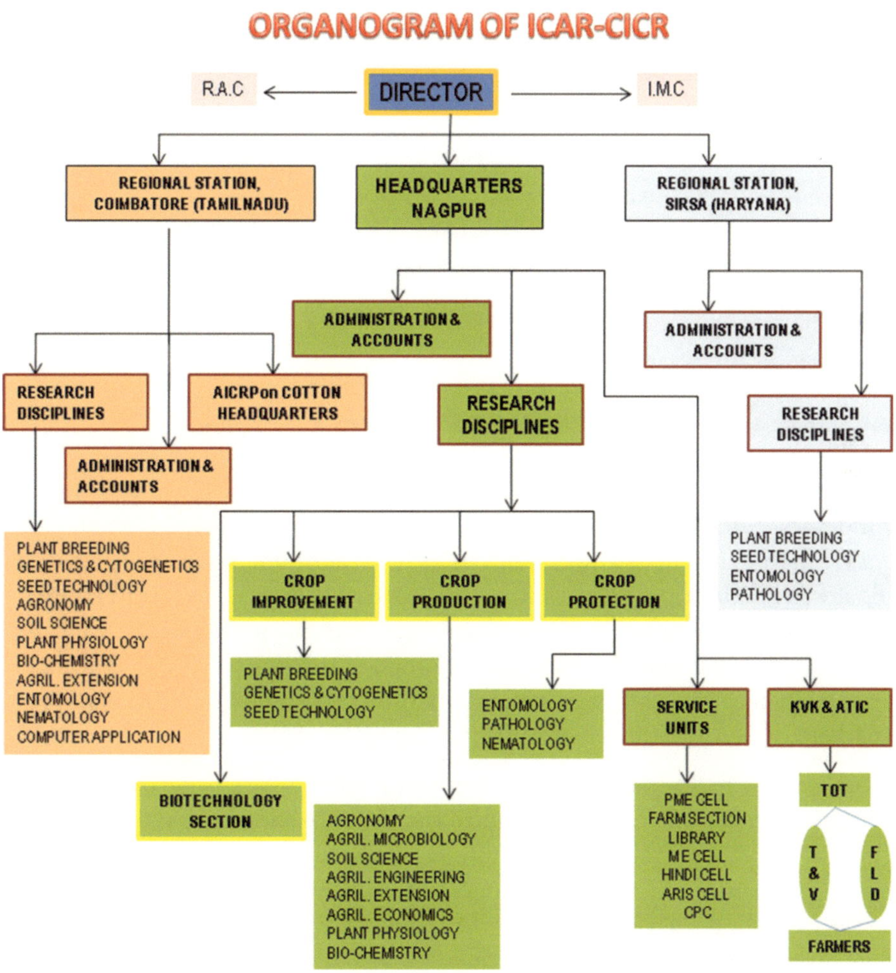

Figure 2. Organogram of ICAR-CICR.

The institute is the custodian of the world's largest germplasm collection on cotton. At present, the repository has 11,543 accessions including 8413 accessions of *G. hirsutum*, 310 accessions of *G. barbadense*, 1936 accessions of *G. arboreum*, 565 accessions of *G. herbaceum* and 40 interspecific derivatives in addition to 26 wild species, 253 accessions of perennials and land races. The collection is being continuously enriched by procuring exotic accessions under the 'Reciprocal Exchange of Germplasm Agreement'. Efforts are underway to characterize them. These serve as valuable resources of biodiversity and are being utilized for developing varieties with economically important traits. All the land races of indigenous cotton are being collected and conserved *ex situ*.

ICAR-CICR has released 30 improved genotypes with high yield potential, excellent adaptability and fibre characteristics (**Table 1**).

Name of species	Name of hybrids/varieties
Intra-*hirsutum* hybrids	'Savitha', 'Suguna', 'Surya', 'Kirthi', 'Omshankar', 'CSHH 198', 'CSHH 238', 'CSHH 243' and 'CSHG 1862'
Interspecific hybrids (*G. hirsutum* × *G. barbadense*)	'HB 224' and 'Shruthi'
Intra-*arboreum* hybrid	'CISAA 2'
G. hirsutum varieties	'MCU 5 VT', 'LRA 5166', 'Supriya', 'Kanchana', 'Anjali', 'CNH36', 'Arogya', 'Surabhi', 'Sumangala', 'CNH 120 MB', 'Suraj', 'CNHO 12', 'CSH-3129' and 'CCH 2623'
G. arboreum varieties	'CISA 310','CISA 614' and 'CNA 1003 (Roja)'
G. barbadense variety	'Suvin'

Table 1. List of hybrids and varieties released by ICAR-CICR for commercial cultivation.

Notable among them are 'LRA 5166', 'LRK 516', 'Surabhi', 'Suraj', 'CISA 2' and 'Suvin'. 'Suvin' is the World's best extra-long staple variety. 'Suraj' has excellent fibre quality and is now being promoted for high-density planting system (HDPS). In addition, researchers have developed 49 genetic stocks (*G. hirsutum*—33, *G. arboreum*—16) that have been registered for their unique, novel and distinct characteristics. For instance, a *G. arboreum* genetic stock with the highest ever fibre strength of 29 g/tex [International Calibration Cotton (ICC mode)] is available. These are being used to develop genotypes with economically important traits and unique morphological markers.

Cytoplasmic genetic male sterile system comprising 137 *Gossypium harknessii*, 15 *Gossypium aridum*, 57 *G. harknessii*–based restorers, and 20 genetic male sterile lines are being maintained at ICAR-CICR. Utilizing male sterility system, 82 genotypes have been converted under cytoplasmic male sterility (CMS) background and, 66 genotypes have been converted under genetic male sterility (GMS) background. To reduce the cost of hybrid seed production, a thermosensitive genetic male sterile line, TGMS 1-1, was identified and characterized in *G. arboreum*. This could be used for hybrid seed production during summer months. Recombinant inbred lines for ginning out turn, fibre quality traits (length, strength, micronaire) and disease

(BLB) resistance have been developed. These are being used in marker-assisted breeding programme for specific traits.

CICR developed, patented and commercialized 'farmer-usable' immunodiagnostic kits for genetically modified (GM) cotton and insecticide quality. The Bt kits are popular among farmers and seed testing agencies in the country, and these helped to curb the spread of illegal and spurious Bt-cotton seeds. The ELISA and dip stick kits to test the quality and residue of pyrethroids and organophosphates are also popular. The institute has developed 'PCR-based kits' to detect various diseases including the dreaded cotton leaf curl virus.

The institute is globally recognized for its pioneering work on fundamental research on insect resistance to insecticides and Bt toxins. It has developed stochastic models and insecticide resistance management (IRM) strategies. The institute provides leadership for national dissemination of the IRM and integrated pest management (IPM) technologies for conventional and Bt cotton. It has won national and international awards for its contribution in development and dissemination of IRM strategies.

Mealy bugs (*Phenacoccus solenopsis*) caused considerable economic damage to cotton during 2005 to 2008, and ICAR-CICR devised a minimum invention strategy to control this pest. Biological formulations, 'MEALY-KILL' and 'MEALY-QUIT' have been developed and found effective for the control of mealy bug. Three novel lectins have been identified having potential to control sap-sucking insect pests (aphids, leaf hoppers, whiteflies).

The agronomists developed several production technologies. Some promising ones include technology for organic cotton production, poly-mulch techniques, multi-tier cropping systems, innovative inter-cropping systems, conservation tillage system, *in situ* soil moisture conservation, water harvesting and recycling, stale seed-bed technique for weed management, foliar nutrition in cotton, integrated nutrient management in cotton-based cropping system, enhance nitrogen use efficiency (NUE) using coated urea, dry seeding and transplanting technology, etc. A cotton crop simulation model InfoCrop-cotton was developed and validated to simulate cotton growth and yield. This is being put to use in land evaluation and climate change studies.

For sustainable cotton production on marginal soils, the institute developed and demonstrated a new concept of HDPS using non-Bt varieties that has potential to improve yields of rainfed cotton, especially in the states of Maharashtra, Madhya Pradesh and Andhra Pradesh. More than 10,000 demonstrations on HDPS technology were conducted. Results showed that HDPS is a viable option to improve the productivity of cotton particularly under rainfed conditions at reduced production costs.

The effect of elevated CO_2 at ambient and increased temperatures and different soil moisture regimes has been researched. Both dry matter production and seed cotton yields were higher at elevated CO_2 (600 ppm) compared to ambient temperature. Elevated levels of CO_2 significantly increased plant height, node number, sympodia number, leaf number, reduced shedding of bud and bolls and delayed senescence of leaves. The increased biomass production under elevated CO_2 atmosphere also helps in sequestering more carbon.

ICAR-CICR has recently established a 'voice call' weekly advisory system called 'e-kapas' network and connected more than 0.2 million cotton farmers for technology dissemination and backstopping. Advisories and alert services are being issued to these cotton growers in eight regional languages so as to enable them initiate proactive measures. The institute is also engaged in first-line transfer of technology. These include front-line demonstration (FLD), on-campus/off-campus demonstrations, seed village programme, farmer-scientist interaction and training of farmers and extension personnel.

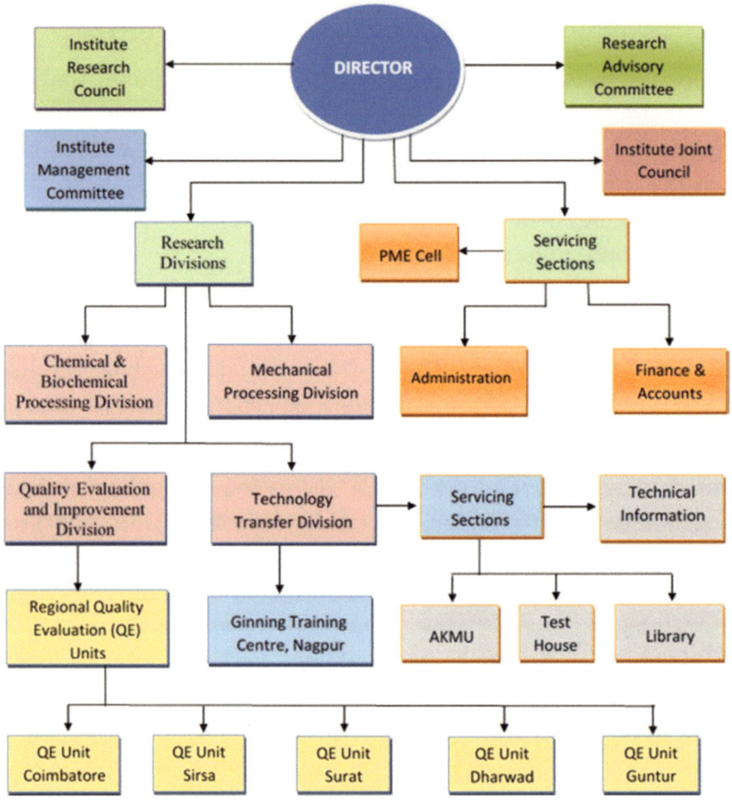

Figure 3. Organizational structure of ICAR-CIRCOT (Source: ICAR-CIRCOT Annual Report 2014–2015 available at [19]).

6.2. ICAR- Central Institute for Research on Cotton Technology (CIRCOT), Mumbai

The ICAR-CIRCOT was established in 1924 for conducting research on all aspects of cotton processing. It houses state-of-the-art research facilities and is notified as a referral laboratory on cotton textile. Its **vision** is to achieve global excellence in cotton technology. Its **mission** is to provide scientific and managerial interventions to post-harvest processing and value addition to cotton and utilization of cotton by-products to maximize economic, environmental and societal benefits. The **mandates** of the ICAR-CIRCOT are as follows: (1) technology development for enhanced utilization of cotton and other natural fibres and their by-products; (2) improve the quality of cotton and other textile products through participatory research in

http://dx.doi.org/10.5772/63798

national programmes; (3) develop human resource and standard reference materials, undertake technology commercialization, consultancy and testing and function as referral laboratory for cotton and allied sectors.

6.2.1. Core areas of current research programmes

1. Pre-ginning and ginning;
2. Mechanical processing, technical textiles and composites;
3. Characterization of cotton and other natural fibres, yarn and textiles;
4. Chemical and bio-chemical processing and biomass and by-product utilization;
5. Entrepreneurship and human resource development along the cotton value chain.

6.2.2. Structure

ICAR-CIRCOT has four research divisions (**Figure 3**). These are the mechanical processing division (MPD), quality evaluation and improvement division (QEID), chemical and biochemical processing division (CBPD) and transfer of technology division (TTD). It has five regional units at Sirsa (Haryana), Surat (Gujarat), Dharward (Karnataka), Guntur (Andhra Pradesh) and Coimbatore (Tamil Nadu). Additionally, the Ginning Training Centre (GTC) situated at Nagpur (Maharashtra) regional unit also provides training to persons employed in ginning-pressing industries.

6.2.3. Research achievements

The institute is constantly engaged in developing new technologies and machineries for better utilization of cotton and other natural fibres. It provides yeomen service to the cotton trade and industry by providing the quality assessment support for fibre, yarn and fabrics. A glimpse on important research achievements of CIRCOT is as follows. This portion has been adapted from CIRCOT Vision 2050 document.

Since its inception, ICAR-CIRCOT has been guiding cotton breeders of India by fixing norms for fibre characteristics. It also evaluates fibre quality parameters of elite cultures sponsored by breeders into AICRP on Cotton and evaluates the spinning potential of pre-release varieties/hybrids. It has also developed a miniature spinning system for assessing the spinning potential of small quantity of cotton available with researchers and preparation of fibre sliver and yarn samples. Research on rotor spinning has proved its utility in Indian spinning sector for the production of quality cotton and blended yarns. Outputs from its research on yarn faults have helped the textile industry to produce yarn with fewer defects at par with world standards.

ICAR-CIRCOT has conducted pioneering research in revealing the basic structure of cotton and other natural fibres. It has also developed a non-destructive infrared technique to determine the cellulose content in fibres. The institute supplies 'calibration cotton', a standard reference material, to spinning mills, cotton-trading houses and various other organizations.

It provides separate sets of standards for conventional fibre testing instruments and for high-volume instrumentation.

The institute undertakes regular cotton ginning and skill training of technicians for ginning industry. The Ginning Training Centre at Nagpur, Maharashtra, with state-of-the-art facility for research and training, is first of its kind in Asia. Designing, development and commercialization of inclined and horizontal pre-cleaners for removal of sticks, bur, etc. for installation in ginning centres was another remarkable achievement. It has also developed an array of pre-cleaning systems for processing machine picked cotton and lowering the trash to 5% in the ginned lint. It was actively engaged in the TMC programme that led to the modernization of over 850 ginneries. This helped in the reduction of trash and other contaminants in Indian cotton.

The institute has developed a variable speed double roller gin where in the speed of both rollers and beaters can be adjusted without any additional demand of power. It has also developed portable ginning machines (Lilliput Gin, CLOY gin, Hipro Gin) for assisting cotton breeders, seed producers, traders and farmers to gin small quantity of seed cotton for assessment of ginning out turn (GOT) and quality of fibres.

The institute has developed a technology for dying of cotton and other cellulosic fabrics using natural (lac) dyes. Its research on the use of natural dyes to achieve uniform shades through machine dyeing has received global appreciation. ICAR-CIRCOT has also developed a technology for bio-scouring of cotton and blended fabrics that saves energy load by 30% and also minimizes the pollution load by 25%.

ICAR-CIRCOT is engaged in basic research on the application of nontechnology, keeping in view the ethical and ecological issues. Research programmes are focusing on the preparation of nano-composites from biopolymers, nano-functional (UV protection, self cleaning, anti-bacterial, file retardant) textiles electro-spinning of nano-fibres for nano-filters and nano-absorbents [3]. It has recently developed a technology for coating of cotton fabrics using zinc oxide nano-particles to impart UV protection and anti-microbial properties.

In the field of bi-product utilization, use of cotton stalks for the production of pulp and paper, kraft paper for the preparation of corrugated boxes, charcoal briquettes and particle boards and bio-methanation from textile waste are some noteworthy achievements. Its technology of aerobic composting of willow dust using NaOH and microbial consortia provides valuable organic manure in 30 days. Solid-state fermentation technology for producing gossypol-free lysine-rich cotton seed cake for feeding non-ruminants has been developed. The institute is also credited with the development of an enzymatic process to prepare peptones from cotton seed meal. Peptones are used for producing enzymes, antibiotics and bio-pesticides.

6.3. All India Coordinated Research Project on Cotton (AICRP on cotton)

The AICRP on Cotton was established in 1967 with Headquarters at Coimbatore. AICRP on Cotton conducts multi-location and multi-disciplinary research with network of centres involving State Agricultural Universities (SAUs) of all the major cotton-growing states of the

http://dx.doi.org/10.5772/63798

country. The centres of AICRP on Cotton, located in all the major cotton-growing states have researchers from different disciplines to facilitate multi-locational evaluation. Its objectives are to identify and facilitate release of best varieties and hybrids for different agro-climatic situation. The centres also validate and fine tune agro technologies and pest/disease management strategies. After a techno-economic feasibility assessment, these technologies are incorporated into the package of practices for cotton production in the respective location [20].

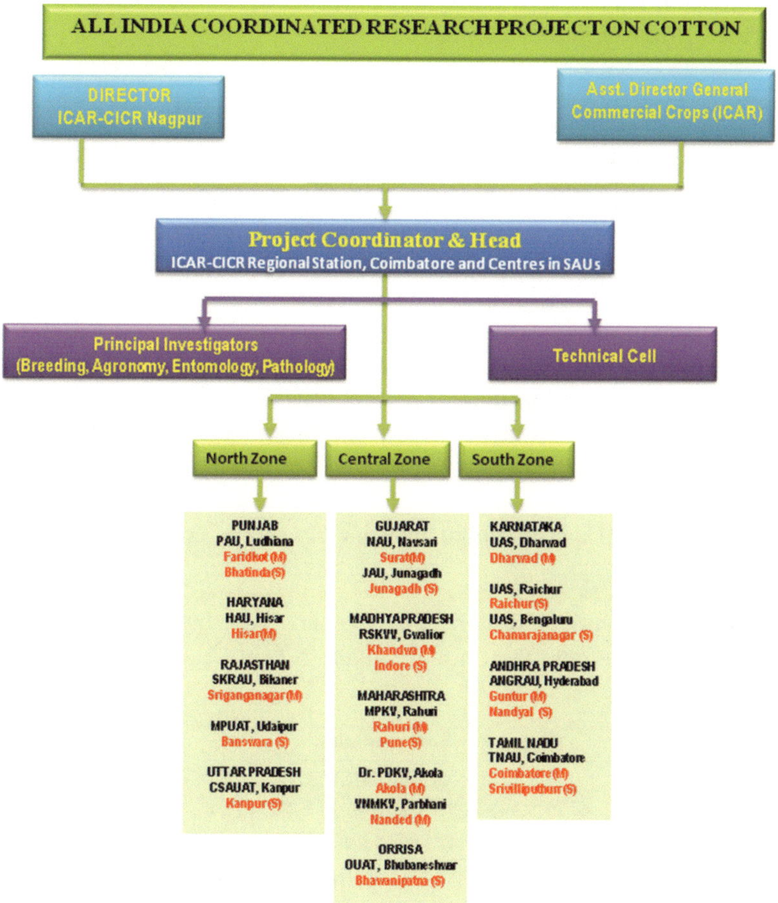

Figure 4. Structure of the AICRP on Cotton network.

6.3.1. Current cotton research programmes

Currently, the research programmes of AICRP on Cotton is focusing on developing high-yielding (1) high-strength, cotton leaf curl virus disease-resistant varieties/hybrids for north zone; (2) early maturing diploid cotton varieties/hybrids with improved fibre quality; (3) short-duration, high-strength *hirsutum* varieties/intra-*hirsutum* hybrids for central zone and south zone and (4) extra-long staple (ELS) *G. barbadense*/*G. hirsutum* × *G. barbadense* hybrids for central and south zone. The breeders are also entrusted with the responsibility of the maintenance of breeding and production of the required quantity of nucleus and breeder seeds of varieties/ parents of hybrids. Agronomists are involved in standardizing planting geometry and fertilizer requirement of pre-release of varieties/hybrids, fine-tuning integrated nutrient management (INM) and integrated weed management strategies, scheduling water delivery through drip and developing production technology for organic cotton production. Entomologists and pathologists are focusing on the seasonal dynamics of pests, pathogens and natural enemies, testing the efficacy of new molecules and fine-tuning of location-specific IPM/IRM strategies and their promotion through FLDs.

6.3.2. Structure

The AICRP on Cotton operates in a multi-locational network mode through 11 main centres and 11 sub-centres involving 17 SAUs (**Figure 4**). This structure facilitates the evaluation of cultures and validation of technologies in different agro-ecological situations.

6.3.3. Research achievements

Since its inception in 1967, the AICRP on Cotton has played a stellar role in shaping the cotton sector in India through the development of several varieties/hybrids and fine tuning agro-eco region-specific cotton production and protection technologies. Detailed account on its past and recent achievements have been published elsewhere [21, 22] and is also available in [23]. The AICRP on Cotton also acts as a nodal centre for transfer of technologies through FLDs. A complete account of the FLDs is available in [20]. Only salient achievements are presented in this section.

Around 250 high-yielding varieties and hybrids of cotton have been developed by the network partners and released. Some popular ones are given in **Table 2**.

Name of species	**Name of hybrids/varieties**
G. hirsutum varieties	'LRA 5166', 'Anjali', 'MCU 5', 'MCU 7', 'SVPR 2', 'H 777', 'Abhadita', 'Khandwa 2', 'Narasimha', 'NDLH 1938', 'Suraj', 'PKV 081', 'NH 615', 'LH 900', 'Surabhi', 'Pusa 8-6' and 'Sahana'
G. barbadense variety	'Suvin'
G. arboreum varieties	'HD 123', 'HD 324', 'PA 255', 'AKH 4', 'AKA 7', 'AKA 8' and 'AKA 8401'
Intra-*hirsutum* hybrids	'NHH 44', 'LHH 144', 'Shresth', 'HHH 287', 'DHH 11', 'H 6', 'H 8', 'PKV Hy 2' and 'JK Hy 2'
Interspecific hybrids (*G. hirsutum* × *G. barbadense*)	'DCH 32', 'TCHB 213' and 'DHB 105'
Intra-*arboreum* hybrid	'AAH 1', 'RAJ DH 9' and 'CISAA 2'
Interspecific hybrids (*G. herbaceum* × *G. arboreum*)	'G cot DH 7' and 'G cot DH 9'

Table 2. Prominent hybrids and varieties released through AICRP on Cotton for commercial cultivation.

The breeding and varietal release priorities changed with time to meet the changing quality requirements of the textile industry and also to suit specific requirements of the region in terms of maturity, agronomic traits tolerance to biotic and abiotic stresses, etc. The production and distribution of breeder seed of all the varieties and parents of hybrids released by the public sector based on the indent received from the Government of India is coordinated and monitored by AICRP on Cotton. The production has kept pace with the demand.

Location-specific agro-technologies—INM (organic, bio-fertilizers, Azospirillum, Azotobacter) for nutrient management, prevention of boll shedding using naphthalic acetic acid (40 ppm), weed management through pre-emergence application of pendimethalin @ 1.5 kg a.i./ha or fluchloralin @ 1.0 kg a.i./ha, soil moisture conversation using ridges/furrow system, microirrigation and fertigation using drip system, canopy managements using de-topping, diversification through innovative crop rotation/inter cropping, production technology of Bt hybrids (spacing, fertilizer requirement, water management, micro nutrient nutrition through foliar sprays) etc. were standardized, demonstrated and approved for subsequent incorporation into the package of practices for cotton production by the respective Agricultural Universities. A recent review by Venugopalan et al. [24] traces the agronomic research during the last six decades.

Screening for pest and disease resistance has been a regular feature of AICRP on Cotton programmes. Lines showing resistance/tolerance to key pest and diseases were recommended for utilizations as donors in breeding programmes (**Table 3**). Several multi-adversity-resistant lines with high yield have been developed.

Studies on seasonal dynamics of key pests and diseases at different locations over several years led to the development of robust pest and disease forecasting models using weather parameters. These modules are used to forewarn farmers through advisories disseminated using mass media. Economic threshold limits (ETLs) of various pests have been worked out to suggest timing of intervention for pest management. A simple symptom-based ETL was developed for major pests replacing the more cumbersome procedure of counting the number of insect pest. AICRP on Cotton is involved in testing the efficacy of new molecules and biological agents against pests and evaluation of their bio-safety. This has resulted in continuous revision of plant protection strategies using more effective and softer molecules. Location-specific IPM, IRM and disease management strategies have been formulated, validated, demonstrated and incorporated into the package of practices for commercial cotton cultivation in respective agro-climatic regions.

Front-line demonstrations on integrated nutrient management, novel inter-cropping systems, drip irrigation system, seed treatment with bio-fertilizers, maintenance of optimum plant density, *in situ* soil moisture conservation techniques, IPM, disease management, residue management techniques helped in bridging yield gaps, increasing yields and improving farm income. New farm implements and plant protection equipment with better ergonomics were demonstrated to reduce drudgery in cotton farming.

Biotic stress	Variety
Whitefly	Abhadita, LK 861, Kanchana and Supriya
Boll worms	Abhadita
Pink bollworms	Bikaneri Narma, H 777, F 414, F 286 and Ganganagar Ageti
Jassids	B 1007, Khandwa 2, Kirti, Mahalakshmi and CNHO 12
Fusarium wilt	G Cot 13, Eknath and Rohini
Bacterial blight	Arogya
Verticillium wilt	MCU 5 VT and Surabhi
Source: CIRCOT annual reports [19]	

Table 3. Varieties conferring resistance to biotic stress.

6.4. Other organizations/societies

Apart from the three institutions discussed earlier, several other government/non-governmental organizations (NGOs) and professional societies are also involved in the development, validation and dissemination of technologies on cotton. Prominent among the government organizations are the Directorate of Cotton Development (DCD), Nagpur, under the Ministry of Agriculture, and Cotton Corporation of India (CCI), Mumbai, under the Ministry of Textiles. While the Cotton Association of India, Mumbai, facilitates cotton testing and trade, its extension unit The Cotton and Allied products (COTAAP) Research Foundation conducts extension programmes to improve cotton productivity. Associations of the textile industries such as Ahmedabad Textile Industry Research Foundation (AITRA), Ahmedabad; Bombay Textile Research Association (BTRA), Mumbai; South India Textile Research Association (SITRA), Coimbatore; Northern India Textile Association (NITRA), Ghaziabad, Uttar Pradesh; and Southern India Mills Association (SIMA) along with Cotton Development and Research Association (CDRA), Coimbatore, are also involved in promoting cotton production and textile research. Three professional societies *viz*. the Indian Society for Cotton Improvement (ISCI), Mumbai; Cotton Research and Development Associations (CRDA), Hisar, Haryana; and the Indian Fibre Society, Mumbai, promote dissemination of research information through its journals and newsletters, and by organizing seminars, conferences and symposia.

7. Institutional mechanisms for transfer of technology, varietal release and seed production

7.1. Transfer of technology

Under the NARES, several institutional arrangements have been made to transfer new products and technologies to cotton farmers. The 'first-line extension system' includes the operational research projects (ORPs), on-farm demonstrations (OFDs), Lab-to-Land Programmes (LLPs), Krishi Vigyan Kendras (KVKs), e-kapas and Institute Village Linkage Programmes (IVLPs). The Directorate of Extension in SAUs also provide a variety of extension services. The General Extension Programmes are sponsored by the Ministry of Agriculture. Government of India comprises package programmes. Training and Visit (T&V), Agriculture Technology Management Agency (ATMA) and Farmer Field Schools (FFS). The 'Special Extension Programmes' with focus on cotton sponsored by the Ministry of Agriculture, Government of India, included 'Grow More Cotton' campaign, Intensive Cotton Development Programme (ICDP), TMC MM-II in the past and IRM—HDPS at present. The ICT-enabled e-kapas is another novel initiative to reach cotton farmers.

Among these institutions, ICDP made remarkable impact in the past [25]. It was launched in 1971/1972 and continued up to 1998/1999. Its objective was to achieve self-sufficiency in raw cotton by improving productivity through the adoption of improved farm practices and modern cotton production technologies. From 2000, these functions were carried out under the TMC MM-II. The ICAR launched Lab-to-Land Programme to transfer latest agro-technologies especially to small and marginal farmers. In cotton, the programme concentrated on promoting the use of improved seeds, IPM, disease management, nutrient management and yield maximization. The FFS, initiated in the 1990s by the Government of India to promote the concept of IPM in cotton through a participatory learning approach was funded by the TMC. The FLD in cotton began in 1996–1997 for demonstrating new cotton technologies and reduce

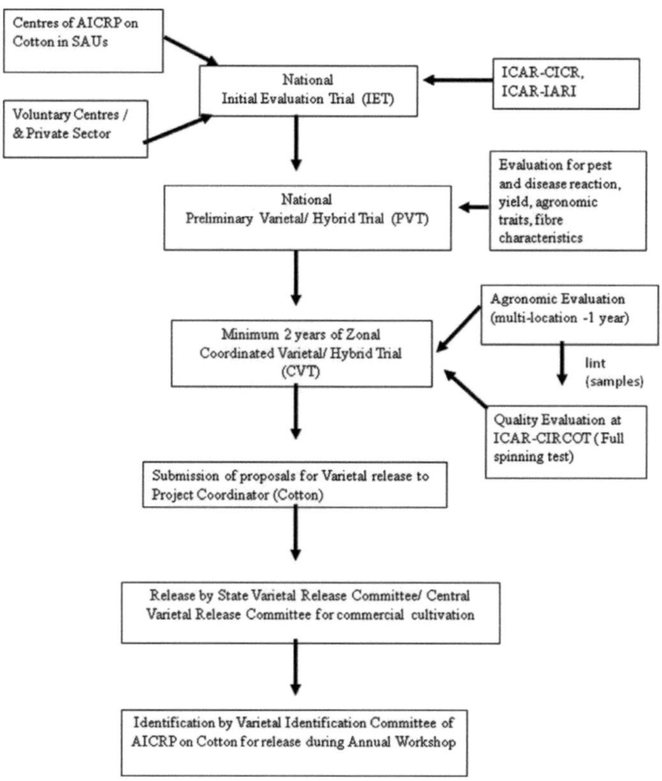

Figure 5. Protocol for testing and release of cotton varieties.

the time gap between technology generation and technology adoption. The AICRP on Cotton is the nodal agency for implementing FLDs, and the funds are provided by Government of India initially through the ICDP and later through the TMC MM-II. In a landmark initiative, the Government of India launched the TMC in 2000, to improve the yield and quality of cotton and increase the income of cotton farmers by reducing the cost of cultivation. Another objective of TMC was to improve the quality of processing of cotton by improving the infrastructure for market yards, for modernizing the existing ginning and pressing units and also to set up new units. Detailed account on the transfer of cotton technology has been discussed by Vithal et al. [25] and Wasnik et al. [26].

7.2. Varietal release

The AICRP on Cotton facilitates the development, evaluation and release of a variety/hybrid of cotton through a multi-location and multi-disciplinary approach. The entire process leading to the release of a variety by the Varietal Identification Committee is given in **Figure 5**. If a variety is indented to be released in a state, it is done by the State Varietal Release Committee. If during the evaluation trials, the variety/hybrid performs well in more than one state, the proposal for release is submitted to the Sub-Committee on Crop Standards Notification and Release of Variety of Central Seed Committee where it is released and notified. Even if a variety is released by the State Committee, it has to be notified by the Central Committee for its notification [27]. The denotification of old/obsolete varieties is also done by the same committee.

7.3. Structure of cotton seed production chain

To meet the requirement of quality seed, it is very much essential to produce large quantity of genetically pure seed which has to be multiplied in the following stages:

1. Nucleus seed is produced by the breeder who developed the variety;

2. Breeder's seed is produced from nucleus seed by the concerned ICAR/Institutes/SAUs as per the state indents;

3. Foundation seed is produced from breeder's seed by National Seed Corporation (NSC)/ State Seed Corporations (SSC)/State Farm Corporation of India (SFCI) subjected to certification by a certification agency;

Certified seed/registered seed is produced from foundation seed by SSC and gets it certified by State Seed Certification agency. Alternatively, in the case of shortage of certified seed, truthfully labelled seeds are multiplied under official supervision.

The R&D divisions of various seed companies in private sector are engaged in developing superior Bt-cotton hybrids. These are also tested in multi-location trials through sponsored trials in SAUs, and the companies own research farms for productivity and adaptability. For approved events, these hybrids are released through the EBAM. The mechanism and functional linkages between the different institutions involved in the approval of Bt cotton for commercial release is available in [28]. The seed quality testing and marketing of these hybrids are also exclusively undertaken by the private seed companies.

8. Linkages and collaborations

The ICAR-CICR and ICAR-CIRCOT are actively involved in guiding, formulating, monitoring and evaluating the research and technology transfer works undertaken by the collaborating centres of AICRP on Cotton. Need-based research collaborations within the NARES system and with other scientific organizations and universities are common. International collaborations and linkages to strengthen research capabilities and enhance human resource capabilities of ICAR-CICR involved the Indo-Australian Project with the Energy and Resources Institute —Centre for Environmental Stress and Adaptation Research, Melbourne (TERI-CEASAR) 'for insect transgenic detection kits, International Plant Genetic Resource Institute (IPGRI)', Rome for augmenting cotton germplasm, International Centre for Genetic Engineering Biotechnology (ICGEB) for the development of gene construct and International Cotton Genome Initiative (ICGI) for the development of cotton genome.

A collaborative programme on the management of *Helicoverpa armigera* was operating with Central Cotton Research Institute, Pakistan, Nanjing Agricultural University, China, and Natural Resources Institute, UK. ICAR-CICR is also closely involved in the activities of the ICAC and International Cotton Researchers Association (ICRA). It collaborates with the C4 countries, Nigeria, Uganda and Malawi under the Cotton Technical Assistance Programme for Africa for capacity building and human resource development. ICAR-CIRCOT has developed close collaboration with international organizations such as ICAC; Common Fund for Commodities (CFC); United Nations Development Programme (UNDP); World Bank Cotton Development Organization (CDO), Uganda; Ministry of Agriculture and Food Security, Malawi; and *Institut National des Recherches Agricoles du Benin* (INRAB), Benin.

9. Future perspectives

The last two decades witnessed the emergence of private sector as a strong partner to public sector research organizations particularly in the development of transgenic Bt hybrids and seed production. There was a rapid adoption of Bt hybrids. Cotton spread to new areas and the production increased, but today several pointers are being raised at the sustainability of the 'hybrid' technology. High cost of inputs (seed, fertilizer, pesticides), increasing production cost, increasing severity of jassids, whitefly, leaf reddening and resistance in pink bollworms to Cry1Ac and Cry2Ab are the challenges evading solutions. Currently, the cotton varietal seed production chain in public sector is almost defunct, and this needs to be revived. Technologies for future must be based on sustainable practices giving high yield at low production cost.

Immediate challenges in cotton production include but not limited to:

1. Development of novel technologies to reduce cost of cultivation and make cotton farming more profitable by reducing the dependence on chemical fertilizers, pesticides and labour.

2. Delineation of areas not suitable for hybrid cotton and replacement of this area with cotton production systems using straight varieties of *G. hirsutum* or *G. arboreum*.

3. Improvement of the management options to delay the development of resistance of bollworms to Cry toxins and manage sucking pests more efficiently.

4. Mechanization of cotton production 'including mechanical picking' to suit small land holding and reduce drudgery among labour.

5. Application of efficient cropping systems (inter and sequential cropping) preferably with pulses/legumes to enhance atmospheric N fixation and increase pulse production.

6. Utilization of climate resilient technologies to realize stable and sustainable yields on marginal soils under rainfed conditions.

7. Intensification of researches on IRM and host plant resistance to whitefly and cotton leaf curl virus disease to combat biotic stress.

8. Development of human resource for improving research infrastructure and research funding to address emerging challenges.

9. Retention of the competitive edge of cotton over other natural and synthetic fibres.

Research and development expertise available in the public and private sector needs to complement each other to deliver the best solutions to the cotton farmer. There is a need to consolidate international linkage activities with International Rice Research Institute (IRRI), ICGEB, International Maize and Wheat Improvement Center (CIMMYT), International Crops Research Institute for the Semi-Arid Tropics (ICRISAT), ICAC, International Board for Plant Genetic Resources (IBPGR), Bio-21 Biodiversity International-Rome, International Food Policy Research Institute (IFPRI), Indo-American Knowledge Initiative, International Centre for Agricultural Research for Dry Area (ICARDA), IITA-International Institute for Tropical Agriculture (legumes, cereals, pulses), Commonwealth Scientific and Industrial Research Organisation (CSIRO), Australia, through collaborative research programmes.

10. Conclusion

The ICAR-CICR, ICAR- CIRCOT and the AICCIP now renamed as AICRP on Cotton form the pillars of public sector R&D in cotton. A strong public sector R&D set-up backed by a vibrant private sector has provided cutting-edge technological support to enable India to emerge from a chronic importer into a global leader in cotton production over the years. The production of a wide variety of cotton provides the desired raw material to the textile industry at competitive price and enables the industry produce apparels and other end-products in a globally competitive environment. The entire value chain of cottonseed to finished products is primarily built on technologies generated by indigenous R&D. The entry of private sector in the development and marketing of Bt hybrids is another feature of Indian cotton sector that enabled it to emerge as the largest cotton producer in the world. Challenges still remain in both cotton production, and processing and these institutions will continue to play a major role in the years ahead.

Acknowledgements

The support, assistance and encouragement provided by the Director Dr. K.R. Kranthi, ICAR-CICR is gratefully acknowledged.

Author details

Mangat V. Venugopalan*, Mahendra Singh Yadav and Vandana Satish

*Address all correspondence to: mvvenugopalan@gmail.com

ICAR-Central Institute for Cotton Research, Nagpur, Maharashtra, India

References

[1] Indian Council of Agricultural Research. ICAR Vision 2050. 1st ed. New Delhi: ICAR; 2015. 34p.

[2] Senthilkumar M. Home grown cotton – the growth driver for the Indian textile industry. In: Souvenir 74th Plenary meeting of ICAC; 6–11 December 2015; Mumbai: ICAC; 2015. pp. 60–63.

[3] Central Institute for Research on Cotton Technology, editor. CIRCOT Vision 2030. 1st ed. Mumbai: CIRCOT; 2011. 29p.

[4] Sethi BL. Advances in cotton production in India during 1947-62. The Indian Cotton Growing Review. 1963;XVII :75–81.

[5] Sikka SM, Joshi AB. Breeding. In: Cotton in India, A Monograph. Vol. I, Bombay, India: Indian Central Cotton Committee; 1960. pp. 137–335.

[6] Santhanam V. Genetic improvement of cotton in India. Indian Journal of Genetics and Plant Breeding. 1974;34:816–821.

[7] Basu AK. Genetic research in cotton in India. Genetica. 1996;97:279–290.

[8] Rajendran TP, Basu AK. Integrated pest management in cotton: Historical perspectives, present scenario and future strategies. In: Sundaram V, Basu AK, Krishna Iyer KR, Narayanan SS, Rajendran TP, editors. Handbook of Cotton in India. Mumbai: Indian Society for Cotton Improvement; 1999. pp. 205–232.

[9] Kranthi KR, Russell D. Changing trends in Cotton Pest Management. In: Peshin R, Dhawan AK, editors. Integrated Pest Management: Innovation-Development Process. The Netherlands: Springer Science+Business; 2009. pp. 499–541.

[10] Kranthi KR. Diagnosis holds the key to "Problem-Solving" in cotton cultivation. In: ICAC, editor. Souvenir 74th Plenary Meeting of ICAC; 6–11 Dec. 2015; Mumbai. India: ICAC; 2015. pp. 25–30.

[11] Suresh A, Ramasundaram P, Samuel S, Wankhade S. Impact of Technology and Policy on Growth and Instability of Agricultural Production: The Case of Cotton in India. Indian Journal of Agricultural Sciences. 2013;83(8):939–948.

[12] Rajendran TP, Venugopalan MV, Prahraj CS. Cotton research towards sufficiency to Indian textile industry. Indian Journal of Agricultural Sciences. 2005;75:699–705.

[13] Sethi BL. History of cotton. In: Cotton in India. A Monograph. Vol. I ed. Indian Central Cotton Committee, Bombay, India; 1960. pp. 1–39.

[14] Santhanam V, Sundaram V. Agri-history of cotton in India–an overview. Asian Agri-History . 1997;1:235–251.

[15] Santhanam V, Sundaram V. Historical perspective of cotton in India. In: Sundaram V, Basu AK, Krishna Iyer KR, Narayanan SS, Rajendran TP, editors. Handbook of Cotton in India. Mumbai: Indian Society for Cotton Improvement; 1999. pp. 1–17.

[16] Sundaram V. Antiquity of Cotton. In: 50 years of research at Cotton Technological Research Laboratory. Indian Council of Agricultural Research, New Delhi, India; 1974. DOI: 212

[17] Current Research Projects in Cotton. International Cotton Advisory Committee; 2012. 140 p.

[18] Central Institute for Cotton Research [Internet]. CICR, Nagpur. 2016. Available from: www.cicr.org.in [Accessed: 2016-014-16].

[19] CIRCOT annual reports [Internet]. CIRCOT, Mumbai. 2016. Available from: http://circot.res.in/circot/publications/circot-annual-reports [Accessed: 2016-014-16].

[20] Rajendran TP, Jain KC. Achievements in Cotton Research in the All India Coordinated Cotton Improvement Project; CICR Regional Station, Coimbatore (TN). 2004. 104 p.

[21] Basu AK, Narayanan SS, editors. Achievements of AICCIP (1967-92). Coimbatore, India: All India Coordinated Cotton Improvement Project (AICCIP); CICR, Nagpur. 1992. 176p.

[22] Gopalakrishnan N, Manickam S, Sabesh M, Usharani S, Pundhir P, Nehra PL, Surulivelu T, Monga D. All India Coordinated Cotton Improvement Project – in the service of Indian cotton farmers. Technical Bulletin No. 2; CICR Regional Station, Coimbatore (TN). 2010. 31p.

[23] All India Coordinated Cotton Improvement Project (AICCIP) [Internet]. CICR Regional Station, Coimbatore (TN). 2016. Available from: http://aiccip.cicr.org.in/ [Accessed: 2016-014-16]

[24] Venugopalan MV, Blaise D, Yadav MS, Vandana S. Advances and milestones in agronomic research on cotton in India. Indian Journal of Agronomy. 2012;57:71–78.

[25] Vithal BM, Barik A. Tranfer of Technology – A strong tool to improve cotton productivity and farmer's income in India. In: Sundaram V, Basu AK, Krishna Iyer KR, Narayanan SS, Rajendran TP, editors. Handbook of Cotton in India . Indian Society for Cotton Improvement, Mumbai; 1999. pp. 508–525.

[26] Wasnik SM, Mayee CD, Singh P. Technology Transfer in Cotton. Technical Bulletin No: 23. CICR, Nagpur; 2002. 11p.

[27] Basu AK. Present scenario and future prospects of cotton seed in India. In: Sundaram V, Basu AK, Krishna Iyer KR, Narayanan SS, Rajendran TP, editors. Handbook of Cotton in India. Indian Society for Cotton Improvement, Mumbai; 1999. pp. 79–103.

[28] Karihaloo J L, Kumar PA. Bt Cotton in India – A Status Report. 2nd ed. Asia-Pacific Consortium on Agricultural Biotechnology (APCoAB), New Delhi, India; 2009. 56p.

Chapter 3

Photoprotection of Cotton in the Field

Ya-li Zhang, Xiao-ping Yi, Wang-feng Zhang,
Wah Soon Chow, Yuan-yuan Hu, Chao Zhang and
Dong-xia Zhan

Additional information is available at the end of the chapter

http://dx.doi.org/10.5772/64049

Abstract

This chapter focuses on the mechanisms by which cotton leaves regulate and use incident light and dissipate the excess light energy when cotton suffers from drought in the field. The photoprotection of non-foliar organs, including bract, capsule wall and stem, will also be considered. This chapter includes a general description of photoprotection from the perspective of leaf movement, drought and non-foliar organs. Leaf diaheliotropic movement and wilting movement can regulate the excess light energy of the photosynthetic apparatus. Besides non-photochemical (heat) energy dissipation, the alternative electron sinks for the electron transport chains are of vital importance for resistance of the photosynthetic apparatus against excess light energy under drought. Thus, the functioning of both photosystem II (PSII) and the photosynthetic electron transport systems of cotton leaves shows a relatively high stability. Compared with leaf, bract mainly relies on high activities of thermal energy dissipation for photoprotection. Nevertheless, capsule wall of bolls is less able to dissipate energy via heat.

Keywords: cotton, leaf movement, thermal dissipation, photochemistry, ROS scavenging

1. Introduction

Sunlight is essential for photosynthesis and supports most life on earth. However, too much sunlight damages the photosynthetic machinery. The amount of light energy encountered by plants in excess of that needed for photosynthetic assimilation is termed excess light energy. When the excess light energy cannot be dissipated safely, the electron transport chain becomes highly reduced, and electron transfer to O_2 increases, producing reactive oxygen species (ROS). ROS is very damaging to the photosynthetic apparatus, primarily photosystem II (PSII), causing photoinhibition [1–3]. To counteract photoinhibition, plants have evolved multiple photoprotective mechanisms to cope with the potentially damaging effects of excess light energy. On the one hand, acclimation to adverse conditions can occur in terms of morphological characteristics such as light avoidance associated with the movement of leaves [4, 5] and chloroplasts [6]. On the other hand, biochemical processes such as photorespiration [7, 8], the Mehler-peroxidase reaction [9], cyclic electron transport [10, 11] and thermal dissipation [12, 13] can help to dissipate excess light energy from the photosynthetic apparatus.

High-light stress is exacerbated by drought. Drought is considered to be the most limiting environment factor [14, 15]. During drought, the process of photosynthetic carbon assimilation is primarily suppressed [15, 16]. As a result, the plant has to dissipate more excess light energy in order to avoid photo-oxidative stress, thereby maintaining photosynthetic productivity under drought.

Cotton (*Gossypium* spp.) is a plant of tropical origin, an oilseed and fibre crop that is cultivated in more than 70 countries worldwide. There are four species of cultivated cotton, *G. hirsutum, G. barbadense, G. arboretum* and *G. herbaceum*, providing the world's most important textile fibre. *G. hirsutum*, commonly referred to as upland cotton, is the most extensively developed species and accounts for about 90% of total world production. *G. barbadense*, referred to as pima cotton, is valued for superior fibre properties. Thus, two cotton species, upland cotton and pima cotton, will be discussed here. In this chapter, we not only focus on the photoprotection of the leaf but also on the photoprotection of non-foliar organs, because photosynthetic production of non-foliar organs significantly contributes to the yield in cotton [17]. In addition, we emphasize results from the field experiments on cotton, not from the lab or greenhouse.

2. Leaf movement and photoprotection

Generally, leaf movement includes three types: leaf diaheliotropic movement, leaf paraheliotropic movement and leaf wilting movement. The first one provides maximum interception of sunlight, whereas both the second and the third give minimum interception of sunlight. Many researchers have reported that leaf paraheliotropic movement is a vital important way to reduce the excess light energy of the leaves generally in leguminous species [18, 19]. However, cotton has leaf diaheliotropic movement and wilting movement depending on the water status of leaves. Actually, leaf wilting movement is quite general in higher plants.

Upland cotton has leaf diaheliotropic movement, but pima cotton has no or only weak diaheliotropic movement [20, 21]. Given their maximum interception of light, the leaves of upland cotton must be accompanied by strong photosynthetic assimilation or dissipation of excess light energy. When leaves of upland cotton are restrained to the horizontal position, carbon assimilation decreases compared to diaheliotropic leaves because of less interception of light [22]. However, there is no difference in the recovery of maximal quantum yield of PSII photochemistry (F_v/F_m) between diaheliotropic and restrained leaves [22]. This means that the leaves of upland cotton have photoprotection mechanisms to trade-off the maximum interception of light and excess light energy. A number of reports have suggested that thermal energy dissipation in the photosynthetic apparatus is involved in photoprotection in upland cotton and pima cotton [22–24]. As mentioned above, leaf diaheliotropic movement is absent or weakly expressed in pima cotton. Pima cotton has lower actual photosynthetic assimilation than upland cotton in the field even if diaheliotropic leaf movement of upland cotton resulting in high incident leaf sunlight is taken into account. However, both cotton species exhibit similar photosynthetic potential [24].

Zhang et al. [25] found that upland cotton preferentially dissipates light energy via electron transport, whereas pima cotton mainly does so through thermal energy dissipation. Indeed, Wise et al. [26] reported that electron transport limits the photosynthesis of field-grown pima cotton. Thus, using different photoprotective mechanisms, both cotton species have a strong capacity for photoprotection to maintain the activity of the two photosystems. Further, some photoprotective mechanisms, such as thermal energy dissipation and photorespiration, mitigate against excess light energy. Interestingly, in young leaves of upland cotton, the photoprotective mechanisms also operated well even when the photosynthetic apparatus was not yet fully assembled [27]. In addition, in an experiment conducted to compare cotton and soybean which differ in leaf movement under drought, cotton and soybean showed different strategies for conferring photoprotection [28].

Leaf wilting movement occurs generally under drought when the water potential of leaves and the osmotic potential of petiole cells exceed the threshold. This leaf movement may have multiple physiological significance for plants because it may reduce both water loss from the leaf and the amount of light incident on the leaf surface, the latter lowering the energy load on a leaf [29]. Leaf wilting movement becomes apparent only after several anatomical and physiological adjustments have occurred as drought develops [30]. In cotton, when leaves are not restrained to the horizontal position, the wilting movement of leaves protects water-stressed cotton plants against photoinhibition and maintains considerable carbon assimilation in the long term [5]. Clearly, passive wilting leaf movement can be a strategy for photoprotection that enables plants to survive under drought.

3. Photoprotection under drought

3.1. Drought and photoinhibition

Drought decreases CO_2 assimilation rate [31], and photosynthesis saturates at a lower PPFD in drought plants. For instance, maximum CO_2 assimilation rates under well-watered conditions are about 42.4 (upland cotton) and 37.1 (pima cotton) μmol m^{-2} s^{-1}, and 25.1 (upland cotton) and 23.9 (pima cotton) μmol m^{-2} s^{-1} under drought, respectively [32]. The light saturation points are 2304 and 1996 μmol m^{-2} s^{-1} in well-watered and drought upland cotton plants, respectively [28]. In field conditions, drought is usually accompanied by other limiting factors, such as high temperature and irradiance. Therefore, when drought stress occurs simultaneously with high irradiance, cotton plants may be exposed to an excess of excitation energy, potentially increasing the susceptibility of PSII to photoinhibition.

Zhang et al. [5] have reported that the diurnal time course of F_v/F_m is similar in both well-watered upland and pima cotton plants; the values of F_v/F_m are ~0.80 in the morning, after which the values decrease to ~0.72 at noon and recover to ~0.80 in late afternoon. Some reports have demonstrated that drought-stressed upland cotton plants are characterized by a higher F_v/F_m [33–35]. For example, Yi et al. [32] have reported that the pre-dawn F_v/F_m is ~0.85 in both upland and pima cotton under well-watered and water-deficit conditions. Sustained photoinhibition of PSII seems not to occur in field-grown cotton plants under drought since no significant decrease in pre-dawn F_v/F_m has been reported. This phenomenon has been observed earlier by Genty et al. [36] who demonstrated that water stress does not induce sensitization to photoinhibition in cotton. Additionally, Yi et al. [37] found that the activities of photosystem II (PSII) and photosystem I (PSI) show almost no changes during water deficit and recovery, though water deficit leads to a reversible reduction in the photosynthetic rate. Therefore, the photosystems of field-grown cotton plants are relatively stable under drought stress.

As describe above, drought stress decreases CO_2 assimilation rate but does not induce sustained photoinhibition of PSII in field-grown cotton plants. Therefore, field-grown cotton plants may possess multiple photoprotective strategies to cope with drought stress (see below).

3.2. Thermal dissipation of absorbed light energy

Plants can dissipate excessive light energy harmlessly as heat [38–40] which is called 'thermal energy dissipation'. Thermal dissipation, measured as non-photochemical quenching of Chl fluorescence (NPQ), is related to the pH gradient across the photosynthetic (thylakoid) membrane and promoted by the activity of the xanthophyll cycle, with conversion of violaxanthin to zeaxanthin, via antheraxanthin, by the catalyst violaxanthin de-epoxidase (VDE) [41]. Demmig-Adams et al. [42] showed that in well-watered sunflower plants, more than 50% of absorbed light is thermally dissipated at midday. In well-watered cotton plants, ~44% of the absorbed light energy is used in photosynthetic electron transport (photosynthesis and photorespiration), and the remaining 56% is dissipated as thermal energy [43]. Kornyeyev et al. [44] and Massacci et al. [33] also reported that non-photochemical energy dissipation serves as the major photoprotective mechanism when light energy absorption becomes excessive in cotton plants. Under moderate and severe drought, thermal dissipation increases up to 70–82% of the total absorbed light in cotton plants [43]. In addition, Zhang et al. [28] and Yi et al. [32] observed that pima cotton has generally higher thermal energy dissipation capacity than upland cotton under well-watered conditions. However, Genty et al. [36] and Yi et al. [32] also found that water deficit does not increase thermal dissipation in upland cotton plants. A similar result was reported by Inamullah and Isoda [45] who found that there is no significant change in photochemical reflectance index (PRI) (which is correlated with the epoxidation state of the xanthophyll cycle) in upland cotton under water deficit. Perhaps different cotton cultivars, studied under different experimental conditions such as temperature and irradiance, exhibit different thermal energy dissipation capacities in response to drought (**Figure 1**).

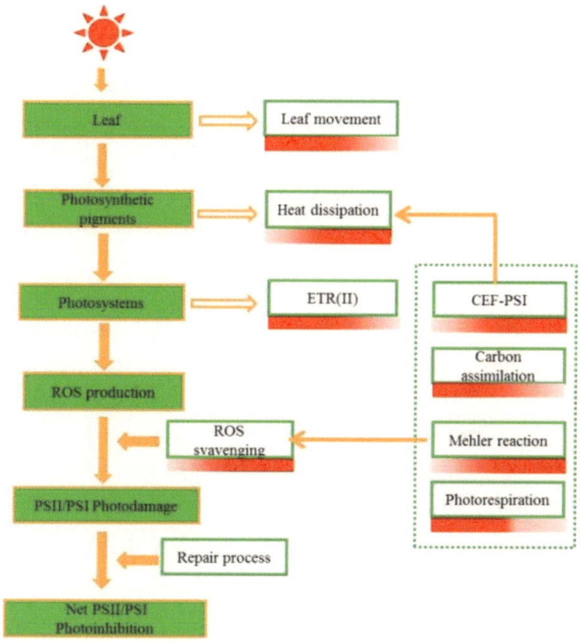

Figure 1. A model of photoprotection mechanisms in field-grown cotton plants under drought. Cotton leaves can utilize diaheliotropic movement and wilting movement to adjust the absorption of light energy. In addition, leaves can dissipate excessive energy through electron transport pathways, including photorespiration, Mehler reaction and cyclic electron transport. Furthermore, ROS scavenging and repair process also have an important role in avoiding sustained photoinhibition in leaves. Arrow indicates the induction processes, and the shades of red indicate the response of biochemical processes to drought.

3.3. Photoprotection through photochemistry

It is well known that under normal conditions much of the photosynthetic electron flow is used to drive the photochemical reaction, with conversion of the absorbed light energy to active chemical energy stored in ATP, NADPH and Fd_{red}. The excitation energy, distributed in favour of photochemical reactions, is mainly used for photosynthetic carbon reduction, photorespiratory carbon oxidation and alternative electron transport. A few studies have reported that when the CO_2 assimilation rate is decreased under drought, cotton plants can dissipate excessive energy through other electron transport pathways, including photorespiration [23, 32–34], Mehler reaction [23, 32] and cyclic electron transport [46, 47].

3.3.1. Photorespiration

Photorespiration is the reaction of O_2 with ribulose-1,5-bisphosphate (RuBP) catalysed by ribulose-1,5-bisphosphate carboxylase/oxygenase (rubisco), producing glycolate-2-P [48]. Photorespiration is second only to photosynthesis as the most important mechanism for utilization of electrons, occurring at high rates in the leaves of C_3 plants [8]. Under well-watered and saturating light conditions, photosynthesis and photorespiration dissipate 20–30%

and 10–20% of absorbed light, respectively [49]. Similarly, Björkman and Schäfer [43] reported that in well-watered cotton plants, 25% of the absorbed light is used for photosynthesis and 19% for photorespiration. Tourneux and Peltier [50] demonstrated that photorespiration is a substantial sink for electrons in leaves at high and low relative water content (RWC). Chastain et al. [34] and Yi et al. [23] concluded that water deficit increases photorespiration since photosynthesis is decreased by stomatal (CO_2) limitation in field-grown cotton plants. However, Cornic and Fresneau [51] pointed that during mild drought, photosynthesis and photorespiration are the main electron sinks for PSII activity. Further, Massacci et al. [33] demonstrated that cotton leaves can increase the capacity for photorespiration to prevent photodamage during the onset of drought stress. A similar result was reported by Yi et al. [32] who showed that under mild water deficit, pima cotton appears to rely on enhanced photorespiration to dissipate light energy while under moderate water deficit, the contribution of photorespiration decreases. Actually, all the results that reported increased photorespiration under conditions of CO_2 limitation have been based on relative values (such as the ratio of photorespiration to photosynthesis or the ratio of oxygenation to carboxylation) or indirect data [23, 32, 33, 43, 52, 53]; the absolute rate of photorespiration decreases [28, 52, 54, 55].

3.3.2. Mehler-peroxidase reaction or the water-water cycle

The Mehler-peroxidase reaction (MPR) is the reduction of O_2 to water in PSI by the electrons generated in PSII from water [56]. The functions of the Mehler-peroxidase reaction for protection from photoinhibition are to scavenge reactive oxygen species (ROS), thereby protecting chloroplasts from the direct effects of ROS [9]. Badawi et al. [57] reported that overexpression of ascorbate peroxidase (APX) in tobacco chloroplasts show enhanced tolerance to salt and drought stresses. In addition, the Mehler-peroxidase reaction can regulate CO_2 fixation and excess energy dissipation through adjustment of the production ratio of ATP/NADPH. Ziem-Hanck and Heber [58] demonstrated that under anaerobic conditions, no CO_2 is fixed in intact chloroplasts because of a low ratio of ATP/NADPH, but the addition of O_2 allows CO_2 assimilation to start by increasing the production of ATP through the Mehler-peroxidase reaction. Osmond [7] indicated that higher ATP/NADPH is required to operate photorespiration, and that the Mehler-peroxidase reaction may supply additional ATP for photorespiration. Neubauer and Yamamoto [59] reported that the Mehler-peroxidase reaction contributes to the generation of a transmembrane proton gradient for thermal dissipation of excess absorbed light energy. Furthermore, the Mehler-peroxidase reaction itself can dissipate excess electrons using O_2 as the electron acceptor.

Wingler et al. [60] suggested that at low water potential, the increased electron flow to O_2 was mainly due to the Mehler reaction. Biehler and Fock [55] observed that 29% of the photosynthetic electrons are consumed in the Mehler-peroxidase reaction in drought-stressed wheat leaves. Our recent results showed that water deficit increases the electron flux for O_2-dependent alternative electron transport in upland cotton plants, which is related to the Mehler-peroxidase reaction activity [23]. However, studies conducted with different species under drought stress provide partly contradictory results on the role of Mehler-peroxidase reaction. Yi et al.

[32] found that the contribution of the Mehler-peroxidase reaction to excess electrons dissipation is very low in water-deficit pima cotton. Similar results were also reported by Haupt-Herting and Fock [61] in tomato and Flexas et al. [53] in grapevines. In addition, Björkman and Schäfer [43] reported that energy dissipation through photorespiration plus the Mehler-peroxidase reaction gradually decreases with increasing water deficit in cotton plants, and the contribution of the Mehler-peroxidase reaction to total dissipation is low or null.

3.3.3. Cyclic electron transport

Cyclic electron flow (CEF) around PSI (CEF-PSI) is the recycling of electrons from PSI to the plastoquinone pool and the cytochrome b6f complex via reduced Fd or NADPH [10, 62–65]. It is well known that CEF-PSI is essential for protecting PSII against excess excitation pressure because CEF-dependent build-up of a ΔpH across the thylakoid membrane helps the activation of NPQ [10, 66–70] and prevents the inhibition of the repair of photodamaged PSII [3, 11]. The result can be explained by the fact that NPQ suppresses the production of ROS [71].

A number of studies indicated that CEF-PSI plays a significant physiological role in plant responses to drought or desiccation [11, 68, 70, 72, 73]. Singh et al. [46] demonstrated that CEF-PSI plays an important role in tolerance under drought stress in upland cotton plants, which are grown in a growth chamber. A similar result was also observed in our recent experiment on greenhouse-grown upland cotton, using the method of Kou et al. [70] to estimate CEF-PSI (data not shown). In addition, Singh et al. [47] compared the activity of CEF-PSI in drought stress upland and pima cotton plants and concluded that drought increases the activity of CEF-PSI in both cotton species, but that pima cotton showed lower CEF-PSI under drought as well as well-watered condition in comparison to upland cotton. However, our recent studies with field-grown cotton under water-deficit conditions showed that pima cotton possessed a higher CEF-PSI capacity compared with upland cotton (data not shown). Different grown conditions and methods may result in different conclusions, and so far, there is still a considerable lack of knowledge about the photoprotective functions of CEF-PSI in field-grown cotton. Therefore, CEF-PSI in cotton requires further study.

3.4. Scavenging of reactive oxygen species

Drought may induce an oxidative stress due to the inhibition of photosynthesis, resulting in the production and accumulation of reactive oxygen species (ROS) at the photosystems [9]. ROS can damage the photosynthetic apparatus, through oxidation of lipids, proteins, carbohydrates and nucleic acids [74, 75]. The major antioxidative systems in the plant, including superoxide dismutases (SOD), ascorbate peroxidase (APX), peroxidase (POD) and catalase (CAT), together with carotenoids, ascorbate (AsA) and glutathione (GSH), provide cells with highly efficient machinery for detoxifying O_2 and H_2O_2 [76]. Additionally, some osmolytes such as proline and glycine betaine can also contribute to the relief of oxidative stress [77].

Mahan and Wanjura [78] reported that the content of AsA and the activity of APX are increased in response to water stress, but the GSH amount and form are not. Further, there is no significant change in the levels of malondialdehyde (MDA), an indicator of cell-membrane damage. Therefore, they concluded that antioxidative metabolism in field-grown cotton plants exposed to drought stress is sufficient to protect against oxidative damage. A similar result was also observed in our experiment [37]. Over-expression of APX improves the antioxidative system and enhances tolerance of cotton plants against low temperature [79]. In addition, our results also showed that the activities of SOD and POD are increased under water deficit [23, 37] and that the activities of SOD and APX increase under water deficit in upland cotton, while those enzymes do not response to water deficit in pima cotton [32]. However, Kawakami et al. [80] also reported that the activity of SOD in water-stressed cotton plants is significantly decreased compared to the well-watered plants. It appears that the levels of the antioxidative systems may increase, decrease or remain unchanged depending on plant species, the period and the intensity of water deficit and plant age or developmental stage [81]. Additionally, De Ronde et al. [82] and Yi et al. [37] reported that with increasing water deficit there is a progressive increase in free proline in cotton plants.

3.5. Repair of photodamage

Although there are multiple photoprotective mechanisms, photo-oxidative damage to the photosynthetic apparatus is an inevitable process under drought. Takahashi and Badger [3] reported that net photoinhibition only occurs when the rate of damage exceeds the rate of repair. Chow and Aro [83] reported that during the course of a sunny day, the entire population of PSII could be photoinactivated if repair is inhibited. Aro et al. [84] suggested that fast recovery of damaged PSII helps the plant reduce the susceptibility to photoinhibition. Lee et al. [85] and Kato et al. [86] indicated that a higher rate of turnover of D1 protein plays a crucial role in photoprotection in high light-grown plants. A similar result was also observed by Oguchi et al. [87] in spinach and *Alocasia* leaves. Field-grown cotton plants are often exposed to high irradiance, but there is no sustained net photoinhibition of PSII. It means that the rate of repair must match the rate of damage to avoid the occurrence of net photoinhibition in field-grown cotton plants under water deficit. Indeed, the rate coefficient of repair of upland cotton increases steadily with irradiance up to at least 1300 μmol photons m^{-2} s^{-1}, provided there is no oxidative stress [88].

3.6. Non-foliar organs and photoprotection

Aschan and Pfanz [89] in a review have concluded that photosynthesis of non-foliar organs is an important, additional contribution to carbon acquisition and yield. Examples are the panicles of rice, the ear of wheat [90, 91], the spikes of barley and the fruit in tomato [92]. Besides leaves, many parts of cotton, including stem, bract and boll, contain chlorophyll and, therefore, capture light energy to perform photosynthesis. The stems, bracts and the capsule wall of bolls contribute to carbon gain [93–96]. In cotton, Hu et al. [17] have reported that darkening the non-foliar organs reduced the boll weight by 24.1 (boll) and 9% (main stem) and the seed weight by 35.9 (boll) and 16.3% (main stem). Therefore, we have concluded that non-foliar organs of cotton are of vital importance to the yield at the late growth stage due to leaves tending to senesce earlier than non-foliar organs [17].

Undoubtedly, the leaves are more physiologically active, with greater rates of photosynthesis and respiration than the bracts and capsule walls [17, 93, 95]. As we can see in the field, however, non-foliar organs and leaves are normally exposed to similar irradiance. Therefore, one wonders whether the non-foliars organs have different ways of dissipating the excess light energy safely to confer on photoprotection. Zhang et al. [97] have conducted an experiment to compare the characteristics of PSII behaviour in leaves and non-foliar organs and concluded that lower PSII photochemical activity in non-foliar organs may result from limitations at the donor side of PSII and the acceptor sides of both photosystems. Compared to leaves, the thermal dissipation fraction of light absorbed by the PSII antennae is the highest in the bract and the lowest in the capsule wall of bolls. Furthermore, the capsule wall of bolls is characterized by a smaller combined constitutive thermal dissipation (with little dependence on irradiance) and dissipation as fluorescence emission [97]. Furthermore, Hu et al. [98] suggested that the bract dissipates its absorbed light energy via ΔpH- and xanthophyll-regulated thermal dissipation for photoprotection, aided by the high activities of antioxidative enzymes. The main stem preferentially uses both light-regulated and light-independent non-photochemical quenching to confer photoprotection. The capsule wall of bolls is less able to dissipate energy via heat. Thus, its main photoprotective mechanisms of the capsule wall of bolls seem to be direct quenching of the energy by abundant carotenoids and light-independent constitutive thermal dissipation. Furthermore, because of lower activities of antioxidative enzymes, the capsule wall of bolls is less able to scavenge reactive oxygen species.

In addition, we have proposed that the photosynthesis from non-foliar organs is important for increasing cotton yield especially under drought conditions [98, 99]. Non-foliar organs (bract and capsule wall) show less ontogenetic decrease in photosynthetic capacity, photosynthetic enzyme activity and better antioxidative systems than leaves in response to drought stress. Thus, the relative photosynthetic contribution of the non-foliar organs to the whole plant is expected to increase under drought [98]. In the bract, both photorespiration and energy dissipation appear to alleviate photoinhibition and play important roles in photoprotection [100].

4. Conclusion

A brief review of the photoprotection of cotton in the field has been presented. We included a general description of photoprotection from the perspective of leaf movement, drought and non-foliar organs. Clearly, leaf diaheliotropic movement and wilting movement can regulate the excess light energy of the photosynthetic apparatus. Besides non-photochemical (heat) energy dissipation, the alternative electron sinks for the electron transport chains are of vital importance for resistance of the photosynthetic apparatus against excess light energy in the field. Thus, both the functioning of PSII and the photosynthetic electron transport systems of cotton leaves show a relatively high stability. Compared with leaf, bract mainly relies on high activities of thermal energy dissipation for photoprotection. Nevertheless, the capsule wall of bolls is less able to dissipate energy via heat.

Acknowledgements

This study was financially supported by the National Natural Science Foundation of China (Grant No. 31260295; U1203283), the Shihezi University Funds for Distinguished Young Scientists (Grant No. 2012ZRKXJQ04) and China Scholarship Council fellowship.

Author details

Ya-li Zhang[†1], Xiao-ping Yi[†1], Wang-feng Zhang[1*], Wah Soon Chow[2], Yuan-yuan Hu[1], Chao Zhang[1] and Dong-xia Zhan[1]

*Address all correspondence to: zhwf_agr@shzu.edu.cn; zwf_shzu@163.com

1 The Key Laboratory of Oasis Eco-Agriculture, Xinjiang Production and Construction Group, Shihezi University, Shihezi, Xinjiang, P.R. China

2 Division of Plant Sciences, Research School of Biology, The Australian National University, Acton, ACT, Australia

†These authors contributed equally to this work and should be regarded as joint first authors.

References

[1] Krieger-Liszkay A, Fufezan C, Trebst A. Singlet oxygen production in photosystem II and related protection mechanism. Photosynthesis Research. 2008;98:551–64. DOI: 10.1007/s11120-008-9349-3

[2] Murchie EH, Niyogi KK. Manipulation of photoprotection to improve plant photosynthesis. Plant Physiology. 2011;155:86–92. DOI: 10.1104/pp.110.168831

[3] Takahashi S, Badger MR. Photoprotection in plants: a new light on photosystem II damage. Trends in Plant Science. 2011;16:53–60. DOI: 10.1016/j.tplants.2010.10.001

[4] Isoda A, Wang PW. Leaf temperature and transpiration of field grown cotton and soybean under arid and humid conditions. Plant Production Science. 2002;5:224–8. DOI: 10.1626/pps.5.224

[5] Zhang YL, Zhang HZ, Du MW, Li W, Luo HH, Chow WS, et al. Leaf wilting movement can protect water-stressed cotton (*Gossypium hirsutum* L.) plants against photoinhibition of photosynthesis and maintain carbon assimilation in the field. Journal of Plant Biology. 2010;53:52–60. DOI: 10.1007/s12374-009-9085-z

[6] Kasahara M, Kagawa T, Oikawa K, Suetsugu N, Miyao M, Wada M. Chloroplast avoidance movement reduces photodamage in plants. Nature. 2002;420:829–32. DOI: 10.1038/nature01213

[7] Osmond CB. Photorespiration and photoinhibition. Biochimica et Biophysica Acta (BBA) – Reviews on Bioenergetics. 1981;639:77–98. DOI: 10.1016/0304-4173(81)90006-9

[8] Foyer CH, Bloom AJ, Queval G, Noctor G. Photorespiratory metabolism: genes, mutants, energetics, and redox signaling. Annual Review of Plant Biology. 2009;60:455–84. DOI: 10.1146/annurev.arplant.043008.091948

[9] Asada K. The water-water cycle in chloroplasts: scavenging of active oxygens and dissipation of excess photons. Annual Review of Plant Biology. 1999;50:601–39. DOI: 10.1146/annurev.arplant.50.1.601

[10] Heber U, Walker D. Concerning a dual function of coupled cyclic electron transport in leaves. Plant Physiology. 1992;100:1621–6. DOI: 10.1104/pp.100.4.1621

[11] Huang W, Yang SJ, Zhang SB, Zhang JL, Cao KF. Cyclic electron flow plays an important role in photoprotection for the resurrection plant *Paraboea rufescens* under drought stress. Planta. 2012;235:819–28. DOI: 10.1007/s00425-011-1544-3

[12] Demmig-Adams B, Adams III WW. The role of xanthophyll cycle carotenoids in the protection of photosynthesis. Trends in Plant Science. 1996;1:21–6. DOI: 10.1016/S1360-1385(96)80019-7

[13] Song XS, Shang ZW, Yin ZP, Ren J, Sun MC, Ma XL. Mechanism of xanthophyll-cycle-mediated photoprotection in *Cerasus humilis* seedlings under water stress and subsequent recovery. Photosynthetica. 2011;49:523–30. DOI: 10.1007/s11099-011-0065-4

[14] Boyer JS. Plant productivity and environment. Science. 1982;218:443–8. DOI: 10.1126/science.218.4571.443

[15] Flexas J, Bota J, Galmés J, Medrano H, Ribas-Carbó M. Keeping a positive carbon balance under adverse conditions: responses of photosynthesis and respiration to water stress. Physiologia Plantarum. 2006;127:343–52. DOI: 10.1111/j.1399-3054.2006.00621.x

[16] Chaves M, Flexas J, Pinheiro C. Photosynthesis under drought and salt stress: regulation mechanisms from whole plant to cell. Annals of Botany. 2009;103:551–60. DOI: 10.1093/aob/mcn125

[17] Hu YY, Zhang YL, Luo HH, Li W, Oguchi R, Fan DY, et al. Important photosynthetic contribution from the non-foliar green organs in cotton at the late growth stage. Planta. 2012;235:325–36. DOI: 10.1007/s00425-011-1511-z

[18] Pastenes C, Pimentel P, Lillo J. Leaf movements and photoinhibition in relation to water stress in field-grown beans. Journal of Experimental Botany. 2005;56:425–33. DOI: 10.1093/jxb/eri061

[19] Arena C, Vitale L, Virzo De Santo A. Paraheliotropism in *Robinia pseudoacacia* L.: an efficient strategy to optimise photosynthetic performance under natural environmental conditions. Plant Biology. 2008;10:194–201. DOI: 10.1111/j.1438-8677.2008.00032.x

[20] Lang ARG. Leaf orientation of a cotton plant. Agricultural Meteorology. 1973;11:37–51. DOI: 10.1016/0002-1571(73)90049-6

[21] Ehleringer JR, Hammond SD. Solar tracking and photosynthesis in cotton leaves. Agricultural and Forest Meteorology. 1987;39:25–35. DOI: 10.1016/0168-1923(87)90013-X

[22] Zhang YL, Zhang HZ, Feng GY, Tian JS, Zhang WF. Leaf diaheliotropic movement can improve carbon gain and water use efficiency and not intensify photoinhibition in upland cotton (*Gossypium hirsutum* L.). Photosynthetica. 2009;47:609–15. DOI: 10.1007/s11099-009-0087-3

[23] Yi XP, Zhang YL, Yao HS, Zhang XJ, Luo HH, Gou L, et al. Alternative electron sinks are crucial for conferring photoprotection in field-grown cotton under water deficit during flowering and boll setting stages. Functional Plant Biology. 2014;41:737–47. DOI: 10.1071/FP13269

[24] Zhang YL, Yao HS, Luo Y, Hu YY, Zhang WF. Difference in leaf photosynthetic capacity between pima cotton (*Gossypium barbadense*) and upland cotton (*G. hirsutum*) and analysis of potential constraints. Acta Ecologica Sinica. 2011;31:1803–10.

[25] Zhang YL, Luo Y, Yao HS, Tian JS, Luo HH, Zhang WF. Mechanism for photoprotection of leaves at the bolling stage under field conditions in *Gossypium barbadense* and *G. hirsutum*. Journal of Plant Ecology. 2010;34:1204–12. DOI: 10.3773/j.issn.1005-264x.2010.10.009

[26] Wise R, Olson AJ, Schrader SM, Sharkey TD. Electron transport is the functional limitation of photosynthesis in field-grown pima cotton plants at high temperature. Plant Cell and Environment. 2004;27:717–24. DOI: 10.1111/j.1365-3040.2004.01171.x

[27] Li W, Zhang YL, Hu YY, Yang MS, Wu J, Zhang WF. Research on the photoprotection and photosynthesis characteristics of young cotton leaves under field conditions. Chinese Journal of Plant Ecology. 2013;36:662–70.

[28] Zhang YL, Hu YY, Luo HH, Chow WS, Zhang WF. Two distinct strategies of cotton and soybean differing in leaf movement to perform photosynthesis under drought in the field. Functional Plant Biology. 2011;38:567–75. DOI: 10.1071/FP15247

[29] Chiariello NR, Field CB, Mooney HA. Midday wilting in a tropical pioneer tree. Functional Ecology. 1987;1:3–11. DOI: 10.2307/2389351

[30] Hsiao TC. Plant responses to water stress. Annual Review of Plant Physiology. 1973;24:519–70. DOI: 10.1146/annurev.pp.24.060173.002511

[31] Flexas J, Medrano H. Drought-inhibition of photosynthesis in C_3 plants: stomatal and non-stomatal limitations revisited. Annals of Botany. 2002;89:183–9. DOI: 10.1093/aob/mcf027

[32] Yi XP, Zhang YL, Yao HS, Luo HH, Gou L, Chow WS, et al. Different strategies of acclimation of photosynthesis, electron transport and antioxidative activity in leaves of two cotton species to water deficit. Functional Plant Biology. 2016;43:448–60. DOI: 10.1071/FP15247

[33] Massacci A, Nabiev SM, Pietrosanti L, Nematov SK, Chernikova TN, Thor K, et al. Response of the photosynthetic apparatus of cotton (*Gossypium hirsutum*) to the onset of drought stress under field conditions studied by gas-exchange analysis and chlorophyll fluorescence imaging. Plant Physiology and Biochemistry. 2008;46:189–95. DOI: 10.1016/j.plaphy.2007.10.006

[34] Chastain DR, Snider JL, Collins GD, Perry CD, Whitaker J, Byrd SA. Water deficit in field-grown *Gossypium hirsutum* primarily limits net photosynthesis by decreasing stomatal conductance, increasing photorespiration, and increasing the ratio of dark respiration to gross photosynthesis. Journal of Plant Physiology. 2014;171:1576–85. DOI: 10.1016/j.jplph.2014.07.014

[35] Snider JL, Chastain DR, Meeks CD, Collins GD, Sorensen RB, Byrd SA, et al. Predawn respiration rates during flowering are highly predictive of yield response in *Gossypium hirsutum* when yield variability is water-induced. Journal of Plant Physiology. 2015;183:114–20. DOI: 10.1016/j.jplph.2015.06.003

[36] Genty B, Briantais JM, Vieira Da Silva JB. Effects of drought on primary photosynthetic processes of cotton leaves. Plant Physiology. 1987;83:360–4. DOI: 10.1104/pp.83.2.360

[37] Yi XP, Zhang YL, Yao HS, Luo HH, Gou L, Chow WS, et al. Rapid recovery of photosynthetic rate following soil water deficit and re-watering in cotton plants (*Gossypium herbaceum* L.) is related to the stability of the photosystems. Journal of Plant Physiology. 2016;194:23–34. DOI: 10.1016/j.jplph.2016.01.016

[38] Demmig-Adams B. Carotenoids and photoprotection in plants: a role for the xanthophyll zeaxanthin. Biochimica et Biophysica Acta (BBA) – Bioenergetics. 1990;1020:1–24. DOI: 10.1016/0005-2728(90)90088-L

[39] Horton P, Ruban AV, Walters RG. Regulation of light harvesting in green algea. Annual Review of Plant Physiology and Plant Molecular Biology. 1996;47:655–84. DOI: 10.1146/annurev.arplant.47.1.655

[40] Ahn TK, Avenson TJ, Ballottari M, Cheng YC, Niyogi KK, Bassi R, et al. Architecture of a charge-transfer state regulating light harvesting in a plant antenna protein. Science. 2008;320:794–7. DOI: 10.1126/science.1154800

[41] Niyogi KK. Photoprotection revisited: genetic and molecular approaches. Annual Review of Plant Physiology and Plant Molecular Biology. 1999;50:333–59. DOI: 10.1146/annurev.arplant.50.1.333

[42] Demmig-Adams B, Adams III WW, Barker DH, Logan BA, Bowling DR, Verhoeven AS. Using chlorophyll fluorescence to assess the fraction of absorbed light allocated to thermal dissipation of excess excitation. Physiologia Plantarum. 1996;98:253–64. DOI: 10.1034/j.1399-3054.1996.980206.x

[43] Björkman O, Schäfer C. A gas exchange-fluorescence analysis of photosynthetic performance of a cotton crop under high-irradiance stress. Philosophical Transactions of the Royal Society B Biological Sciences. 1989;323:309–11. DOI: 10.1098/rstb.1989.0012

[44] Kornyeyev D, Logan BA, Allen RD, Holaday AS. Field-grown cotton plants with elevated activity of chloroplastic glutathione reductase exhibit no significant alteration of diurnal or seasonal patterns of excitation energy partitioning and CO_2 fixation. Field Crops Research. 2005;94:165–75. DOI: 10.1016/j.fcr.2005.01.001

[45] Inamullah IA. Adaptive responses of soybean and cotton to water stress: II. Changes in CO_2 assimilation rate, chlorophyll fluorescence and photochemical reflectance index in relation to leaf temperature. Plant Production Science. 2005;8:131–8. DOI: 10.1626/pps.8.131

[46] Singh R, Naskar J, Pathre UV, Shirke PA. Reflectance and cyclic electron flow as an indicator of drought stress in cotton (*Gossypium hirsutum*). Photochemistry and Photobiology. 2014;90:544–51. DOI: 10.1111/php.12213

[47] Singh R, Pandey N, Naskar J, Shirke PA. Physiological performance and differential expression profiling of genes associated with drought tolerance in contrasting varieties of two *Gossypium* species. Protoplasma. 2015;252:423–38. DOI: 10.1007/s00709-014-0686-0

[48] Ogren WL, Bowes G. Ribulose diphosphate carboxylase regulates soybean photorespiration. Nature New Biology. 1971;230:159–60. DOI: 10.1038/newbio230159a0

[49] Flexas J, Medrano H. Energy dissipation in C_3 plants under drought. Functional Plant Biology. 2002;29:1209–15. DOI: 10.1071/FP02015

[50] Tourneux C, Peltier G. Effect of water deficit on photosynthetic oxygen exchange measured using $^{18}O_2$ and mass spectrometry in *Solanum tuberosum* L. leaf discs. Planta. 1995;195:570–7. DOI: 10.1007/BF00195717

[51] Cornic G, Fresneau C. Photosynthetic carbon reduction and carbon oxidation cycles are the main electron sinks for photosystem II activity during a mild drought. Annals of Botany. 2002;89:887–94. DOI: 10.1093/aob/mcf064

[52] Lawlor DW. Water stress induced changes in photosynthesis, photorespiration, respiration and CO_2 compensation concentration of wheat. Photosynthetica. 1976;10:378–87.

[53] Flexas J, Bota J, Escalona JM, Sampol B, Medrano H. Effects of drought on photosynthesis in grapevines under field conditions: an evaluation of stomatal and mesophyll limitations. Functional Plant Biology. 2002;29:461–71. DOI: 10.1071/PP01119

[54] Gerbaud A, André M. Effect of CO_2, O_2, and light on photosynthesis and photorespiration in wheat. Plant Physiology. 1980;66:1032–6. DOI: 10.1104/pp.66.6.1032

[55] Biehler K, Fock H. Evidence for the contribution of the Mehler-peroxidase reaction in dissipating excess electrons in drought-stressed wheat. Plant Physiology. 1996;112:265–72. DOI: 10.1104/pp.112.1.265

[56] Asada K. The water-water cycle as alternative photon and electron sinks. Philosophical Transactions of the Royal Society B Biological Sciences. 2000;355:1419–31. DOI: 10.1098/rstb.2000.0703

[57] Badawi GH, Kawano N, Yamauchi Y, Shimada E, Sasaki R, Kubo A, et al. Over-expression of ascorbate peroxidase in tobacco chloroplasts enhances the tolerance to salt stress and water deficit. Physiologia Plantarum. 2004;121:231–8. DOI: 10.1111/j.0031-9317.2004.00308.x

[58] Ziem-Hanck U, Heber U. Oxygen requirement of photosynthetic CO_2 assimilation. Biochimica Biophysica Acta. 1980;591:266–74. DOI: 10.1016/0005-2728(80)90158-9

[59] Neubauer C, Yamamoto HY. Mehler-peroxidase reaction mediates zeaxanthin formation and zeaxanthin-related fluorescence quenching in intact chloroplasts. Plant Physiology. 1992;99:1354–61. DOI: 10.1104/pp.99.4.1354

[60] Wingler A, Lea PJ, Paul Quick W, Leegood RC. Photorespiration: metabolic pathways and their role in stress protection. Philosophical Transactions of the Royal Society of London. 2000;355:1517–29. DOI: 10.1098/rstb.2000.0712

[61] Haupt-Herting S, Fock HP. Oxygen exchange in relation to carbon assimilation in water-stressed leaves during photosynthesis. Annals of Botany. 2002;89:851–9. DOI: 10.1093/aob/mcf023

[62] Joliot P, Joliot A. Cyclic electron transfer in plant leaf. Proceedings of the National Academy of Sciences of the United States of America. 2002;99:10209–14. DOI: 10.1073/pnas.102306999

[63] Breyton C, Nandha B, Johnson GN, Joliot P, Finazzi G. Redox modulation of cyclic electron flow around photosystem I in C_3 plants. Biochemistry. 2006;45:13465–75. DOI: 10.1021/bi061439s

[64] Joliot P, Joliot A. Cyclic electron flow in C_3 plants. Biochimica Biophysica Acta. 2006;1757:362–8. DOI: 10.1016/j.bbabio.2006.02.018

[65] Johnson GN. Physiology of PSI cyclic electron transport in higher plants. Biochimica et Biophysica Acta (BBA) – Bioenergetics. 2011;1807:384–9. DOI: 10.1016/j.bbabio.2010.11.009

[66] Arnon DI, Tsujimoto HY, Mcswain BD. Ferredoxin and photosynthetic phosphorylation. Nature. 1967;214:562–6. DOI: 10.1038/214562a0

[67] Endo T, Shikanai T, Takabayashi A, Asada K, Sato F. The role of chloroplastic NAD(P)H dehydrogenase in photoprotection. FEBS Letters. 1999;457:5–8. DOI: 10.1016/S0014-5793(99)00989-8

[68] Golding AJ, Johnson GN. Down-regulation of linear and activation of cyclic electron transport during drought. Planta. 2003;218:107–14. DOI: 10.1007/s00425-003-1077-5

[69] Shikanai T. Cyclic electron transport around photosystem I: genetic approaches. Annual Review of Plant Biology. 2007;58:199–217. DOI: 10.1146/annurev.arplant.58.091406.110525

[70] Kou JC, Takahashi S, Oguchi R, Fan DY, Badger MR, Chow WS. Estimation of the steady-state cyclic electron flux around PSI in spinach leaf discs in white light, CO_2-enriched air and other varied conditions. Functional Plant Biology. 2013;40:1018–28. DOI: 10.1071/FP13010

[71] Baroli I, Niyogi KK. Molecular genetics of xanthophyll–dependent photoprotection in green algae and plants. Philosophical Transactions of the Royal Society of London. 2000;355:1385–94. DOI: 10.1098/rstb.2000.0700

[72] Katona E, Neimanis S, Schönknecht G, Heber U. Photosystem I-dependent cyclic electron transport is important in controlling Photosystem II activity in leaves under conditions of water stress. Photosynthesis Research. 1992;34:449–64. DOI: 10.1007/BF00029818

[73] Gao S, Shen SD, Wang GC, Niu JF, Lin AP, Pan GH. PSI-driven cyclic electron flow allows intertidal macro-algae *Ulva* sp. (Chlorophyta) to survive in desiccated conditions. Plant and Cell Physiology. 2011;52:885–93. DOI: 10.1093/pcp/pcr038

[74] Monk L, Fagerstedt K, Crawford R. Superoxide dismutase as an anaerobic polypeptidea: a key factor in recovery from oxygen deprivation in *Iris pseudacorus*? Plant Physiology. 1987;85:1016–20. DOI: 10.1104/pp.85.4.1016

[75] Sharma P, Jha AB, Dubey RS, Pessarakli M. Reactive oxygen species, oxidative damage, and antioxidative defense mechanism in plants under stressful conditions. Journal of Botany. 2012;2012:1–26. DOI: 10.1155/2012/217037

[76] Smirnoff N. The role of active oxygen in the response of plants to water deficit and desiccation. New Phytologist. 1993;125:27–58. DOI: 10.1111/j.1469-8137.1993.tb03863.x

[77] Ashraf M, Foolad MR. Roles of glycine betaine and proline in improving plant abiotic stress resistance. Environmental and Experimental Botany. 2007;59:206–16. DOI: 10.1016/j.envexpbot.2005.12.006

[78] Mahan JR, Wanjura DF. Seasonal patterns of glutathione and ascorbate metabolism in field-grown cotton under water stress. Crop Science. 2005;45:193–201. DOI: 10.2135/cropsci2005.0193

[79] Kornyeyev D, Logan BA, Allen RD, Holaday AS. Effect of chloroplastic overproduction of ascorbate peroxidase on photosynthesis and photoprotection in cotton leaves subjected to low temperature photoinhibition. Plant Science. 2003;165:1033–41. DOI: 10.1016/S0168-9452(03)00294-2

[80] Kawakami EM, Oosterhuis DM, Snider JL. Physiological effects of 1-methylcyclopropene on well-watered and water-stressed cotton plants. Journal of Plant Growth Regulation. 2010;29:280–88. DOI: 10.1007/s00344-009-9134-3

[81] Reddy AR, Chaitanya KV, Vivekanandan M. Drought-induced responses of photosynthesis and antioxidant metabolism in higher plants. Journal of Plant Physiology. 2004;161:1189–202. DOI: 10.1016/j.jplph.2004.01.013

[82] de Ronde J, van der Mescht A, Steyn HSF. Proline accumulation in response to drought and heat stress in cotton. African Crop Science Journal. 2000;8:85–91. DOI: 10.4314/acsj.v8i1.27718

[83] Chow WS, Aro EM. Photoinactivation and mechanisms of recovery. In: Wydrzynski T, Satoh K, Freeman J, editors. Photosystem II. The Light-Driven Water: Plastoquinone Oxidoreductase Advances in Photosynthesis and Respiration. 1st ed. The Netherlands: Springer; 2005. pp. 627–48. DOI: 10.1007/1-4020-4254-X_28

[84] Aro EM, Mccaffery S, Anderson JM. Photoinhibition and D1 protein degradation in peas acclimated to different growth irradiances. Plant Physiology. 1993;103:835–43. DOI: 10.1104/pp.103.3.835

[85] Lee HY, Hong YN, Chow WS. Photoinactivation of photosystem II complexes and photoprotection by non-functional neighbours in *Capsicum annuum* L. leaves. Planta. 2001;212:332–42. DOI: 10.1007/s004250000398

[86] Kato MC, Hikosaka K, Hirose T. Photoinactivation and recovery of photosystem II in Chenopodium album leaves grown at different levels of irradiance and nitrogen availability. Functional Plant Biology. 2002;29:787–95. DOI: 10.1071/PP01162

[87] Oguchi R, Jia HS, Barber J, Chow WS. Recovery of photoinactivated photosystem II in leaves: retardation due to restricted mobility of photosystem II in the thylakoid membrane. Photosynthesis Research. 2008;98:621–9. DOI: 10.1007/s11120-008-9363-5

[88] Hu YY, Fan DY, Losciale P, Chow WS, Zhang WF. Whole-tissue determination of the rate coefficients of photoinactivation and repair of photosystem II in cotton leaf discs based on flash-induced P700 redox kinetics. Photosynthesis Research. 2013;117:517–28. DOI: 10.1007/s11120-013-9822-5

[89] Aschan G, Pfanz H. Non-foliar photosynthesis – a strategy of additional carbon acquisition. Flora – Morphology, Distribution, Functional Ecology of Plants. 2003;198:81–97. DOI: 10.1078/0367-2530-00080

[90] Araus JL, Brown HR, Febrero A, Bort J, Serret MD. Ear photosynthesis, carbon isotope discrimination and the contribution of respiratory CO_2 to differences in grain mass in durum wheat. Plant Cell and Environment. 1993;16:383–92. DOI: 10.1111/j.1365-3040.1993.tb00884.x

[91] Li XJ, Wang HG, Li HB, Zhang LY, Teng NJ, Lin QQ, et al. Awns play a dominant role in carbohydrate production during the grain-filling stages in wheat (*Triticum aestivum*). Physiologia Plantarum. 2006;127:701–9. DOI: 10.1111/j.1399-3054.2006.00679.x

[92] Xu HL, Gauthier L, Desjardins Y, Gosselin A. Photosynthesis in leaves, fruits, stem and petioles of greenhouse-grown tomato plants. Photosynthetica. 1997;33:113–23. DOI: 10.1023/A:1022135507700

[93] Wullschleger SD, Oosterhuis DM. Photosynthetic and respiratory activity of fruiting forms within the cotton canopy. Plant Physiology. 1990;94:463–9. DOI: 10.1104/pp.94.2.463

[94] Wullschleger SD, Oosterhuis DM. Photosynthesis, transpiration, and water-use efficiency of cotton leaves and fruit. Photosynthetica. 1991;25:505–15.

[95] Wullschleger SD, Oosterhuis D, Hurren R, Hanson P. Evidence for light-dependent recycling of respired carbon dioxide by the cotton fruit. Plant Physiology. 1991;97:574–9. DOI: 10.1104/pp.97.2.574

[96] Zhang YL, Feng GY, Hu YY, Yao YD, Zhang WF. Photosynthetic activity and its correlation with matter production in non-foliar green organs of cotton. Acta Agronomica Sinica. 2010;36:701–8. DOI: 10.3724/SP.J.1006.2010.00701

[97] Zhang YL, Luo HH, Hu YY, Strasser RJ, Zhang WF. Characteristics of Photosystem II behavior in cotton (*Gossypium hirsutum* L.) bract and capsule wall. Journal of Integrative Agriculture. 2013;12:2056–64. DOI: 10.1016/S2095-3119(13)60343-3

[98] Hu YY, Zhang YL, Yi XP, Zhan DX, Luo HH, Chow WS, et al. The relative contribution of non-foliar organs of cotton to yield and related physiological characteristics under water deficit. Journal of Integrative Agriculture. 2014;13:975–89. DOI: 10.1016/S2095-3119(13)60568-7

[99] Zhan DX, Zhang C, Yang Y, Luo HH, Zhang YL, Zhang WF. Water deficit alters cotton canopy structure and increases photosynthesis in the mid-canopy layer. Agronomy Journal. 2015;107:1947–57. DOI: 10.2134/agronj14.0426

[100] Zhang C, Zhan DX, Luo HH, Zhang YL, Zhang WF. Photorespiration and photoinhibition in the bracts of cotton under water stress. Photosynthetica. 2016;54:12–8. DOI: 10.1007/s11099-015-0139-9

Chapter 4

Nutritional Status of Cotton Plant Assessed by Compositional Nutrient Diagnosis (CND)

Ademar Pereira Serra, Marlene Estevão Marchetti,
Manoel Carlos Gonçalves, Simone Cândido Ensinas,
Bendaly Labaied Mouna, Eulene Francisco da Silva,
Elaine Reis Pinheiro Lourente,
Anamari Viegas de Araujo Motomiya,
Alessandra Mayumi Tokura Alovisi and
Flávia de Araújo Matos

Additional information is available at the end of the chapter

http://dx.doi.org/10.5772/64388

Abstract

The use of compositional nutrient diagnosis (CND) to assess the nutritional status of cotton crop is quite important to improve knowledge on plant nutritional requirement and assist the fertilizer recommendation. The aim of this chapter is to introduce the possibility of using CND for cotton crop. This method has scarcely been used to assess the nutritional status of cotton plant although a few results have indicated that it can be promising. In fact, CND methodology seems to be better in the nutritional diagnosis than traditional methods such as sufficient range (SR) and critical value approach (CVA). Its efficiency has increased with the possibility of applying multivariate analysis, principal component analysis (PCA), canonical correlation, and so on. The application of PCA possibility to note some interactions among the nutrients is important for understanding the dynamics of nutrients in plants.

Keywords: multivariate analysis, nutritional balance, nutrient concentration, PCA, plant nutrition, soil science, *Gossypium hirsutum* L

1. Introduction

The knowledge of nutritional status of cotton is essential to understand plant nutritional requirement and to help the fertilizer recommendations to improve crop production. Without understanding cotton nutrient requirement, it is difficult to know about plant response to fertilizers. The traditional methods to assess plant nutrient status are the sufficiency range (SR) and critical value approach (CVA); however, these methods do not allow the diagnosis of the nutritional balance of the plant, and their usage is dependent on sampling time and plant development stage [1]. Additionally, in SR and CVA, it is not possible to know which nutrient is more or less required by plant, because there is no interaction among nutrients in these traditional diagnoses.

In order to improve nutritional diagnosis by conventional methods (CVA and SR), Beaufils [2] developed the diagnosis and recommendation integrated system (DRIS), which was based on "minimum law." Through the DRIS index, it is possible to observe the plant nutritional requirement, and the most deficient nutrient is limiting the plant development and production. It is possible to consider DRIS as an early attempt to analyze the compositional space of leaf analysis results [3]. Parent and Dafir [4] developed the compositional nutrient diagnosis (CND) that is conformed to be a multivariate analysis and can combine other refined analysis to improve the nutritional diagnosis. CND uses the row-centered log ratio instead of dual ratios between nutrients [5]. CND consists in the relation between each individual nutrient concentration with the geometric mean of the other nutrients in composition. Thus, CND comprises multiple interactions among all nutrients in diagnosis. Therefore, CND method has more advantages than DRIS method due to the interaction among all nutrients instead of dual ratios mentioned above [4].

For cotton crop, Serra et al. [6, 7] have compared CVA and SR diagnosis with CND method and observed that CND shows more precise diagnosis results than CVA and SR, and the authors have reported that the use of SR may generate wide nutrient range that can disturb the accurate diagnosis.

The aim of this chapter is to introduce the CND applications to assess the nutritional status of cotton plant as a more precise method of plant diagnosis than the widely applied traditional CVA and SR methods.

2. Nutritional diagnosis in cotton plant

CVA or SR method has been defined as an interventionist approach because the production variability is explained by the variation on nutrient supply or availability of the nutrients under analysis. In CVA and SR, the other production factors are remained under unlimited levels. The understanding of the principles, considered by different diagnosis methods, and the comparison of their results are important to the application of these diagnosis tools.

In cotton and most grain crops, usually, the nutritional diagnoses are conducted using SR and CVA, which measure only individual leaf nutrient concentration of a nutrient in diagnosis without any relationship with other nutrients in the sample of leaf tissue. These traditional methods do not report the nutritional balance in plant tissue. Bates [1] noted the nutritional diagnosis through CVA was affected by the interaction of nutrients in plant tissue and other factors related to plant growth depending on the age of plant.

In the last decade, the interests for bivariate and multivariate methods of nutritional diagnosis, as DRIS and CND, increased. DRIS is based on the dual ratio between nutrients, as N/P, N/K, etc., which is considered to have a bivariate relation. DRIS method allows the assessment of the nutritional equilibrium of a plant, ranking the nutrient contents in relative order of nutritional requirement, from the most deficient nutrient to the most excessive [2].

In DRIS results, in order to express the relative nutrient balance into the plant tissue, the DRIS index is calculated through the comparison of dual nutrient ratios (N/P, P/K, K/Ca, Ca/Mg, etc.) in the sample with the DRIS norms from a reference population (N/P′, P/K′, K/Ca′, Ca/Mg′, etc.). Besides, in the DRIS, there are other bivariate methods such as modified DRIS (M-DRIS) [8] and multivariate method like the CND, which was developed by Parent and Dafir [4].

3. Steps to develop CND norms

3.1. Obtaining leaf nutrient concentration and cotton crop yield to compose the database

The first step to develop CND norms is to obtain leaf nutrient concentration and cotton yield (database). The leaf sampling may be conducted in commercial or experimental cotton field, but it is recommended that the number of samples cannot be under 30 samples of complete leaves (blade + petiole) per plot, which must be combined to form just 1 composed sample [9].

One leaf sample per plant should be taken from the fifth leaf on the main stem, during flowering of the cotton crop (stages F1–F4), according to classification of Marur and Ruano [10]. The cotton yield is assessed at the end of plant cycle, which is usually accomplished with a combine harvester in commercial field or manually in experimental plots.

In the leaf samples, the total concentrations of N, P, K, Ca, Mg, S, B, Zn, Cu, Mn, and Fe are usually determined. Nevertheless, there are cases where authors used just five nutrients (N, P, K, Ca, and Mg) [4, 11] or more, as the case of Anjaneyulu and Raghupathi [12], who used ten nutrients (N, P, K, Ca, Mg, S, Fe, Mn, Zn, and Cu).

The leaf nutrient concentration must follow normal distribution. That is why, it is necessary to transform the data of nutrient concentration from leaf tissue. However, with CND method, the calculation of row-centered log ratio corrects the non-normal distribution. As observed by Serra et al. [6], the multinutrient variable (Zi) showed 100% normal distribution in data of leaf nutrient concentration of cotton.

The size of the database (leaf nutrient concentration and yield) is not well defined in the literature. Serra et al. [6, 7] used 65 sampling from commercial plots to develop CND norms in the Western region of Bahia State, in Brazil, whereas Serra et al. [13] used 108 sampling in the database for DRIS. Khiari et al. [11] used 240 observations of commercial plots of sweet corn and five nutrient determinations, and Parent et al. [5] collected 1117 samples in potato crop to establish the database. More than quantity, the quality of the database might be more far reaching to obtain profitable CND norms. In fact, the essential to have an effective database is to acquire plots with high-yield and healthy leaves with no damage to make possible the development of the CND or DRIS norms.

3.2. Selecting the high-yielding subpopulation to develop CND norms

In order to develop the CND norms, it is necessary to define the high-yielding subpopulation into the database. The database might be divided into two subpopulations, using the mean + 0.5 standard deviation (SD) as criterion to separate the populations into a high-yielding group and low-yielding group [6].

Serra et al. [13] published a paper about the criterion of population selection for cotton crops to separate low-yielding from high-yielding population to develop DRIS norms; nevertheless, it is possible to apply these criteria for CND norms. In this criterion, they used the mean and standard deviation of the yield in the database to separate the high-yielding from low-yielding subpopulation.

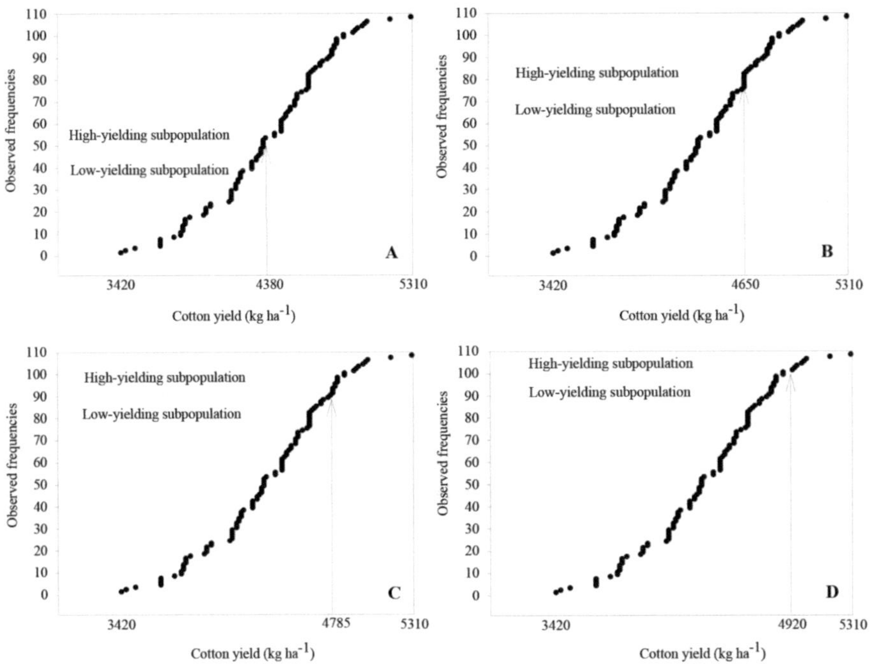

Figure 1. Graphic representation of the observed frequency of yields. The criteria for establishing the high-yield subpopulations were plots with (A) yield above average (4380 kg ha^{-1}), (B) yield above average + 2/3 standard deviation (above 4650 kg ha^{-1}), (C) yield above average + 1 standard deviation (above 4785 kg ha^{-1}), and (D) yield above average + 4/3 standard deviation (above 4920 kg ha^{-1}).

As shown in **Figure 1**, Serra et al. [13] used as criteria for determining the high-cotton-yield subpopulation plots with yields above the population mean (**Figure 1A**), yield above mean + 2/3 standard deviation (SD) (**Figure 1B**), yield above mean + 1 SD (**Figure 1C**), and yield above mean + 4/3 SD (**Figure 1D**). They concluded that the increasing of rigor to select the high-yielding subpopulation increases the capacity to discriminate low yielding from high-yielding subpopulation.

For other crops as well as for cotton crop, the selection of the high-yielding reference subpopulation may be carried across multiple ratios using a cumulative variance function fit to cubic [11] or Boltzmann [14] equations.

3.3. Calculation of the CND norms

The nutrient leaf tissue composition is defined by the simplex S where the sum of all components is constrained to 100%, which forms a d-dimensional nutrient arrangement, i.e., simplex (S^d) made of $d + 1$ nutrient proportions including d nutrients and a filling value (R_d) [4]:

$$S^d = [(N, P, K, Ca, Mg, S, B, Zn, Cu, Fe, Mn, \dots, R_d): N > 0, P > 0, K > 0, \dots R_d > 0; N + P + K + \dots + R_d = 100]$$

where 100 is the dry matter concentration (%); N, P, K, etc., are nutrient proportions (%); and R_d is the filling value computed as follows:

$$R_d = 100 - (N + P + K + Ca + Mg + S + B + Zn + Cu + Fe + Mn + \cdots)$$

The geometric mean (G) is computed as follows [4]:

$$G = (NxPxKx \dots xR_d)^{\frac{1}{d+1}}$$

After calculation of the geometric mean (G), the new expression for the multinutrient is log-transformed to generate a row-centered log ratio as follows [4]:

$$V_N = log\left(\frac{N}{G}\right), V_P = log\left(\frac{P}{G}\right), V_K = log\left(\frac{K}{G}\right), \dots, V_{R_d} = log\left(\frac{R_d}{G}\right)$$

The sum of all row-centered log ratios must be equal to zero ($V_N + V_P + V_K + \dots + V_{R_d} = 0$. CND norms are the means and standard deviations (SD) of row-centered log ratios of high-yielding subpopulation from the database.

Following the procedure above, Serra et al. [6] developed the CND norms for cotton crop in the Western region of Bahia State, Brazil (**Table 1**).

Row-centered log ratios	Mean	SD
V_N	3.136	0.0696
V_P	0.456	0.1432
V_K	2.4282	0.2256
V_{Ca}	2.6399	0.1554
V_{Mg}	1.4709	0.1769
V_S	0.9033	0.2539
V_{Fe}	−2.0931	0.046
V_{Zn}	−2.8972	0.042
V_{Cu}	−5.0268	0.0812
V_{Mn}	−3.6224	0.1641
V_B	−3.8234	0.0464

[1]CND norms based on the high-yield subpopulation (>4250 kg ha^{-1}) of cotton crop in the Western region of Bahia state in Brazil [6].

Table 1. Compositional nutrient diagnosis (CND) norms [mean and standard deviation (SD) of row-centered log ratio][1].

4. CND index and interpretation

4.1. Procedure to calculate CND index in cotton crop

As reported in Section 3.3, from the leaf nutrient concentration of the high-yielding subpopulation (>4250 kg ha^{-1}), CND norms were defined (**Table 1**), which are the means, and standard deviations of row-centered log ratios of the nutrients concentration in leaf tissue, denoted as $'V_N + 'V_P + 'V_K + \dots + 'V_{R_d}$ and $'SD_N$, $'SD_P$, $'SD_K$,.... $'SD_{Rd}$, respectively, were then calculated.

The CND indices, denoted as I_N, I_P, I_K,..., I_{Rd}, were calculated from the row-centered log ratios as follows [4]:

$$I_N = \frac{V_N - 'V_N}{'SD_N}, I_P = \frac{V_P - 'V_P}{'SD_P}, I_K = \frac{V_K - 'V_K}{'SD_K}, \dots, I_{R_d} = \frac{V_{R_d} - 'V_{R_d}}{'SD_{R_d}},$$

The nutrient imbalance index (NII) of a diagnosed specimen, which is its CND r^2, followed the recommendation of Parent and Dafir [4]:

$$r^2 = I_N^2 + I_P^2 + I_K^2 + \dots + I_{R_d}^2$$

The interpretation of CND is based on CND index. CND index is defined as the distance of a given nutrient X_i from its geometric mean [4], which is relative to the distance of the same nutrient from the geometric mean of the target population (reference population with high yield).

From this point of view above, it is expected that when CND index is closer to zero, X_i nutrient is less imbalanced than others in analysis. Serra et al. [6, 7] observed CND index close to zero showed higher nutritional balance. This may be related to nutrient leaf concentration and result in high relationship in cotton crop.

4.2. Interpretation of CND index by nutrient application potential response (NAPR)

Wadt [15] developed the nutrient application potential response (NAPR), which was originally used to interpret the DRIS index. However, the use of this method was extended to interpret CND index for cotton crop [6, 7]. This method proved to be efficient to accomplish the interpretation of CND index. Besides the interpretation of CND index in cotton crop, the methodology has already been applied in other crops to interpret the DRIS index, such as *Eucalyptus grandis* [16], coffee [17], and "cupuaçu" trees [18].

The NAPR consists in defining five groups of crop response (**Table 2**). The use of this methodology enables to obtain the most responsive nutrient in the case of fertilizer recommendation; however, this recommendation might be carried with the soil physical and chemical analysis to guide the decisions.

Nutritional status	Criteria	Type of nutrient application potential response[1]
Deficiency	IA < 0, |IA| > NIIa[2], and IA is the index of lower value	Positive, with higher probability (p)
Deficiency prone	IA < 0 and |IA| > NIIa	Positive, with low probability (pz)
Sufficient	|IA| ≤ NIIa	Null (z)
Excess prone	IA > 0 and |IA| > NIIa	Negative, with a low probability (nz)
Excess	IA > 0, |IA| > NIIa, and IA is the index of higher value	Negative, with a higher probability (n)

[1]The NAPR was calculated based on Wadt [17].
NIIa = nutritional imbalance index average. IA = CND index for nutrient A.
Adapted with permission from Wadt [17].

Table 2. Criteria to interpret the CND index by nutrient application potential response (NAPR).

The practical interpretation for the nutritional status of the plant in **Table 2** is that "deficiency" means this nutrient shows high probability to positive response if applied in soil, which expects higher cotton yields. On the other hand, "excess" means the application of the nutrient in soil may result in luxury consumption and no response ought to be shown in terms of yield or food quality [15].

Nutrients	Method of diagnosis	Nutrient application potential response (NAPR)[1] (%)				
		p	pz	z	nz	n
N	DRIS	0	16.92	64.62	13.85	4.62
	CND	1.54	24.62	47.69	9.23	16.92
P	DRIS	7.69	12.31	49.23	6.15	24.62
	CND	6.15	9.23	58.46	4.62	21.54
K	DRIS	23.08	13.85	40	7.69	15.38
	CND	20	7.69	53.85	9.23	9.23
Ca	DRIS	23.08	10.77	50.77	9.23	6.15
	CND	21.54	7.69	56.92	9.23	4.62
Mg	DRIS	6.15	6.15	41.54	32.31	13.85
	CND	3.08	4.62	60	23.08	9.23
S	DRIS	9.23	12.31	50.77	12.31	15.38
	CND	7.69	10.77	60	13.85	7.69
Fe	DRIS	3.08	4.62	86.15	1.54	4.62
	CND	6.15	10.77	61.54	16.92	4.62
Zn	DRIS	0	4.62	89.23	6.15	0
	CND	0	7.69	75.38	12.31	4.62
Cu	DRIS	7.69	18.46	61.54	9.23	3.08
	CND	10.77	16.92	56.92	10.77	4.62
Mn	DRIS	18.46	15.38	46.15	9.23	10.77
	CND	13.85	15.38	50.77	10.77	9.23
B	DRIS	1.54	10.77	76.92	6.15	4.62
	CND	6.15	13.85	58.46	13.85	7.69

[1](p) positive, with higher probability; (pz) positive, with low probability; (z) null; (nz) negative, with a low probability; (n) negative, with a higher probability.

Table 3. Percentage of nutrient application potential response (NAPR) in cotton crop in Western region of Bahia State, Brazil [6].

The use of CND index interpretation for cotton crop can be a useful tool in association with soil analysis and experience of the agronomist to recommend fertilizer for cotton crop. Furthermore, the absence of nutritional diagnosis can result in excess of fertilizer as the case of P fertilizer observed by Serra et al. [6] in cotton crop in Western region of Bahia State, Brazil. In some specific plots where 180 kg P_2O_5 ha^{-1} was applied, Serra et al. [6] noted that by using NAPR the P In some specific leaf tissue was higher than plant requirement and it could be reduced by the P fertilizer doses (**Table 3**).

5. Nutrient interactions through principal component analysis on CND multivariable

In order to calculate the principal components analysis (PCA) of the row-centered log ratio in the high-yielding subpopulation, it was used the database (leaf nutrient content and crop yield) from Serra [19]. As reported by Parent and Dafir [4], the row-centered log ratios are compatible with PCA; based on it, this section aims at observing some interaction among the nutrients in PCA.

Row-centered log ratio	High-yield subpopulation (n = 40)		
	PC1	PC2	PC3
V_N	**0.6288**	**0.4875**	−0.0093
V_P	**−0.5588**	**−0.5935**	−0.2575
V_K	−0.2150	−0.1672	**−0.7761**
V_{Ca}	−0.1868	**0.7223**	−0.0605
V_{Mg}	0.2401	0.0017	**0.6842**
V_S	**−0.4352**	−0.2937	**0.5691**
V_{Fe}	**0.8159**	**−0.4529**	−0.0919
V_{Zn}	**0.8078**	**−0.4037**	−0.0469
V_{Mn}	**0.3879**	**0.6686**	−0.1689
V_B	**0.2892**	−0.0871	0.0494
V_{Cu}	−0.2150	0.1026	−0.1148
Eigenvalues	3.11	2.06	1.5192
Explained variance (%)	28.25	18.72	13.81
Accumulated variance (%)	28.25	46.97	60.78
Selection criterion (SC)	0.2836	0.3484	0.4056

Values in boldface are the dominant in the PC loadings by setting the level of significance defined according the selection criterion (SC).
Database from Serra [19].

Table 4. Correlations between the row-centered log ratio and the first three principal components (PC) for the high-yield subpopulation (40 observations).

One of the major objectives of the PCA is to reduce the number of interdependent variables into smaller numbers of independent principal component (PC), which are linear combinations of original variables. According to Parent and Dafir [4], CND is the multivariate expansion of CVA and DRIS and fully compatible to PCA.

Based on the PCA, it was obtained three PCs with eigenvalues above 1 and accumulated variance equal 60.78% (**Table 4**). The definition of the loading significance was defined according to Ovalles and Collins [20]. PC loadings or correlations between row-centered log ratios and the first three principal components must have values greater than the selection criterion (SC) for significant acceptation. SC proposed by Ovalles and Collins [20] was defined as follows:

$$SC = \frac{0.50}{\sqrt{PCeigenvalues}}$$

The three PCs combined explained 60.78 % of the total variance (**Table 4**). The first principal component was positively correlated with V_N, V_{Fe}, V_{Zn}, V_{Mn}, and V_B and negatively correlated to V_P, S, and V_{Cu} (**Table 4**). The second principal component was positively correlated with V_N, V_{Ca}, and V_{Mn} and negatively correlated with V_P, V_{Fe}, and V_{Zn} (**Table 4**). Finally, the third principal component showed positively correlated with V_{Mg} and V_S and negatively correlated with V_K (**Table 4**).

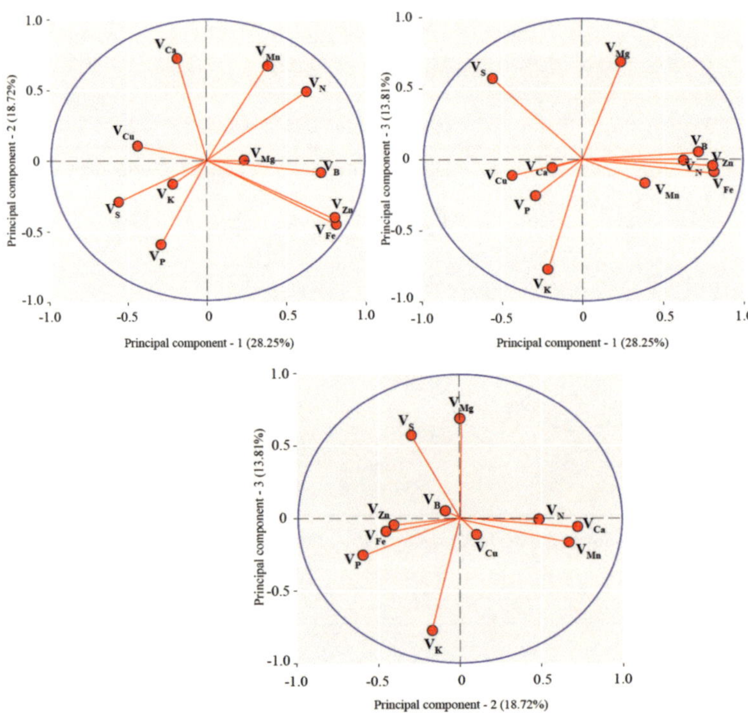

Figure 2. Distribution of principal component analysis (PCA) for row-centered log ratios. PC = principal components. Database from Serra [19].

The structures obtained by PC-1 (N+P-S-Fe+Zn+Cu-Mn+B+), PC-2 (N+P-Ca+Fe-Zn-Mn+), and PC-3 (K-Mg+S+) are supported by some rules of plant nutrition relative to interaction between nutrients, but other structures should be studied carefully for a better understanding (**Figure 2**).

In PC-1, it is feasible to observe positive interaction among N, Fe, and Zn; this result may be explained as reported by Marschner [21] that Fe, Zn, and protein are very highly correlated, which infer that protein is a sink for Fe and Zn. In PC-2, the inverse relation between P and Ca may be explained because of dilution and accumulation effects with plant age. The PC-3 showed the opposite direction for K and Mg inferring the antagonism effects between these nutrients (**Figure 2**).

N and S showed to be highly correlated with the first PC; however, S was negatively correlated with N (**Figure 2A**). It is important to have N availability in soil in balance with S, since this nutrient is a component of amino acids and proteins. Cysteine is the first stable compost of the assimilatory reduction of S that is the precursor of all compounds, in which S makes part in the plants [21]. Thus, S deficiency compromised the formation of amino acids. Furthermore, the N and S show essential functions in the activity of chlorophyll molecule. The S deficiency may deplete the action of chlorophyll and consequently reduction of photosynthesis [22].

The second PC was strongly influenced by positive and negative eigenvectors V_N, V_{Ca}, and V_{Mn} and V_P, V_{Fe}, and V_{Zn}, respectively (**Figure 2C**). In positive and negative quadrant, the nutrients are grouped according to the relationship among them in the plant metabolism, as example, the Zn affects the metabolism of Fe [23], or interactions among nutrients in the rhizosphere. V_{Mg} (positive) and V_K (negative) affected the third PC, which showed opposite directions between these variables inferring the excessive application of K source in soil, inhibit the uptake of Mg by plant roots [21].

6. Conclusion

Being an effective diagnosis tool for the nutritional status of cotton, CND may improve the diagnosis with the application of multivariate analysis. The development of CND norms including means and standard deviation of row-centered log ratios in high-yielding subpopulation can be accomplished based on field trials or experimental database. This information in database is comprised at least by the concentration of leaf nutrients and cotton yield in well-defined plots. CND, due to its interactions with multi-nutrients, can improve the nutritional diagnosis in cotton crop better than traditional methods as CVA and SR. In literature, there are not many results published about CND in cotton crop, but researches should be encouraged worldwide to use this method because of CND importance, to know the plant nutritional requirement, and to direct the decision on fertilizer management. Moreover, the row-centered log ratio is fully compatible with principal component analysis (PCA) that can expand the results of nutrient interaction in leaf tissue of cotton crops.

Author details

Ademar Pereira Serra[1*], Marlene Estevão Marchetti[2], Manoel Carlos Gonçalves[2], Simone Cândido Ensinas[3], Bendaly Labaied Mouna[4], Eulene Francisco da Silva[5], Elaine Reis Pinheiro Lourente[2], Anamari Viegas de Araujo Motomiya[2], Alessandra Mayumi Tokura Alovisi[2] and Flávia de Araújo Matos[2]

*Address all correspondence to: ademar.serra@embrapa.br

1 Brazilian Agricultural Research Corporation (EMBRAPA), Campo Grande, Brazil

2 Federal University of Grande Dourados (UFGD), Dourados, Brazil

3 The Mato Grosso do Sul State University (UEMS), Cassilândia, Brazil

4 Department of Agronomy and Vegetal Biotechnology, National Agronomy Institute of Tunisia, Mahragène, Tunisia

5 Federal Rural University of the Semi-arid Region (UFERSA), Mossoró, Brazil

References

[1] Bates TE. Factors affecting critical nutrient concentrations in plants and their evaluation: a review. Soil Science. 1971; 112: 116-130.

[2] Beaufils, E.R. Diagnosis and recommendation integrated system (DRIS). A general scheme of experimentation and calibration based on principles developed from research in plant nutrition. 1st ed. South Africa: University of Natal, Pietermaritzburg; 1973. 132 p.

[3] Parent LE, Natale W, Ziadi N. Compositional nutrient diagnosis of corn using the Mahalanobis distance as nutrient imbalance index. Canadian Journal of Soil Science. 2009; 89: 383-390. DOI: 10.4141/cjss08050

[4] Parent LE, Dafir MA. Theoretical concept of Compositional Nutrient Diagnosis. Journal of American Society for Horticultural Science. 1992; 117: 239-242. DOI: 117/2/239.full.pdf

[5] Parent LE, Cambouris AN, Muhawenimana A. Multivariate diagnosis of nutrient imbalance in potato crops. Soil Science Society of American Journal. 1994; 58: 1432-1438. DOI: 10.2136/sssaj1994.03615995005800050022x

[6] Serra AP, Marchetti ME, Vitorino ACT, Novelino JO, Camacho MA. Development of DRIS and CND norms and evaluation of nutritional status of cotton. Revista Brasileira de Ciência do Solo. 2010; 34: 97–104. DOI: 10.1590/ 7 S0100–06832010000100010.

[7] Serra AP, Marchetti ME, Vitorino ACT, Novelino JO, Camacho MA. Determination of normal nutrient ranges for cotton by the ChM, CND and DRIS methods. Revista Brasileira de Ciência do Solo. 2010; 34: 105–113. DOI: 10.1590/S0100–06832010000100011

[8] Hallmark WB, Walworth JL, Sumner ME, Mooy CJ, Pesek J, Shao KP. Separating limiting from non-limiting nutrients. Journal of Plant Nutrition.1987; 10: 1381–1390. DOI: 10.1080/01904168709363670

[9] Malavolta E. Mineral nutrition of plants manual. 1st ed. São Paulo: Agronômica Ceres: 2006. 638p.

[10] Marur CJ, Ruano O. A reference system for determination of developmental stages of upland cotton. Revista Brasileira de Oleaginosas e Fibrosas. 2001; 5: 313-317

[11] Khiari L, Parent L, Tremblay N. Critical compositional nutrient indexes for sweet corn at early growth stage. Agronomy Journal. 2001; 93: 809–814. DOI: 10.2134/agronj2001.934809x

[12] Anjaneyulu K, Raghupathi HB. CND and PCA approaches for multivariate diagnosis of nutrient imbalance in papaya (*Carica papaya* L.). Acta Horticulture. 2010; 851: 363-368. DOI: 10.17660/ActaHortic.2010.851.55

[13] Serra AP, Marchetti ME, Rojas EP, Morais HSD, Conrad VDA, Guimarães FCN. Establishing DRIS norms for cotton with different selection criteria for the reference population. Pesquisa Agropecuária Brasileira. 2013; 48: 1472- 1480. DOI: 10.1590/S0100-204X2013001100008

[14] Hernandez-Caraballo EA, Rodrıguez-Rodrıguez O, Rodrıguez-Perez V. Evaluation of the Boltzmann equation as an alternative model in the selection of the high-yield subsample within the framework of the compositional nutrient diagnosis system. Environmental and Experimental Botany. 2008; 64: 225–231. DOI: 10.1016/j.envexpbot.2008.05.010

[15] Wadt PGS. The method of mathematic chance and diagnosis and recommendation integrated system (DRIS) in nutritional evaluation of Eucalyptus planting [Thesis].Viçosa: Universidade Federal de Viçosa; 1996.

[16] Silva GGC, Neves JCL, Alvarez VH, Leite, FP. Evaluation of the universality of DRIS, M-DRIS, and CND norms. Revista Brasileira de Ciência do Solo. 2005; 29: 755–761. DOI: 10.1590/S0100-06832005000500011

[17] Wadt PGS. Relationships between soil class and nutritional status of coffee crops. Revista Brasileira de Ciência do Solo. 2005; 29: 227-234. DOI: 10.1590/S0100-06832005000200008

[18] Dias JRM, Wadt PGS, Perez DV, Silva LM, Cleigiane OL. DRIS formulas for evaluation of nutritional status of cupuaçu trees. Revista Brasileira de Ciência do Solo. 2011; 35: 2083–2091. DOI: 10.1590/S0100-06832011000600023

[19] Serra AP. Evaluation of nutritional status and determination of optimal ranges for cotton [Thesis]. Dourados: Universidade Federal da Grande Dourados; 2008.

[20] Ovalles FA, Collins ME. Variability of northwest Florida soils by principal component analysis. Soil Science Society of America Journal. 1988; 52: 430–1435. DOI: 10.2136/sssaj1988.03615995005200050042x

[21] Marschner H. Mineral nutrition of higher plants. 3rd ed. London: Academic Press; 2012. 651 p.

[22] Nikiforova VJ, Kopka J, Tolstikov V, Fiehn O, Hopkins L, Hawkesford MJ, Hesse H, Hoefgen R. Systems rebalancing of metabolism in response to sulphur deprivation, as revealed by metabolome analysis of arabidopsis plants. Plant Physiology. 2005; 138: 304-318. DOI: 10.1104/pp.104.053793

[23] Rout GR, Sahoo S. Role of iron in plant growth and metabolism. Reviews in Agricultural Science. 2015; 3: 1-24. DOI: 10.7831/ras.3.1

Chapter 5

Farming and Cultivation Technologies of Cotton in China

Jianlong Dai and Hezhong Dong

Additional information is available at the end of the chapter

http://dx.doi.org/10.5772/64485

Abstract

Cotton production in China has developed rapidly during the last 60 years. Using only 15% of the world's cotton land, China currently has produced 30% of the world's cotton. Such a great achievement is largely attributed to adoption of intensive farming technologies and cultural practices, including seedling transplanting, plastic mulching, double cropping, plant pruning, and super-high plant density technique. However, the intensive technologies are labor intensive and involve large input of materials such as fertilizers, pesticides, and plastic films. Thus, there are increasing challenges from labor shortage, soil pollution, and low competitiveness. Here, the achievements, challenges, countermeasures, and prospects for intensive cotton cultivation in China are reviewed. An important conclusion from this review is to reform the current intensive technology to be more light and simplified. Sustainable development of cotton production in China will be supported by the light and simplified farming and cultural system, and China cotton has a bright prospect.

Keywords: cotton, challenges and countermeasures, intensive farming technologies, sustainable development

1. Introduction

China is one of the largest cotton producers and consumers in the world [1]. The planting area of cotton in China was 4.35 million hectares in 2014 with an average lint yield of 1484 kg ha^{-1} and total production of 6.53 million tons (mt). Currently, there are three major cotton-growing regions, including the northwest inland cotton region, the Yellow River valley region, and the Yangtze River valley region (**Table 1**). These three main cotton regions account for 99.5% of output and 99.3% of growing area in the nation [2].

Cotton agroecological zones	Provinces and regions	Planting area (million hectares)	Total output (million tons)	Lint yield (kg ha^{-1})
Northwest inland cotton region	Xinjiang and Gansu	1.76	3.64	2068
Yellow River valley region	Shandong, Hebei, Henan, Shanxi, Shanxi, Tianjin	1.45	1.61	1110
Yangtze River valley region	Hubei, Hunan, Anhui, Jiangsu, Jiangxi, Sichuan	1.11	1.25	1126
Source [3].				

Table 1. Main cotton planting areas, total output, and average lint yield for 2014/2015 in China.

Although cotton cultivation has a long history in China, scientific cultivation was not adopted until the founding of People's Republic of China in 1949. As a result, average unit yield increased by 3.12% annually, from 160 kg ha^{-1} in 1949 to 1280 kg ha^{-1} in 2009 [4]. Many factors have contributed to the increased average yield, including adoption of improved varieties and intensive farming technologies. Although such intensive farming technologies meet the need of a growing population under limited arable land in China, they are labor-intensive and involve large input of various kinds of chemical products like fertilizers, pesticides, and plastic films. Therefore, a transition has been occurring from intensive farming to light and simplified cotton cultivation to cope with the increasing challenges of soil pollution and labor shortage. The achievements, challenges, and the occurring transition of intensive cotton cultivation in China are reviewed in this chapter.

2. Intensive farming technologies and achievements

Intensive farming technologies have supported China to be one of the countries with the highest unit yield of cotton in the world. In 2014/2015, the average lint yield was 768 kg ha^{-1} in the world, while it was 1484 kg ha^{-1} in China, being 58%, 189%, 90%, and 93% higher than the yield in the US, India, Pakistan, and the world average **(Table 2)**. These technologies include double cropping, seedling transplanting, plastic mulching, plant training, and "short-dense-early" high-yielding cultivation pattern in northwest inland which have played more important roles than cotton varieties and other contributors to the significant increase in lint yield for the past 60 years.

2.1. Double cropping

There has existed a strong competition for land between grain crops and cotton in China. The grain-cotton double cropping can ease such a competition by improving farmland and solar energy use efficiency, thus it becomes to be one of the most popular cropping systems in the nation. It ensures higher total output than monocropping, particularly the cotton-wheat double cropping system [6], because it meets the need of farmers to grow a profitable cash crop and secure food supply [7]. According to seeding time (season) of cotton, the double cropping system consists of spring cotton (full-season cotton) double cropping and summer cotton (short-season cotton) double cropping. Of the double cropping, the summer cotton double cropping exhibits obvious advantages in alleviating plant diseases and insect pests by using short-season cotton varieties. Thus it was once widely adopted from the 1980s to the 1990s [8]. It was noted that double cropping of summer cotton and wheat was relatively lower in lint yield and fiber quality of short-season cotton. Therefore, double cropping of spring cotton and wheat began to replace summer cotton and wheat system from the 2000s [9], and currently occupies a dominant position in the cropping system in China **(Figure 1)**. According to the different planting modes of cotton-wheat, three kinds of planting modes (3–1 planting modes: 3 rows wheat and 1 row cotton; 3–2 planting modes: 3 rows wheat and 2 rows cotton; and 4–2 planting modes: 4 rows wheat and 2 rows cotton) were commonly adopted in Huang-Huai-Hai Plain of China.

Country	Area (million hectares)	Average yield (kg ha^{-1})	Total lint yield (million tons)
World	33.83	768	26.4
United States	3.78	939	3.55
India	12.7	514	6.53
Pakistan	2.95	782	2.18
Brazil	0.98	1563	1.52
China	4.35	1484	6.53

Source [5].

Table 2. Cotton area, average yield, and total lint yield for 2014/2015 in the world.

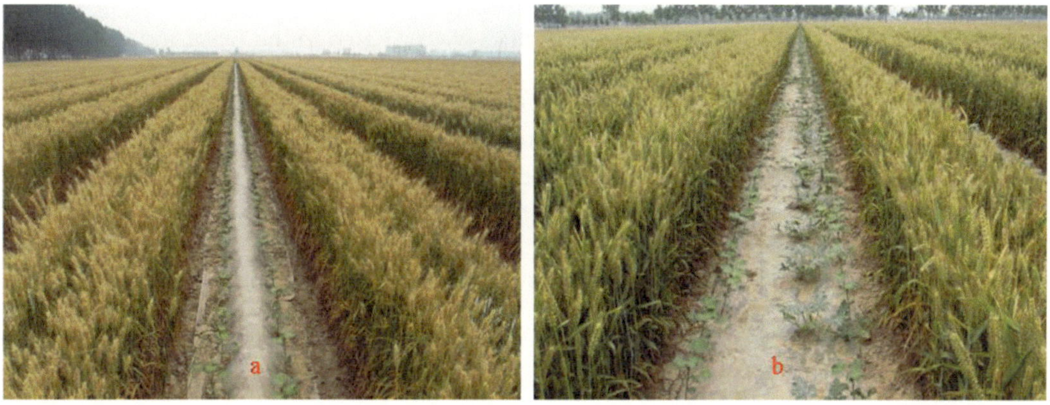

Figure 1. Double cropping systems in China. (a) Double-cropping of cotton-wheat; (b) multicropping of cotton-wheat-watermelon.

As a popular intensive cultivation technology, wheat-cotton intercropping significantly increases multiple crop index and reduces the competition between grain and cotton for land compared with monoculture. For example, the average seed cotton yield under wheat-cotton system in Huang-Huai-Hai Plain in China since 1959 was 2836 kg ha^{-1}, being roughly 88% of that under monocropping, but an extra harvest of 3861 kg wheat per hectare was also obtained compared to monocropping [10]. Thus the total output and economic benefits were significantly raised.

However, the planting area and the proportion of cotton-wheat double cropping system to traditional monocropping system was sharply reduced owing to the following disadvantages: (a) relatively low lint yield and poorer fiber quality owing to delaying seedlings growth at intergrowth stage of wheat-cotton and late senescence either in spring cotton double cropping system or summer cotton double cropping system; (b) relay intercropping of cotton into wheat being not conducive to mechanization; (c) decreased comparative benefits due to high labor input.

2.2. Seedling transplanting

In double cropping system of wheat-cotton, wheat is harvested in early or mid June, while cotton is directly sown in late April. Both crops overlap for approximately 7 weeks. The two crops in the system interact directly during the overlapping period, which usually delays plant growth and maturity, as well as reduces cotton yield due to shading and competition for water and nutrients between the two crops [11]. An investigation of the relationship between boll weight in wheat-cotton double cropping and meteorological factors showed that hours of sunshine was the key meteorological factor in most wheat-cotton double cropping patterns and position of most bolls in the plant; temperature had an important influence on upper and top bolls, especially for double cropped short-season cotton [12]. Although a wider cotton belt may reduce crop interaction, it will definitely decrease wheat yield and not be adopted by farmers. Transplanting cotton seedlings into field just before or after wheat harvest can solve or alleviate the interaction effects of both crops [13].

The technology of seedling transplanting in cotton was initiated in the 1950s and was widely adopted from the 1980s in China [14]. It once accounted for 18% of the nation's total cotton growing areas in the 1980s. Traditionally, seedling nursery in the bed, transplanting seedlings to the fields, and field management after transplanting are the three main steps of seedling transplanting [15]. Seedlings were nursed in "columned soil blocks" (4–6 cm in diameter and 8–12 cm high) made of soil and organic fertilizer (9:1, w/w) in a 50 cm-high arciform hut. After emergence, the seedlings were allowed to grow in the hut until transplanting. Seedlings should experience cold acclimation by keeping the hut open for at least a week before transplanting. Soil blocks along with seedlings were then transplanted to the fields manually. Generally, seedling transplanting can be conducted about 35 days before wheat harvest with spring (full-season) cotton or soon after wheat harvest with summer (short-season) cotton, when the mean soil temperature at the 5 cm depth reaches 17–19°C and cotton seedlings have 2–4 true leaves on the main stem. Soon after transplanting, seedlings were watered to recover normal growth quickly. Intertillage and irrigation are conducted timely after transplanting [16].

Seedling transplanting has several advantages compared with direct seeding: (a) it reduces the quantity of seeds; (b) the growing process is accelerated and cotton maturity is fully guaranteed [17]; (c) water and nutrient uptake was improved with promoted lateral root growth. Also, the root weight and lateral root number of soil-cubes transplanting were 43.4% and 18.8% higher than those in direct seeding cotton [18]; (d) cotton germination, emergence, and early seedling growth are sensitive to salinity stress. Stand establishment was greatly improved by seedling transplanting with nonsaline soil as nursery substrate relative to direct seeding in saline soils [19]. Seedling transplanting is thus used as an efficient practice to increase stand establishment of cotton in saline soils.

Compared with direct-seeded cotton after wheat harvest, the yield of transplanted seedlings was increased by 20–30% [20]. Moreover, seed yield and quality parameters were significantly improved in the transplanting system through the increased number of bolls per square meter and earlier blooming; the net revenue for producers was also increased relative to direct planting. About 2 million hectares of cotton were covered with the seedling transplanting technology in the 1990s.

However, traditional seedling nursery and transplanting is considerably labor-intensive. The intensive process can be simplified by replacing nutrient soil clay with medium, and by transplanting naked seedling rather than soil-clay combined seedling to fields, and by mechanized transplanting instead of manual transplanting [21]. Because simplified seedling transplanting decreases labor cost and increases working efficiency, it is a promising alternative for transplanting.

2.3. Plastic mulching

Low temperature and drought at sowing as well as soil salinity stress and disease during the seedling stage usually decrease the rate of seed emergence and stand establishment [22, 23]. Low temperature combined with salinity stress can further reduce cotton emergence and stand establishment in saline fields [24]. Although late sowing may reduce environmental stress of early season chilling and disease incidence, cotton yield was decreased by shortening of growth period. Fortunately, all these problems can be solved by plastic mulching, because it functions well in increasing soil temperature, water conservation, salinity control in the root zone, and weed control [25].

Plastic mulching has been widely adopted for cotton production since the 1980s. Currently, about 70% of total cotton fields, equivalent to 2.7 million hectares, are covered with plastic film each year, especially in the arid and semi-arid regions of northern China and coastal saline-alkali areas. Plastic mulching increases soil temperature through greenhouse effect and conserves moisture through preventing direct evaporation of moisture from the soil, finally leading to improved seedling establishment, plant growth, and economical yield. Moreover, plastic mulching in saline field could effectively reduce the accumulation of salts in the surface soil by suppressing evaporation and salinity stress is thus decreased [26].

Plastic film coverage (mulching) is usually conducted soon after sowing manually or mechanically in the Yellow River and the Yangtze River valley region **(Figure 2a)**. Seedlings are freed from mulching cover by cutting film above hills at emergence **(Figure 2b)**, and thinned to the planned population density by leaving one vigorous plant per hill at the two-leaf stage. It should be noted that with the development of cotton's whole-course mechanization, plastic film coverage (mulching) before sowing can be interactively conducted with machine in the northwest inland cotton region (**Figure 2c**), which can avoid the process of seedling freed under rainless sowing stage (**Figure 2d**).

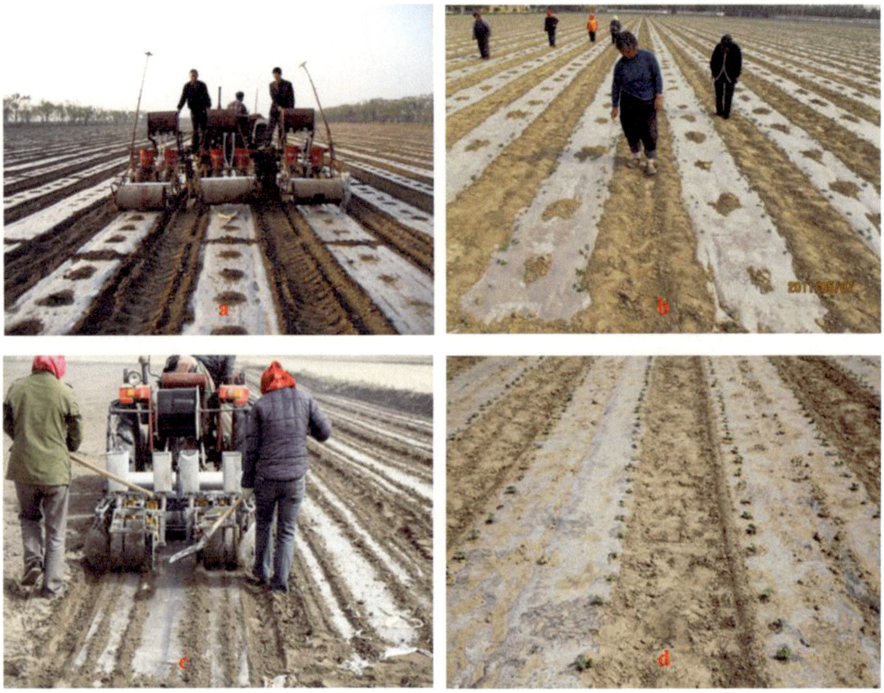

Figure 2. Row covering with plastic mulching. (a) Plastic mulching after sowing conducted with machine;(b) manually freeing seedlings from mulching cover at emergence; (c) plastic film coverage (mulching) before sowing conducted with machine; (d) avoiding the process of seedling freed.

Treatment	**Biomass (g/plant)**	**Na^+ (mg/g)**	**Stand establishment (%)**	**Lint yield (kg ha^{-1})**	**Earliness (%)**
No-mulching	1.47c	11.3a	47.8c	900c	64.0b
Conventional mulching	1.71b	10.0b	59.5b	1000b	71.4a
Early mulching	1.88a	9.2c	66.3a	1071a	73.0a

Source [27].

Table 3. Effects of early and conventional mulching on biomass, Na^+ content, stand establishment, lint yield, and earliness of cotton.

Large evaporation usually occurs in naked land without coverage before sowing in spring, and a large quantity of salts would accumulate in the surface layer of saline soils. Plastic film mulching before sowing would reduce salt accumulation in soil surface layer and improve stand establishment in saline soils. As indicated in a previous report, row covering with plastic film 30 days before sowing (early mulching) greatly improved stand establishment, and increased lint yield by 19.0% and earliness by 14.1% relative to no-mulching (**Table 3**). Compared with conventional post-sowing coverage, early mulching reduced leaf Na^+ levels by 8.0% and increased stand establishment by 11.4%, plant biomass by 9.9%, and lint yield by 7.1% in the saline Yellow River Delta. Furthermore, furrow seeding with plastic mulching was also a suitable cultural practice for enhancing cotton production in saline field owing to increase stand establishment, especially in moderate and high levels of saline-alkaline soil. Compared with flat-seeded cotton without mulching, the stand establishment and lint yield under furrow seeding with plastic mulching was increased by 92% and 22% in saline field with ECe of 12.8 dS m^{-1}.

Plastic film mulching in combination with seedling transplanting was recommended because it had dual advantages of increasing soil temperature and promoting early maturity. In such a way, cotton seedlings are transplanted to film-covered fields rather than open fields. An integration of mulching and transplanting was demonstrated to significantly improve plant growth and development, yield, and earliness compared with transplanting or plastic mulching alone [28]. Lint yields were increased with a combination of both practices by 17.4% and 14.6% compared with individual use of plastic mulching and transplanting

2.4. Plant pruning

Plant pruning has been widely applied for more than 70 years in China. It mainly includes vegetative branch removal, plant topping, and excising empty fruit branches and old leaves. It is generally believed that plant training can reduce the nutrient consumption of surplus organs, decrease the number of boll abscission and boll rot, and increase cotton yield and fiber quality [29].

2.4.1. Removal of vegetative branches

Vegetative branches of cotton plants do not set fruit directly, thus they excessively consume nutrients and result in boll shedding especially at a medium plant population density of 4.5–7.5 plants m^{-2}. Vegetative branches can manually be removed after the first fruit branch appears in mid June **(Figure 3a)**. It was reported that removal of vegetative branches decreased boll shedding rate of cotton plants by 9% and increased the boll weight by 7% and seed cotton yield by 8.7% [30]. It also improved the number of fruiting nods per leaf area (31.1%) and dry mass of fruiting parts per leaf area (88.9%) [31].

2.4.2. Plant topping

Removal of growth tips on the main stem by hand (topping) inhibits apical dominance and vegetative growth, allowing more nutrients to be partitioned to reproductive organs, leading to more squares, flowers, bolls, and lint yield. It is critical to identify the best topping time in practice. Topping later always caused an increase in ineffective fruit branches and ineffective flower buds in upper fruit branches; topping earlier always increases the abscission of squares and bolls in the upper fruit branches. It was suggested that topping should be conducted by mid- or late-July when the number of fruit branches achieve 8–10 per m^2 ground area. Plant topping is also suggested to be done in windless and clear day to facilitate wound healing (**Figure 3b**).

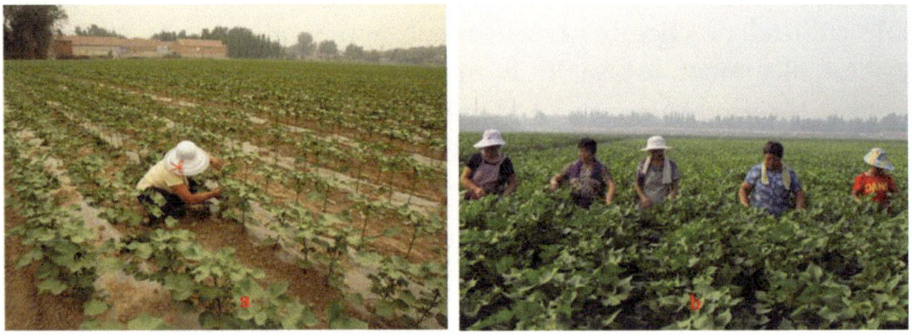

Figure 3. Intensive plant training measures. (a) Removal of vegetative branches; (b) manual plant topping.

2.4.3. *Removal of early fruit branches*

Fruit shedding or loss appears necessary to ensure normal development of retained bolls that are carried through to maturity because cotton produces many more fruits than they can mature [32]. Loss of early fruiting forms can elicit compensatory growth [33]. Early-fruit removal enhances vegetative growth and development, thus it can be used to coordinate relationship between vegetative and reproductive growth [34]. Removal of early fruiting forms is currently used in early squaring cotton to mitigate premature senescence because it increased levels of total nitrogen (N), soluble protein, as well as glutamic-pyruvic transaminase (GPT) activity in leaves [35], and lint yield was thus increased [36]. It was also reported that removal of early squares reduced the *verticillium* wilt disease indexes and early senescence indexes [37]. The lowermost two or three fruiting branches on the main stem are manually removed 5 days after squaring.

2.5. Super-high plant density technique

Northwest inland cotton region occupies abundant light and heat resources, but cotton growing season is very short due to low temperature in spring and autumn in this region. In order to avoid such a limitation, a cultivation pattern called "short-dense-early" was developed in the 1990s and has been widely adopted in the northwest inland cotton region. In this pattern, plant density is greatly increased as one of the most important practices. Plant height is reduced and early maturity is improved with the help of drip irrigation under plastic mulching.

In the "short-dense-early" pattern, the plant density usually ranges from 200,000 to 300,000 plants ha^{-1}, and the plant height is controlled to a range of 60–75 cm through chemical regulation, water and fertilizer management as well as using early-maturity variety, early planting and drip irrigation under plastic film mulching. The average lint yield in this region reached 1927 kg ha^{-1}. Currently, it is not difficult for farmers in Xinjiang to produce 2250 kg ha^{-1} of lint yield with "short-dense-early" pattern [38]. It was also reported that a lint yield record of 4900 kg ha^{-1} was obtained in a small area in Xinjiang in 2009 [39].

The northwest inland of China is an arid inland with little precipitation but high evaporation, thus drip irrigation under film mulching is well adopted in the region. In the drip irrigation system, one tube can be responsible for two or four rows of cotton. Currently, the most commonly used pattern is four rows of cotton per drip irrigation tube **(Figure 4)**. On the one hand, drip irrigation under film effectively reduces moisture loss and improves water and nutrient use efficiency [40]. Compared with flood irrigation, the water saving and yield increase with drip irrigation under film were improved by 20–50% and 10–30%, respectively [41], and water and nitrogen use efficiency were also greatly improved in Southern Xinjiang; on the other hand, it effectively alleviates weeds, diseases, and insect pests; decreases the number of boll rots; and improves seed cotton yield and fiber quality.

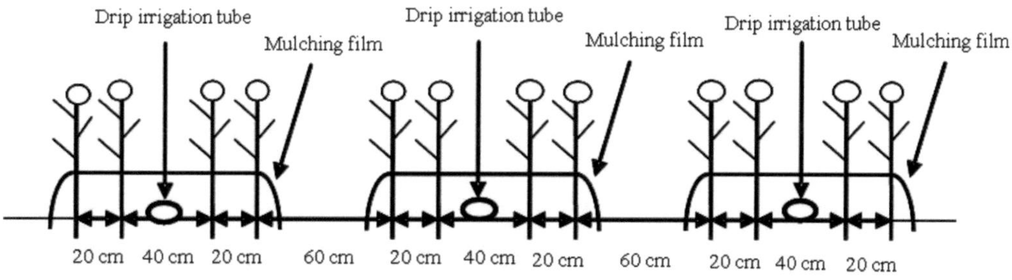

Figure 4. Drip irrigation system with four rows per drip irrigation tube.

In saline fields, drip irrigation under film could induce low salinity distribution around the root zone, which significantly alleviated salinity stress and enhanced seedling establishment and plant growth [42]. It was reported that cotton roots were mainly distributed in the mulched area [43]. Unequal salt distribution decreased Na^+ concentration in leaves owing to higher root Na^+ efflux in the low salinity side, and increased leaf photosynthesis, transpiration and water and nutrient uptake. It thus greatly improved cotton biomass, lint yield, and earliness compared with equal salt distribution in the root zone [44].

3. Problems and challenges

Even though intensive farming technologies have played crucial roles in supporting China to become the largest cotton producer in the world, it is currently facing great challenges, such as soil pollution caused by plastic film and chemicals, labor shortage due to urbanization and competition for land from grain crops.

3.1. Soil pollution

In cotton fields, soil pollutants mainly come from plastic mulch, fertilizers, and pesticides.

3.1.1. Plastic pollution

Plastic mulching has been one of the most important intensive farming and cultural measures, but its residue in the soil destroys soil structure and inhibits crop growth, and has become a common soil pollution phenomenon in China.

As plastic coverage is used year after year, more and more plastic film residues accumulate in the plow layer, which destroys soil integrity and permeability, inhibits the infiltration of soil capillary and free water, and impairs microbial activity and plant growth [45]. It was reported that the germination rate, number of plants at harvest and cotton yield in film-polluted soil were decreased by 9.9–19.1%, 7.3–16.5%, and 7.3–21.6%, respectively [46]. Thus, plastic pollution is a big challenge for intensive farming of cotton in China.

3.1.2. Fertilizer pollution

Nitrogen (N) as an essential macronutrient is more required consistently and in larger amounts than other nutrients for cotton production [47]. Nitrogen fertilization had significant impacts on cotton growth, lint yields, and fiber quality, making it be excessively applied by cotton growers in China. In the northwest inland cotton regions, an overdose of 450 kg N ha^{-1} was applied to cotton fields, leading to excessive vegetative growth and delayed maturity [48]. In addition, excessive nitrogen application decreases the uptake of other nutrient elements and use efficiency of nitrogen; it also destroys the granular soil structure and compact soil, which finally leads to decreases in cotton yield and fiber quality. An overdose of nitrogen fertilizer and the resulting pollution also commonly exist in saline-alkali cotton fields [49].

3.1.3. Pesticide pollution

Cotton is considered a high pesticide consumer crop; about 25–30% of total pesticides produced in China is used for cotton [50]. Pesticide is so indispensable to cotton production, yet while only 1% of the sprayed pesticides is effective, 99% of pesticides applied is released to nontarget soils, water bodies, and atmosphere [51]. Although Bt (*Bacillus thuringiensis*) transgenic cotton has effectively helped to control cotton bollworm (*Helicoverpa armigera* Hübner), other pests like mirid bugs (Heteroptera: Miridae) have progressively increased in population sizes in association with a regional increase in Bt cotton adoption [52]. Organochlorined pesticides (OCPs) such as HCH, DDT, HCB, aldrin, endrin, and chlordane, were commonly used to control pests in China, and were still detected in some cotton fields although OCPs have been banned since 1983. In addition, much more herbicide was excessively applied to control weed in cotton fields, resulting in soil, water, and atmospheric pollution [53].

3.2. Labor shortage

Intensive farming and cultivation is depending on a huge labor power. With the rapid urbanization in the nation, more and more rural laborers have migrated to cities and towns to work in secondary and tertiary industries, leaving only the elderly, women, and children to be engaged in agriculture. According to the statistics, about 0.24 billion rural laborers migrated to cities from 1996 to 2007 in China. Thus, the intensive cultivation techniques are facing severe challenges of labor shortage and low level of mechanization for cotton production in China.

3.3. Food safety and climate change

Rapid urbanization has gradually reduced the total cultivated land in China. The Chinese government is facing a growing pressure of "food security" and pays more attention to grain crops than cotton. A lot of supporting policies and measures such as improving grain price and providing grain subsidy were taken in China to stimulate grain production. This resulted in more cotton fields being converted to grain fields in China. Intensive farming techniques of cotton also have to face a challenge from relatively extensive and simple cultivation techniques of food crops.

Global warming has also resulted in temperature change in the cotton production area of China, especially in fall and winter seasons. As the temperature increases, cotton plants grow and develop more quickly than before. As a result, on the one hand, cotton is subject to premature senescence; on the other hand, more rainfall occurred with increases in water evaporation owing to temperature increase. "*The pollination of cotton is influenced by high rainfall during the reproductive growth stage, which causes more bud, flower and boll abscission. High and/or prolonged rainfall duration also causes plant lodging and serious boll spoiling diseases, further decreasing seed cotton yield and fiber quality*" [4]. Therefore, the increasing area of waterlogging, more serious pest incidence and premature senescence resulting from climate change are also strong challenges which the intensive farming must face.

4. Countermeasures and prospects

In order to support sustainable and green production of cotton in China, the traditional intensive farming technologies should be reformed.

4.1. Reducing soil pollution

Measures to decrease plastic film residues in soils include (a) plastic film recovery. Timely removal of plastic film could effectively increase its residual recovery. This may be achieved by increasing the current film thickness of 0.004–0.006 mm to 0.012 mm or above. It was reported that the recovery of plastic film residues with 0.012 mm was higher (69.2%) than that with 0.006 mm [54]; (b) mechanic collection of plastic film residues after harvest or before planting. Plastic film residues in the soil can be greatly reduced with the help of a cleaning machine. This is usually conducted in combination with tillage; (c) application of degradable plastic film. Photodegradable or biodegradable films have attracted wide interests of researchers and farmer. Once the photodegradable or biodegradable films get to be commercialized, the pollution problems will be solved.

Sustainable development of cotton production also needs to reduce pesticide-and fertilizer-caused soil pollution. Application of Bt transgenic cotton and transgenic herbicide-resistant cotton is an effective alternative to reduce pesticide contamination; Applying low-toxicity and low-residue pesticides can be another effective way to reduce chemical contamination. Appropriate application of fertilizers, especially nitrogen fertilizer inputs, is able to decrease fertilizer contamination of soil. Application of organic fertilizer, increasing plant density as well as fertilization improvement favor lower input of fertilizers without cotton yield reduction.

4.2. Simplifying field management

Cotton is intensively cultivated currently in China with more than 40 procedures during the whole growth period. The amount of labor input for cotton is 3.5 and 3 times that for wheat and corn, respectively. Only simplifying the intensive farming technologies and mechanization of the whole production process can effectively deal with the challenges of the current labor shortage for cotton production.

Year	Seeding patterns	Experimental sites				Means
		Linqing	Xiajin	Huimin	Dongying	
2011	Conventional seeding	3445a	3741a	3673a	3805a	3666a
	Precision seeding	3403a	3720a	3665a	3264b	3513b
2012	Conventional seeding	3295a	3877a	3845a	3639a	3664a
	Precision seeding	3258a	3850a	3632b	3615a	3589a
2013	Conventional seeding	3514a	3445a	3370a	3287a	3404a
	Precision seeding	3490a	3366a	3328a	3232a	3354a

Source [56].

Table 4. Effects of precision seeding on seed cotton yield at four experimental sites from 2011 to 2013.

4.2.1. Precision seeding without thinning

Traditionally, the seeding rate of cotton is usually 35–45 kg ha^{-1} in China, and the resulting number of seedlings is always much larger than the targeted plant density. It thus requires one or two times of manual thinning to remove the extra seedlings after emergence. It is known that cotton yield is not influenced within a certain plant density range owing to its broader adaptability to plant density [55], thus precision seeding can be an important simplification measure. Compared with conventional seeding, the precision seeding on the one hand, significantly reduced the seeding rate without decreasing yield (**Table 4**) and fiber quality; on the other hand, the labor input is also reduced by eliminating the process of thinning. Precision seeding is usually conducted soon after mulching in the northwest inland of China because of dry weather in spring there, while it should be conducted before plastic mulching in the Yellow River valley to avoid interference of raining weather in spring.

Additionally, a precision seeding with double mulching **(Figure 5)**, in which seeds were inserted into the mulched soil and re-covered by plastic film above the first mulch and the re-coverage was removed soon after full emergence. Double mulching is an important practice to improve stand establishment in case of rainfall after seeding in the Yellow River valley of China.

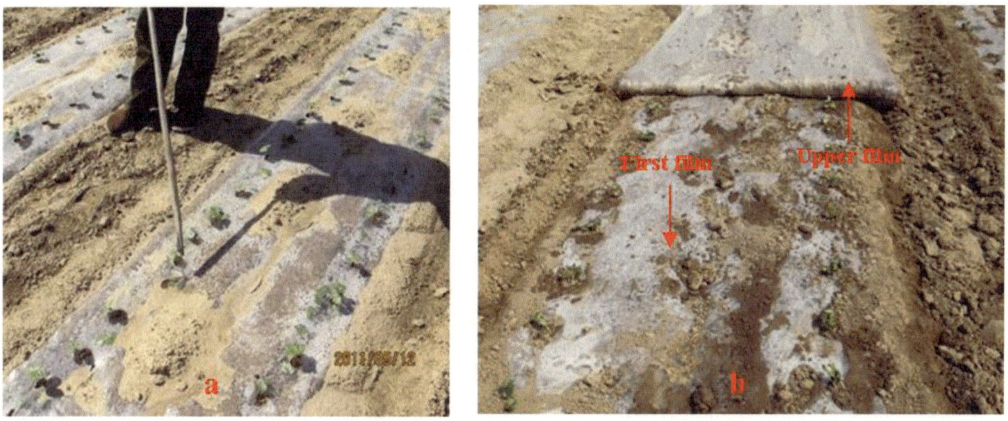

Figure 5. Conventional seeding (a) and precision seeding with double mulching (b).

4.2.2. Application of controlled-release fertilizer

Cotton is traditionally fertilized at least three times with rapid release fertilizers in China. The conventional split fertilization with rapid release fertilizer always results in a great deal of labor input and fertilizer loss. Application of slow- or controlled-release fertilizer reduces labor input and fertilizer loss, because it can be applied only once before planting (basal application) without yield loss [57].

4.2.3. Simplified plant pruning technology

Plant pruning including removal of vegetative branches, old leaves and redundant buds and growth terminals of the main stem is labor intensive. In practice, removal of vegetative branches can be replaced without yield reduction either by retaining vegetative branches at lower plant density or by inhibiting their growth with high plant density [58]. The application of chemical substitutes instead of manual pruning can effectively regulate the relationship between vegetative and reproductive growth without decreasing yield and fiber quality, especially the application of chemicals in plant topping [59].

4.2.4. *Reduced intertillage*

Intertillage is traditionally conducted 5–10 times from seedling to harvest in cotton in China. Some recent studies have shown that the reduced number of intertillage did not affect final lint yield. It can be reduced to two times, the first at full emergence and the second at full squaring, in the whole season without yield reduction. Intertillage can be conducted in combination with weeding, earthing up, plastic film uncovering, and fertilization with the help of machinery at full squaring.

4.2.5. *Harvest-aid application technology*

Cotton is a perennial plant that will shed its mature leaves naturally as the growing season progresses and the crop matures. With the demonstration and extension of machine-harvested cotton, harvest-aid application technologies play an important role in stimulating defoliation and boll opening. Harvest-aid application decisions largely are based on crop maturity, crop condition, weather conditions, desired harvest schedule, and harvest-aid choices and rate. Ethephon is effective in accelerating the opening of mature cotton bolls. Though not labeled as defoliants, satisfactory defoliation may result from applications made under favorable weather conditions or at higher use rates. Commonly, in order to enhance the efficacy of harvest-aid products, ethephon was tank-mixed with defoliants, such as tribufos, thidiazuron, and dimethipin. In cotton with a dense canopy, ethephon can be applied at the boll-opening rate with a low rate of defoliant to achieve both boll opening and leaf drop.

Thorough spray coverage is necessary for good defoliation, because harvest aids are not able to be translocated from one leaf to the other. Each leaf must be sprayed to initiate the abscission process. A second application is usually needed on rank cotton with dense foliage. Additionally, adjuvants were usually added to harvest-aid chemical formulation or tank mixes to enhance performance by improving leaf-surface wetting and penetration and uniformity of deposit.

4.2.6. *Development of mechanization*

Because of high labor input and labor shortage, intensive cotton farming will inevitably be reformed with mechanization. There exist large differences in mechanization rate among regions in China. The northwest inland cotton region is the highest in the integrated ratio of mechanized cotton farming, while the Yangtze River valley cotton region is the lowest.

A full mechanization for cotton production mainly consists of mechanical tillage, soil preparation, seeding, plant protection, intertillage and fertilization, harvesting, and straw returning. At present, some machineries for soil preparation, seeding, intertillage, plant protection, and straw returning have been developed and widely used in cotton production in China. Although cotton pickers from abroad basically meets the mechanic harvest demand of cotton in China, other supporting measures or equipments such as adaptive varieties, techniques of cultivation and defoliation and machine-picked cotton cleaning lines need to be further developed. The integration of agricultural machinery and agronomic measures should be strengthened to accelerate mechanized cotton harvesting. These measures include: (a) improving cotton picker performance and seed cotton quality through developing more efficient harvesting machinery and equipment suitable for different cotton regions; (b) development of cotton varieties suitable for mechanized harvesting; (c) development of new agricultural cultivation technologies well matched to mechanic harvesting; (d) establishment of quality standards for machine-picked cotton.

4.3. Reform of planting system in double cropping

In a traditional double-cropping system, it is mainly implemented through direct seeding or transplanting before harvest of wheat, garlic, or rape (intercropping). This not only takes a large amount of labor input, but also inhibits mechanization. Traditional plant system should be reformed to meet the demands of mechanization and reduced labor inputs **(Figure 6)**. The first alternative is cotton seedling transplanting after wheat or rape. Traditional seedling nursery and transplanting is labor-intensive. The intensive process can be simplified by replacing nutrient soil clay with commercialized medium, and by transplanting naked seedlings rather than soil-clay combined seedlings to fields, and by mechanized transplanting instead of manual transplanting. The second alternative is to use direct seeding of short-season cotton after the harvest of wheat, garlic, or rape instead of intercropping.

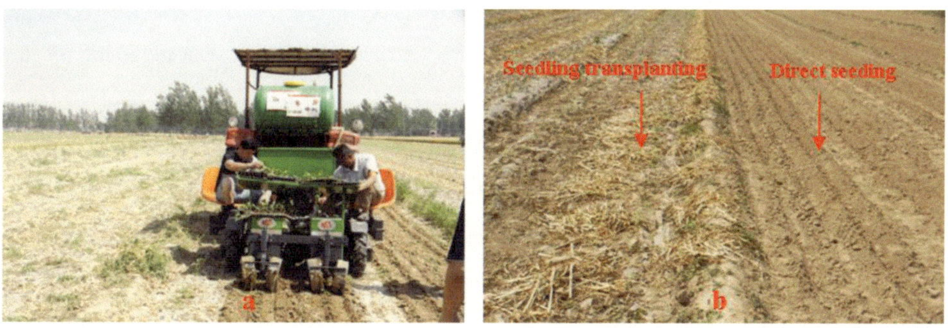

Figure 6. Mechanized transplanting of full-season cotton after harvest of garlic (a) and direct seeding of short-season cotton after harvest of garlic (b).

5. Conclusions

Intensive farming technologies including seedling transplanting, plastic mulching, plant pruning, double cropping, and "short-dense-early" have been widely applied for the past 50 years in China. These intensive technologies have played key roles in supporting China to be the largest cotton producer in the world. However, it should be noted that current cotton production in China is facing a series of challenges, such as soil pollution, labor shortage, and intense competition for land from food crops. Therefore, it is essential to reform the traditional intensive farming technologies. New farming and cultural technologies should be established to reduce soil pollution through rational use of plastic film and chemicals, save labor through simplifying managements and intensifying mechanization, and increase benefit through reforming the cropping system and management mode. It is believed that China cotton has a good prospect with the support of new farming technologies (**Table 5**).

Measures	Present	Prospect
Planting and thinning	Conventional seeding, 30–45 kg seed per hectare, and 2–3 times of manual thinning	Precision seeding, 15–18.75 kg seed per hectare, and no-thinning
Intertillage	8–10 times during the whole growth season	2–3 times at the full post emergence and full squaring or flowering stage
Fertilization	3–4 times at planting, squaring, or flowering stage and after topping with rapid release fertilizers. With more labor input and lower fertilizer use efficiency	One time at planting with slow- or controlled-release fertilizer. Labor saving and higher fertilizer use efficiency
Plant training	Manual removal of vegetative branches, old leaves and redundant buds and growth terminals of the main stem	Retaining vegetative branches at lower plant density or inhibit growth of vegetative branches through increased plant density, or using chemical substitutes for plant training
Plastic mulching	Film thickness of 0.004–0.006 mm, lower film residual recovery	≥0.012 mm in film thickness for recovery, or using film substitutes instead of conventional plastic film
Planting pattern	Double-cropping through direct seeding or transplanting before harvest of wheat/garlic/rape	Direct seeding of short-season cotton after the harvest of wheat/rape, or transplanting after wheat/garlic /rape
Management mode	Scattered distribution and small-scale plantation	Concentrated distribution and scaling up plantation
Mechanization	40% level, including tillage, sowing, fertilization and intertillage, straw returning	≥70% level in ten years, including tillage, sowing, fertilization and intertillage, harvesting, and straw returning

Table 5. Current status and prospect of cotton cultivation measures in China.

Acknowledgements

This work was supported by the earmarked fund for China Agricultural Research System (CARS-18-21), the special fund for Taishan Scholars (NO. tspd20150213), and the National Natural Science Foundation of China (30971720, 31371573).

Author details

Jianlong Dai and Hezhong Dong*

*Address all correspondence to: donghz@saas.ac.cn

Key Laboratory of Cotton Breeding and Cultivation in Huang-Huai-Hai Plain, Ministry of Agriculture, Cotton Research Center, Shandong Academy of Agricultural Science, Jinan, P.R. China

References

[1] Chen XM, Zhang HB, Dong HZ. Understanding on the adjustments of national policy for cotton industry as well as the countermeasures and suggestions. China Cotton. 2015;42: 1–4. DOI:10.11963/issn.1000-632X.201505003.

[2] Yang HQ, Cui WG. Cotton industry in China, status and development strategies. Crops. 2010;5: 13–17. DOI:10.16035/j.issn.1001-7283.2010.05.038 (in Chinese).

[3] Cotton Economic Information System, Cotton Production Statistics [Internet]. 2016. Available from: http://cceis.org/SELECT.aspx?s=year [accessed: 2016-03-24].

[4] Dai JL, Dong HZ. Intensive cotton farming technologies in China: achievements, challenges and countermeasures. Field Crops Research. 2014;155: 99–110. DOI:http://dx.doi.org/10.1016/j.fcr.2013.09.017.

[5] United States Department of Agriculture, Cotton Area Harvested and Production of World [Internet]. 2016. Available from: http://apps.fas.usda.gov/psdonline/psdQuery.aspx [accessed: 2016-03-27].

[6] Zhang LZ, Werf WVD, Zhang S, Li B, Spiertz JHJ. Growth, yield and quality of wheat and cotton in relay strip intercropping systems. Field Crop Res. 2007;103: 178–188. DOI: 10.1016/j.fcr.2007.06.002.

[7] Zhang LZ, Werf WVD, Bastiaans L, Zhang S, Li B, Spiertz JHJ. Light interception and utilization in relay intercrops of wheat and cotton. Field Crop Res. 2008;107: 29–42. DOI: 10.1016/j.fcr.2007.12.014.

[8] Lu P. Wheat-cotton double cropping enhances cotton and wheat yield. China Cotton. 1991;2: 6–7 (in Chinese).

[9] Smith CW, Varvil JJ. Double cropping cotton and wheat. Agron J. 1982;74: 862–865.

[10] Cotton Research Institute (CRI). Chinese Academy of Agricultural Sciences. Cultivation of Cotton in China. 1st ed. Shanghai: Shanghai Science and Technology Press; 2013. p. 309–374 (in Chinese).

[11] Pan XB, Deng SH, Wang YQ. Effects of PAR penetration on the fallow rows remained for cotton in the wheat field. Acta Gossypii Sinica. 1994;6: 109–113 (in Chinese, with English abstract).

[12] Zhou ZG, Meng YL, Shi P, Shen YQ, Jia ZK. Study of the relationship between boll weight in wheat–cotton double cropping and meteorological factors in boll period. Acta Gossypii Sinica. 2000;12: 122–126. DOI:1002-7807(2000)03-0122-05 (in Chinese, with English abstract).

[13] Song MZ. Application and development prospects of cotton cultivation techniques in China. Agr Outlook. 2010;2: 50–55 (in Chinese).

[14] Cao YL, Chen Y, Lu SM, Yang L, Ke XS, Tu QJ, Li J. Review on cotton seedling transplanting technology. China Cotton. 2015;42: 12–14. DOI:1000-632X(2015)01-0012-03 (in Chinese).

[15] Dong HZ, Li WJ, Li ZH, Tang W, Zhang DM. Enhanced plant growth, development and fiber yield of Bt transgenic cotton by an integration of plastic mulching and seedling transplanting. Ind Crop Prod. 2007;26: 298–306. DOI: 10.1016/j.indcrop.2007.03.008.

[16] Sun XZ, Shi P, Zhang H, Zhou ZG. Research process of seedling transplantation and film mulching cultivation technique in China. Chinese Agr Sci Bull. 1999;15: 42–46 (in Chinese).

[17] Dong HZ, Li WJ, Tang W, Zhang DM. Increased yield and revenue with a seedling transplanting system for hybrid seed production in Bt cotton. J Agron Crop Sci. 2005;191: 116–124. DOI:10.1111/j.1439-037X.2004.00130.x.

[18] Mao SC, Li PC, Han YC, Wang GP, Li YB, Wang XH. Preliminary observation on morphological parameters of root system of the root-naked transplanting cotton (*Gossypium hirsutum* L.). Cotton Sci. 2008;20: 76–78. DOI:1002-7807(2008)01-0076-03 (in Chinese, with English abstract).

[19] Zhang JL, Jia YZ, Zhu ZM, Wu MT. Measures of promoting the establishment of cotton in saline soil. J Henan Agr Sci. 1982;5: 1–3 (in Chinese).

[20] Gao Q, Shang YZ. Development base for early mature of seedling transplantation cotton. China Cotton 1982;2: 29-31(in Chinese).

[21] Mao SC, Han YC, Wang GP, Li YB, Dong CW, Feng L, Li XX. To extend technique of industrial seedling raising and mechanized transplanting, and speed up development of modern cotton planting industry. China Cotton. 2012;39: 1–5. DOI: 1000-632X(2012)08-0001-05 (in Chinese).

[22] Meryl N, Rowland C, Rowland RA. Germination and stand establishment. In: Mauney JRJ, Stewart MD, editors. Cotton Physiology. The Cotton Foundation, Memphis, TN; 1986, p. 535–541.

[23] Ahmad S, Khan N, Iqbal MZ, Hussain A, Hassan M. Salt tolerance of cotton (*Gossypium hirsutum* L.). Asian J Plant Sci. 2002;1: 715–719. DOI:10.3923/ajps.2002.715.719.

[24] Dong HZ, Li WJ, Li ZH, Zhang DM. Furrow seeding with plastic mulching increase stand establishment and lint yield of cotton in a saline field. Agron J. 2008;100: 1640–1646. DOI:10.2134/agronj2008.0074.

[25] Mahajan G, Sharda R, Kumar A, Singh KG. Effect of plastic mulch on economizing irrigation water and weed control in baby corn sown by different methods. Afr J Agr Res. 2007;2: 19–26.

[26] Dai JL, Dong HZ, Duan LS. Technology and mechanism in control of salt injury in cotton. Cotton Sci. 2010;22: 486–494. DOI:1002-7807(2010)05-0486-09 (in Chinese, with English abstract).

[27] Dong HZ, Li WJ, Li ZH, Zhang DM. Early plastic mulching increases stand establishment and lint yield of cotton in saline fields. Field Crop Res. 2009;111: 269–275. DOI: 10.1016/j.fcr.2009.01.001.

[28] Wu FA. Studies on super-effective cotton cultivation techniques of double plastic mulching in Shandong province. China Cotton. 1996;23: 11–13 (in Chinese).

[29] Zhou BY, Yang HY. Techniques of plant training on cotton high yield. New Agri. 1999;7: 16 (in Chinese).

[30] Yuan WX. Yield increase effect and application of plant training on cotton. Cotton Sci. 1982;2: 22–26 (in Chinese, with English abstract).

[31] Dong HZ, Niu YH, Li WJ, Tang W, Li ZH, Zhang DM. Regulation effects of various training modes on source-sink relation of cotton. Chinese J. Appl. Ecol. 2008;19: 819–824. DOI:10.13287/j.1001-9332.2008.0206 (in Chinese, with English abstract).

[32] Malik MNA, Edwards DG, Evenson JP. Effects of flower bud removal and nitrogen supply on growth and development of cotton (*Gossypium hirsutum* L.). Aust Plant Physiol. 1981;8: 285–291.

[33] Sadras VO. Compensation growth in cotton after loss of reproductive organs. Field Crop Res. 1995;40: 1–8.

[34] Dong HZ, Niu YH, Kong XQ, Luo Z. Effects of early-fruit removal on endogenous cytokinins and abscisic acid in relation to leaf senescence in cotton. Plant Growth Regul. 2009;59: 90–101. DOI 10.1007/s10725-009-9392-x.

[35] Zhang DM, Li WJ, Tang W, Dong HZ. Fruiting-branch removal enhances endotoxin expression and lint yield in Bt cotton. Acta Agr Scand B-S P. 2009;59: 424–430. DOI: 10.1080/09064710802322147.

[36] Dong HZ, Tang W, Li WJ, Li ZH, Niu YH, Zhang DM. Yield, leaf senescence, and *Cry1Ac* expression in response to removal of early fruiting branches in transgenic Bt cotton. Agr Sci China. 2008;7: 692–702 (in Chinese, with English abstract).

[37] Zhu HQ, Feng ZL, Song XX, Jian GL, Liu XY. Effect of removal of early squares on *verticillium wilt* and premature senescence in Bt transgenic cotton. Cotton Sci. 2008;20: 414–417. DOI:1002-7807(2008)06-0414-04 (in Chinese, with English abstract).

[38] Wang LP. Discussion on the cotton high-yield cultivation techniques under high-density. Anhui Agr Sci Bull. 2009;15: 119–120 (in Chinese).

[39] Maimaiti MM, Li XY, Ai XT, Zheng JY, Wang JD, Tu XJ, Duo LK, Liang YJ. The characteristic analysis of super-high yield cotton field in Xinjiang. Cotton Sci. 2012;34: 31–35. DOI:10.3969/j.issn.2095-3143.2012.05.007 (in Chinese).

[40] Liu XY, Tian CY, Ma YJ, Liu HP. Water consumption characteristics and scheduling of drip irrigation under plastic film for cotton in south Xinjiang. Agr Res Arid Areas. 2006;24: 108–112. DOI:10.3321/j.issn:1000–7601.2006.01.023 (in Chinese, with English abstract).

[41] Liu ZH. Review of the effect of drip irrigation under mulch applied technology in cotton field. Mech Rural Pastoral Area. 2008;3: 27–28 (in Chinese, with English abstract).

[42] Zhou HP, Xu XB, Lan YJ. Review of research on soil water and salt transportation under the condition of drip irrigation under film in Xinjiang area. Water Saving Irrig. 2006;4: 8–13. DOI:10.3969/j.issn.1007-4929.2006.04.003 (in Chinese, with English abstract).

[43] Yan YY, Zhao CY, Sheng Y, Li JY, Peng DM, Li ZL, Feng SL. Effects of drip irrigation under mulching on cotton root and shoot biomass and yield. Chinese J Appl Ecol. 2009;20: 970–976. DOI:10.13287/j.1001-9332.2009.0134 (in Chinese, with English abstract).

[44] Kong XQ, Luo Z, Dong HZ, Eneji AE, Li WJ. Effects of non-uniform root zone salinity on water use, Na^+ recirculation, and Na^+ and H^+ flux in cotton. J Exp Bot. 2012;63: 2105–2116. DOI:10.1093/jxb/err420.

[45] Zhi JH, Zheng DM, Zhu YJ. Effect of leftover film contamination on cotton production and its administration. J Tarim Univ. 2007;19: 66–70. DOI:10.3969/j.issn. 1009-0568.2007.03.015 (in Chinese, with English abstract).

[46] Jiang YJ, Zheng DM, Zhu ZY. Effects of remnant plastic film in soil on growth and yield of cotton. Agro-Environ Prot. 2001;20: 177–179. DOI:1000-0267(2001)03-0177-03 (in Chinese, with English abstract).

[47] Hou Z, Li P, Li B, Gong Z, Wang Y. Effects of fertigation scheme on N uptake and N use efficiency in cotton. Plant Soil. 2007;290: 115–126. DOI:1001-4330(2008)S2-0065-12.

[48] Bondada BR, Oosterhuisan DM, Norman RJ, Baker WH. Canopy photosynthesis, growth, yield, and boll ^{15}N accumulation under nitrogen stress in cotton. Crop Sci. 1996;36: 127–133. DOI:10.2135/cropsci1996.0011183X003600010023x.

[49] Chen WP, Hou ZN, Wu LS, Liang YC, Wei CZ. Effect of salinity and nitrogen on cotton growth in arid environment. Plant Soil. 2010;326: 61–73. DOI:10.1007/s11104-008-9881-0.

[50] Wu KM, Guo YY. The evolution of cotton pest management practices in China. Annu Rev Entomol. 2005;50: 31–52. DOI:10.1146/annurev.ento.50.071803.130349.

[51] Zhang WJ, Jiang FB, Ou JF. Global pesticide consumption and pollution: with China as a focus. Proc Int Acad Ecol Environ Sci. 2011;1: 125–144.

[52] Lu YH, Wu KM, Jiang YY, Xia B, Li P, Feng HQ, Wyckhuys KAG, Gao YY. Mirid bug outbreaks in multiple crops correlated with wide-scale adoption of Bt cotton in China. Science 2010;328: 1151–1154. DOI:10.1126/science.1187881.

[53] Faircloth WH, Patterson MG, Monks CD, Goodman WR. Weed management programs for glyphosate-tolerant cotton (*Gossypium hirsutum* L.). Weed Technol. 2001;15: 544–551. DOI:10.1614/0890-037X(2001)015.

[54] Cao J. Effect of plastic film thickness on remnant plastic film recovery. Xinjiang Agr Sci Technol. 2012;6: 38–39 (in Chinese).

[55] Dai JL, Li WJ, Tang W, Zhang DM, Li ZH, Lu HQ, Eneji AE, Dong HZ. Manipulation of dry matter accumulation and partitioning with plant density in relation to yield stability of cotton under intensive management. Field Crop Res. 2015;180: 207–215. DOI: 10.1016/j.fcr.2015.06.008.

[56] Dai JL, Li ZH, Luo Z, Lu HQ, Tang W, Zhang DM, Li WJ, Xin CS, Dong HZ. Effects of precision seeding without thinning process on yield and yield components of cotton. Acta Agronomica Sinica. 2014;40: 2040–2045. DOI:10.3724/SP.J.1006.2014.02040 (in Chinese, with English abstract).

[57] Yang GZ, Tang HY, Tong J, Nie YC, Zhang XL. Effect of fertilization frequency on cotton yield and biomass accumulation. Field Crop Res. 2012;125: 161–166. DOI:10.1016/j.fcr.2011.08.008.

[58] Dong HZ, Li WJ, Eneji AE, Zhang DM. Nitrogen rate and plant density effects on yield and late-season leaf senescence of cotton raised on a saline field. Field Crop Res. 2012;126: 137–144. DOI:10.1016/j.fcr.2011.10.005.

[59] Zhao Q, Zhou CJ, Zhang JS, Li SL, Yun YL, Tian XL. Effect of chemical detopping on the canopy and yield of cotton (*Gossypium hirsutum* L.) in south Xinjiang. Cotton Sci. 2011;23: 329–333. DOI:1002-7807(2011)04-0329-05 (in Chinese, with English abstract).

Chapter 6

Cover-Crop Management Influences Residue Biomass and Subsequent Weed Suppression in a Conservation Agriculture Corn and Cotton Rotation

Andrew J. Price, Edzard van Santen and Lina Sarunaite

Additional information is available at the end of the chapter

http://dx.doi.org/10.5772/64132

Abstract

The use of winter cover crops is an integral component of conservation systems in a corn and cotton conservation agriculture rotation. Field experiments were conducted from the autumn of 2003 through cash crop harvest in 2006 at three locations. The treatments were five cover-crop-planting timings each fall and four cover-crop termination timings each spring. Five crimson clover or cereal rye planting timings occurred: on the average first 0°C temperature date, 4 and 2 weeks prior and 4 and 2 weeks after the average 0°C temperature date. Termination dates were 1–4 weeks prior to the average optimum soil temperature date for the establishment of each cash crop. Results showed that biomass production by winter covers decreased with even a week's delay in winter cover-crop seeding and resulted in a corresponding increase in summer annual weed biomass. More than 10 times difference in biomass produced by clover was observed when clover was planted on the earliest date and terminated on the last date compared to late planting and early termination, rye eight times. Correspondingly, weed biomass was 556 kg ha^{-1} in the treatment with least rye biomass, eight times higher compared to the treatment with greatest rye biomass.

Keywords: alternative weed control, conservation tillage, cover crops, crop rotation, weed biomass

1. Introduction

Resistance management has become the dominating weed science research and extension focus. In the Southeastern and Mid-South United States, questions concerning management of herbicide resistant *Amaranthus* species, horseweed (*Conyza Canadensis* L.), and Italian ryegrass (*Lolium multiflorum* Lam.), comprise the majority of Cooperative Extension Service (CES) calls in these regions. Conservation agriculture (CA) practices are especially threatened by the emergence and rapid spread of glyphosate-resistant Palmer amaranth (*A. palmeri* S. Wats.). Hundreds of thousands of CA hectares are at risk of being converted to higher-intensity tillage systems due to the inability to reliably control herbicide-resistant weeds in CA systems, especially dry land systems where soil applied herbicides risk non-activation [1]. Currently, the integration of high-residue cover-crop systems, inversion of the soil profile facilitating burial of the surface seedbank, and overlapping residual herbicides are increasingly being recommended by state CES throughout the Southeastern Coastal Plain and Mid-South Delta for herbicide-resistance management [1–3]. The CES in the Southeastern and Mid-South United States is also more frequently recommending tillage to enable increased pre-planting and pre-emergence herbicide use [3–5]. Between-row cultivation is also a proven method of controlling many troublesome and resistant weed species [4, 6]. However, conventional tillage practices decrease soil and water quality and may exclude producers from participating in government loan, insurance, and incentive programs designed to promote soil conservation stewardship. With the rapid spread of acetolactate synthase (ALS) and glyphosate-resistant Palmer amaranth, the hectares in CA could potentially decline further without the development of new, effective weed-control strategies [1].

In the 2012 Weed Science special issue "Herbicide Resistant Weeds", authors describe the need to understand a diverse best management practices (BMPs), including "emphasizing cultural management techniques that suppress weeds by using crop competitiveness" and "using mechanical and biological management practices where appropriate" [7]. Specific examples among many BMPs include crop rotation and cover-crops mulches, respectively. Interest in utilizing high-residue cover crops as a weed management tool is continually increasing from both producers and conservation organizations such as the Soil and Water Conservation Society and USDA Natural Resource Conservation Service among others who both actively support conservation practices through outreach programs and fiscal incentives. This special issue manuscript also states that the appropriate time for cover-crop termination is complex and that the optimum planting and termination timing will be regional and often farm-specific, and concludes "the greatest challenge to the use of any cover crop is the added complexity associated with integration into existing cropping systems."

To reduce the use of intensive tillage practices in integrated weed management systems for controlling problematic weeds, further evaluation of alternative control strategies is necessary. High-residue cover crops, which have been shown to provide early-season weed control, may be utilized in cotton along with other management tactics to suppress *Amaranthus* growth [8–18]. Although early-season weed control is possible with cover crops, season-long control has required the use of herbicides [14, 16, 19–21]. In addition, the quantity of mulch needed to physically suppress weeds has been evaluated [22].

In the past, cover-crop termination has been facilitated utilizing pre-plant (PP) burndown herbicides before planting. The CES recommends terminating winter covers relatively early in the spring, due to concerns for excessive cover-crop biomass interfering with planting operations or excessive soil moisture depletion [23, 24]. However, planting into residue is commonplace (**Figure 1**) and it is well known that planting date affects subsequent residue cover [25].

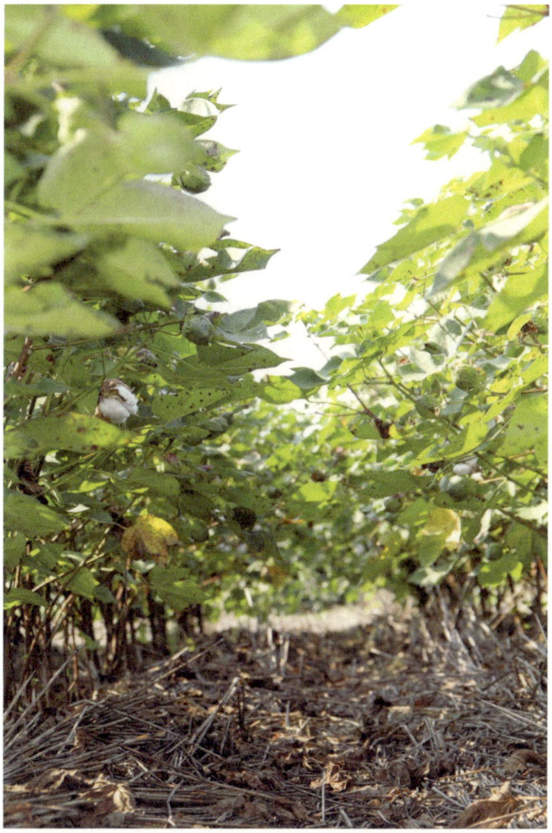

Figure 1. Cotton planted into cereal rye cover crop for weed suppression.

Cooperative extension service recommendations also generally recommend waiting approximately 2–4 weeks after desiccating cereal winter covers before planting cotton to avoid allelopathic effects [26, 27]. However, little research has been conducted evaluating how management of high-residue cover-crop biomass production in situ affects biomass amounts attained as well as weed and crop response. Thus, the objective of this research was to determine how cover-crop planting and termination timing influence subsequent residue and weed biomass and crop yield responses.

2. Materials and methods

Field experiments were conducted at the Alabama Agricultural Experiment Station's E.V. Smith Research Center at Shorter, AL, and Tennessee Valley Research and Extension Center at Belle Mina, AL, from autumn of 2003 through cash crop harvest in 2006. The experiment was also conducted at the University of Florida West Florida Education and Research Center at Jay, FL, from autumn of 2004 to cash crop harvest in 2006. The three locations were selected due to their relatively distant latitude positions and differing soil types, which, according to previous observations concerning forage biomass yield, would influence winter cover-crop growth. Latitude ranged from Belle Mina at 34.689595, E.V. Smith at 32.427626 to Jay, FL, at 30.777618. The soil types were Compass loamy sand (coarse-loamy, siliceous, subactive, thermic Plinthic Paleudults) at E.V. Smith, Decatur silty loam (fine, kaolinitic, thermic, Rhodic Paleudult) at Tennessee Valley, and a Dothan sandy loam (fine-loamy, siliceous, thermic Plinthic Kandiudults) at Jay.

The treatments were five cover-crop-planting timings each fall and four cover-crop termination timings each spring. The five crimson clover or cereal rye-planting timings occurred on the average 30 year first 0°C temperature date, 4 and 2 weeks prior and 4 and 2 weeks after the average 30 year 0°C temperature date. Termination dates were 1–4 weeks prior to the average 30-year optimum soil temperature date for the establishment of corn or cotton (**Table 1** and **2**). Termination dates were 4, 3, 2, and 1 week prior to the chosen date for corn and cotton establishment, which we based on the long-term average date of the minimum soil temperature ideal for corn (*Zea mays L.*) or cotton (*Gossypium hirsutum* L.) seeding as recommended by the Auburn University CES recommendations (**Tables 1** and **2**).

Belle Mina, AL			**Shorter, AL**		**Jay, FL**		
2003/2004	**2004/2005**	**2005/2006**	**2003/2004**	**2004/2005**	**2005/2006**	**2004/2005**	**2005/2006**
Seeding dates							
25-Sep	27-Sep	25-Sep	09-Oct	08-Oct	12-Oct	29-Oct	04-Nov
09-Oct	11-Oct	11-Oct	20-Oct	21-Oct	25-Oct	10-Nov	17-Nov
22-Oct	26-Oct	24-Oct	10-Nov	10-Nov	07-Nov	29-Nov	02-Dec
04-Nov	08-Nov	07-Nov	21-Nov	03-Dec	22-Nov	13-Dec	12-Dec
18-Nov	18-Nov	18-Nov	08-Dec	16-Dec	07-Dec	20-Dec	22-Dec
Termination dates							
23-Feb	23-Feb	22-Feb	23-Feb	23-Feb	22-Feb	03-Feb	10-Feb
01-Mar	01-Mar	01-Mar	01-Mar	01-Mar	01-Mar	10-Feb	17-Feb
08-Mar	09-Mar	08-Mar	08-Mar	09-Mar	08-Mar	17-Feb	24-Feb
15-Mar	18-Mar	15-Mar	15-Mar	18-Mar	15-Mar	24-Feb	03-Mar

Table 1. Crimson clover seeding and termination dates.

The experiment for each location was a randomized complete block design ($r = 3$) with a split-block restriction on randomization. This design was chosen for practical reasons because it enabled us to handle seeding and termination operations for the cover crop efficiently. We assigned cover-crop-planting dates (5) to horizontal and termination dates (4) to vertical strips. For each location x-year combination, therefore, we had three different sizes of experimental units (Steel and Torrie, 1987). The largest experimental unit (TD) equals one-quarter of the block size, the second largest (PD) equals one-fifth of the block size, and the smallest (PD × TD combinations) equals 1/20 of the block size. This design also led to three different sources of experimental errors catering to each experimental unit. Depending on location, the smallest experimental unit (henceforth called plot) was 4 m wide and 8 m long containing four rows of corn and cotton with a 1-m row spacing.

Belle Mina, AL			**Shorter, AL**		**Jay, FL**		
2003/2004	**2004/2005**	**2005/2006**	**2003/2004**	**2004/2005**	**2005/2006**	**2004/2005**	**2005/2006**
Seeding dates							
25-Sep	27-Sep	25-Sep	09-Oct	08-Oct	12-Oct	29-Oct	04-Nov
09-Oct	11-Oct	11-Oct	20-Oct	21-Oct	25-Oct	10-Nov	17-Nov
22-Oct	26-Oct	24-Oct	10-Nov	10-Nov	07-Nov	29-Nov	02-Dec
04-Nov	08-Nov	07-Nov	21-Nov	03-Dec	22-Nov	13-Dec	12-Dec
18-Nov	18-Nov	18-Nov	08-Dec	16-Dec	07-Dec	20-Dec	22-Dec
Termination dates							
02-Apr	04-Apr	05-Apr	23-Mar	23-Mar	22-Mar	10-Mar	16-Mar
09-Apr	11-Apr	10-Apr	31-Mar	30-Mar	29-Mar	17-Mar	24-Mar
16-Apr	18-Apr	17-Apr	07-Apr	06-Apr	04-Apr	24-Mar	31-Mar
22-Apr	28-Apr	24-Apr	13-Apr	13-Apr	12-Apr	29-Mar	07-Apr

Table 2. Cereal rye seeding and termination dates.

Winter cover crops included crimson clover (*Trifolium incarnatum* L.) cv. AU Robin preceding corn and cereal rye (*Secale cereale* L.) cv. Elbon preceding cotton. Both the phases of rotation were present on adjacent areas within the same field tier. Crimson clover and cereal rye were established with a no-till drill at a seeding rate of 28 and 100 kg ha^{-1}, respectively, at the times described previously. In the spring, cover-crop biomass samples were collected immediately prior to termination by clipping all aboveground plant parts close to the soil surface from one randomly selected 0.25-m^2 section in each plot. Plant material was dried at 60°C for 72 h and weighed. Each plot was mechanically rolled/crimped at the timings described previously immediately prior to chemical termination, as described by Ashford and Reeves [28], to aid in cover-crop desiccation and the process leaves a uniform mat of residue on the soil surface. Clover was then sprayed with glyphosate (N-(phosphonomethyl) glycine) at 1.12 kg ae ha^{-1} plus 2,4-D amine (2,4-D-dimethylammonium) at 0.20 kg ai ha^{-1}, while rye was terminated with glyphosate alone, utilizing a compressed CO_2 backpack sprayer delivering 140 L ha^{-1} at 147 kPa.

Because the central Alabama and West Florida sites had a well-developed hardpan, the experimental areas were in-row subsoiled within the week prior to corn and cotton planting with a narrow-shank parabolic subsoiler equipped with pneumatic tires to close the subsoil channel (KMC, Tifton GA, USA). Corn hybrid cv. Dekalb 69-72RR and cotton cultivars DP 444 BG/RR, ST 5242 BR and DP555BRR were planted at Shorter, Belle Mina, and Jay Florida, respectively. Each cash crop was planted 1 week after the final termination date for winter cover crops at each location with a four-row planter equipped with row cleaners and double-disk openers (Great Plains Mfg., Inc. Salina, KS, USA).

At the corn eight-leaf or cotton four-leaf growth stage, all aboveground biomass for all weeds were harvested from two between the row randomly selected 0.25-m^2 sections per plot and treated in a similar manner as to cover-crop samples described above. Immediately after weed sampling, glyphosate was applied at 1.12 kg ae ha^{-1}. Plots were then kept weed-free until harvest utilizing Alabama CES-recommended herbicide applications. For the determination of corn grain yield, the two center rows of each plot were harvested with a plot combine, dried to constant moisture (150 g H_2O kg^{-1}), and weighed. Seed cotton yield was determined by machine harvesting the middle two rows of each plot with a spindle picker.

Data were analyzed separately for each location using generalized linear-mixed models methodology as implemented in SAS® PROC GLIMMIX. Year, planting date and termination date, and all their interactions were considered fixed effects. Interaction of reps with planting date and termination date was considered random effects. Interaction effects were considered to be important whenever the calculated P-value was less than 0.10. Treatment differences were calculated by Dunnett's single degree-of-freedom contrasts.

3. Results and discussion

3.1. Crimson clover cover-crop biomass

Climatic conditions encountered at the three locations resulted in large differences in biomass production. The maximum biomass production (5447 kg ha^{-1}) was observed at Shorter, AL, when crimson clover was seeded 4 weeks prior to the average first 0°C temperature and terminated 1 week prior to planting the corn cash crop (data not shown). The least biomass production (24 kg ha^{-1}) was observed at Belle Mina, AL, when the clover was seeded at the last establishment date (4 weeks post 0°C temperature) and terminated 1 week prior to corn planting (data not shown).

The most general model for this type of study is a classification model that treats seeding and termination dates as categorical variables resulting in a 5 by 4 factorial arrangement. The three-way interaction was significant ($P = 0.051$) only for the Bella Mina location (data not shown). The two-way interactions termination date by year was significant for the northern and southernmost locations only ($P \leq 0.001$), whereas seeding date interacted significantly with years for all three locations ($P < 0.0001$). The seeding by termination date interaction was significant only for Belle Mina and Jay ($P < 0.026$). Main effects for seeding and termination dates were significant at all locations except for termination date at Shorter.

Cover crop seeding date	**Growing season**		
	2003–2004	**2004–2005**	**2005–2006**
	Clover biomass (kg ha^{-1})		
	Belle Mina, AL		
−4 weeks	2861	1928	1904
−2 weeks	1435	2336	1753
Median date	604	945	757
+2 weeks	304	263	381
+4 weeks	76	121	85
SE	172		
Dunnett's *P* versus median-seeding date			
−4 weeks	<0.0001	<0.0001	<0.0001
−2 weeks	<0.0001	<0.0001	<0.0001
+2 weeks	<0.0001	0.009	0.265
+4 weeks	<0.0001	0.001	0.010
	Shorter, AL		
−4 weeks	1808	4750	4511
−2 weeks	2135	3827	3935
Median date	1223	1061	1958
+2 weeks	1321	359	805
+4 weeks	914	414	425
SE	332		
Dunnett's *P* versus median-seeding date			
−4 weeks	0.462	<0.0001	<0.0001
−2 weeks	0.117	<0.0001	<0.0001
+2 weeks	0.998	0.302	0.030
+4 weeks	0.884	0.373	0.002
	Jay, FL		
−4 weeks	NA	601	2123
−2 weeks	NA	468	979
Median date	NA	230	465

Cover crop seeding date	Growing season		
	2003–2004	2004–2005	2005–2006
	Clover biomass (kg ha^{-1})		
	Belle Mina, AL		
+2 weeks	NA	103	205
+4 weeks	NA	90	132
SE	86		
Dunnett's *P* versus median-seeding date			
−4 weeks	NA	0.011	<0.0001
−2 weeks	NA	0.164	<0.0001
+2 weeks	NA	0.683	0.113
+4 weeks	NA	0.605	0.026

Table 3. Clover biomass (kg ha^{-1}) by location and year as influenced by cover-crop seeding date, which were based on the 30-year average day of first frost at each location. Further seeding dates were either 2 or 4 weeks prior (−) or later (+) than that date. Data are averaged over termination dates.

Crimson clover dry biomass yield was significantly reduced by the delay in seeding date at all locations and years (**Table 3**).

In 2003–2004 at Belle Mina, crimson clover planted 4 and 2 weeks prior to the average 0°C date yielded 2257 and 831 kg ha^{-1} higher, respectively, than plots planted on the average 0°C date (604 kg ha^{-1}), and 2785 and 1359 kg ha^{-1} higher, respectively, than the latest planting date. Similar trends were observed in 2004–2005 and 2005–2006 except for one comparison. Belle Mina is the coldest of the three experiment locations with an average temperature of 10, 5.5, and 3.8°C during November, December, and January, respectively. These observations indicate that it is very important to plant a legume cover crop such as crimson clover early enough to get sufficient growth before cooler temperatures reduce growing degree days. Less than 400 kg ha^{-1} of biomass was produced when crimson clover was seeded 2 weeks after the average 0°C temperature at Belle Mina in any year. At Belle Mina in 2003–2004 and 2005–2006, clover biomass was maximized by waiting until 1 week prior to planting to terminate the cover crop gaining an additional 521 and 195 kg ha^{-1}, respectively, compared to terminating at the CES recommended 2 weeks prior to planting.

At Shorter, the variability in crimson clover biomass production among the years was very pronounced; biomass production was less in 2003 compared to 2004 and 2005. Significant reduction in crimson clover biomass production was observed with an advanced seeding date only in 2004 and 2005, as indicated by contrasts. If the seeding of crimson clover was delayed by 4 weeks compared to the earliest date, 3689 and 2553 kg ha^{-1} less biomass were produced in 2004 and 2005, respectively. No significant differences in crimson clover biomass production were, however, observed with early or delayed termination in 2004 and 2005 (**Table 4**).

Cover crop seeding date	Growing season		
	2003–2004	2004–2005	2005–2006
	Clover biomass (kg ha^{-1})		
	Belle Mina, AL		
−1 week prior	1637	1015	1323
−2 week prior	1116	1364	1131
−3 week prior	832	1119	833
−4 week prior	639	977	617
SE	144		
Dunnett's *P* versus first termination date			
−1 week prior	<0.0001	0.991	<0.0001
−2 week prior	0.022	0.059	0.007
−3 week prior	0.550	0.729	0.431
	Shorter, AL		
−1 week prior	1860	2348	2827
−2 week prior	1315	2005	2385
−3 week prior	1691	1813	2389
−4 week prior	1054	2162	1706
SE	335		
Dunnett's *P* versus first termination date			
−1 week prior	0.187	0.956	0.039
−2 week prior	0.891	0.972	0.310
−3 week prior	0.360	0.781	0.306
	Jay, FL		
−1 week prior	NA	474	1144
−2 week prior	NA	217	945
−3 week prior	NA	201	588
−4 week prior	NA	300	446
SE	77		
Dunnett's *P* versus first termination date			
−1 week prior	NA	0.264	<0.0001
−2 week prior	NA	0.787	<0.0001
−3 week prior	NA	0.687	0.426

Table 4. Clover biomass (kg ha^{-1}) by location and year as influenced by cover-crop termination date, which were 4, 3, 2, and 1 week prior to corn planting. Termination dates were based on a 30-year average soil temperature. Data are averaged over seeding dates.

Dry biomass accumulation was maximized if crimson clover was allowed to grow until 1 week prior to corn planting compared in 2006.

At the southernmost location Jay, except the three-way interaction, all other main and interaction effects were significant for crimson clover biomass production. Significant differences among years were observed, with biomass production less in 2004–2005 compared to 2005–2006. In 2004–2005 and 2005–2006, the earliest planting date resulted in 601 and 2123, respectively. With every 2-week delay in seeding, the cover-crop biomass production was reduced by more than half in almost all comparisons (**Table 3**). Significantly high biomass was accumulated when crimson clover was terminated only a week or 2 prior to the corn planting in 2005–2006 compared with the earliest termination date (**Table 4**).

3.2. Weed biomass in corn

The three-way interaction (year by PD by KD) was not significant for any location. The interaction of termination date with year was significant for both Belle Mina and Shorter locations ($P \leq 0.04$). Interactions of seeding date with year as well as with termination date were not significant ($P \geq 0.11$). Years did not have a significant effect at any of the locations ($P \geq 0.12$). The effect of termination date ($P \leq 0.05$) and seeding date ($P = 0.09$) was significant at Belle Mina and Shorter only.

At Belle Mina, weed biomass was only 81 kg ha^{-1} in 2003/2004 growing season corresponding to crimson clover biomass of 2861 kg ha^{-1} when the cover crop was seeded 4 weeks prior to the average 0°C temperature (data not shown). Weed biomass increased with delay in cover-crop seeding date indicating that a greater amount of crimson clover residue produced by earlier seeding dates suppressed early-season weed biomass production in corn. However, contrasts indicate no significant reduction in weed biomass if crimson clover was planted 4 or 2 weeks after the average 0°C temperature. In the 2004–2005 growing season, weed biomass production was significantly reduced by seeding crimson clover 4 and 2 weeks prior to the average 0°C temperature; again, the higher biomass production resulted in less weed biomass. No significant differences in weed biomass production were observed if crimson clover was seeded on the average 0°C temperature or thereafter. In 2005/2006, seeding dates had no significant effect on weed biomass production. No significant effect of delayed termination on weed biomass production was observed in 2003–2004 and 2004/2005 growing seasons compared to the first termination date (4 weeks prior to average 0°C temperature). However, in 2005/2006 growing season, a significant reduction in weed biomass was observed with only a week's delay in crimson clover termination. This could be attributed to the increase in crimson clover biomass production with delayed termination, which in turn resulted in early season weed suppression.

At Shorter location, no significant increase or decrease in weed biomass production was observed with seeding of crimson clover earlier or later than the average 0°C temperature date. However, weed biomass production in general increased with delay in crimson clover seeding date; in 2003/2004 and 2005/2006 growing seasons, weed biomass ranged from 16 to 28 kg ha^{-1} for the first two crimson clover seeding dates, whereas the final seeding date plots averaged nearly 109 kg ha^{-1} weed biomass during both the growing seasons. The effect of termination dates was pronounced only in 2005/2006; significantly less weed biomass was produced if the termination was delayed by even a week (data not shown).

At Jay location, our southernmost location, no definite trend in weed biomass production was observed with earlier seeding or termination of the crimson clover (data not shown). This could be due to rapid decomposition of residue due to warmer temperatures and higher rainfall at this location compared to the northern locations.

3.3. Corn grain yield

Corn grain yield was not affected by crimson clover seeding and termination dates at Belle Mina. Though no statistically significant differences were observed, plots with the earliest seeding of the crimson clover yielded numerically highest at this location. At both Shorter and Belle Mina, significant differences in corn grain yield were observed across years (**Tables 5** and **6**).

Cover crop seeding date	**Growing season**		
	2003–2004	**2004–2005**	**2005–2006**
	Corn grain yield (kg ha^{-1})		
	Belle Mina, AL		
−4 weeks	10,471	9262	4646
−2 weeks	9474	8712	4686
Median date	9963	8684	5228
+2 weeks	10,054	8434	4607
+4 weeks	9344	8414	4831
SE	370		
Dunnett's *P* versus median-seeding date			
−4 weeks	0.501	0.386	0.380
−2 weeks	0.534	1.000	0.445
+2 weeks	0.998	0.919	0.324
+4 weeks	0.326	0.897	0.702
	Shorter, AL		
−4 weeks	11,986	7631	5703
−2 weeks	11,701	7701	5709
Median date	12,429	7333	5629
+2 weeks	11,325	7363	5840

Cover crop seeding date	Growing season		
	2003–2004	2004–2005	2005–2006
	Corn grain yield (kg ha^{-1})		
	Belle Mina, AL		
+4 weeks	11,533	7864	5296
SE	379		
Dunnett's *P* versus median-seeding date			
−4 weeks	0.592	0.847	0.999
−2 weeks	0.175	0.731	0.999
+2 weeks	0.015	1.000	0.949
+4 weeks	0.065	0.431	0.792
	Jay, FL		
−4 weeks	NA	5582	13520
−2 weeks	NA	6259	14328
Median date	NA	5236	12982
+2 weeks	NA	6318	12083
+4 weeks	NA	6432	12694
SE	945		
Dunnett's *P* versus median-seeding date			
−4 weeks	NA	0.972	0.878
−2 weeks	NA	0.446	0.216
+2 weeks	NA	0.397	0.560
+4 weeks	NA	0.310	0.986

Table 5. Corn grain yield (kg ha^{-1}) by location and year as influenced by cover-crop seeding date, which were based on the 30-year average day of first frost at each location. Further seeding dates were either 2 or 4 week prior (−) or later (+) than that date. Data are averaged over termination dates.

Grain yield decreased with the progression of the experiment. Weather conditions were different among the years, 2004 being a normal rainfall year whereas in 2005 majority of the rainfall was received in July at Belle Mina (6 in.) and Shorter (8.5 in.); 2006 was a drought year at both the locations throughout the summer. These differences in rainfall events can likely explain some of the yield differences observed among years at both the locations. Corn is most sensitive to water stress during silking or flowering, and pollination stages of growth and drought stress during this period can result in poor grain development and yield losses.

Cover crop seeding date	Growing season		
	2003–2004	2004–2005	2005–2006
	Corn grain yield (kg ha^{-1})		
	Belle Mina, AL		
−1 week prior	9880	8389	4946
−2 week prior	9707	8392	5201
−3 week prior	10,117	9196	4842
−4 week prior	9741	8827	4209
SE	425		
Dunnett's *P* versus first termination date			
−1 week prior	0.988	0.745	0.370
−2 week prior	1.000	0.748	0.155
−3 week prior	0.818	0.827	0.491
	Shorter, AL		
−1 week prior	10,916	7579	4382
−2 week prior	12,094	7424	5949
−3 week prior	12,453	8225	6933
−4 week prior	11,717	7085	5278
SE	500		
Dunnett's *P* versus first termination date			
−1 week prior	0.482	0.797	0.392
−2 week prior	0.895	0.920	0.616
−3 week prior	0.547	0.209	0.037
	Jay, FL		
−1 week prior	NA	5615	12,565
−2 week prior	NA	5867	12,872
−3 week prior	NA	6225	13,468
−4 week prior	NA	6155	13,581
SE	784		
Dunnett's *P* versus first termination date			
−1 week prior	NA	0.926	0.673
−2 week prior	NA	0.987	0.853
−3 week prior	NA	1.000	0.999

Table 6. Corn grain yield (kg ha^{-1}) by location and year as influenced by cover-crop termination date, which were 4, 3, 2, and 1 week prior to corn planting. Termination dates were based on 30-year average soil temperature. Data are averaged over seeding dates.

3.4. Cereal rye cover-crop biomass

When analyzed by location, the three-way interaction was not significant at Belle Mina. The interaction of experiment years with seeding date was significant. The main effect of seeding date, termination date, and year was also significant. In general, rye biomass production declined with every 2-week delay in seeding the cover crop (**Table 7**).

Cover crop seeding date	Growing season		
	2003–2004	2004–2005	2005–2006
	Rye biomass (kg ha^{-1})		
	Belle Mina, AL		
−4 weeks	8878	5062	6396
−2 weeks	7852	5232	4078
Median date	6584	2863	2479
+2 weeks	4500	2149	3085
+4 weeks	2649	913	2066
SE	611		
Dunnett's *P* versus median-seeding date			
−4 weeks	0.004	0.006	<0.0001
−2 weeks	0.200	0.003	0.070
+2 weeks	0.010	0.701	0.788
+4 weeks	<0.0001	0.018	0.933
	Shorter, AL		
−4 weeks	5566	5331	6177
−2 weeks	5053	4893	6269
Median date	4344	2610	5372
+2 weeks	2779	518	2553
+4 weeks	1276	213	1370
SE	356		
Dunnett's *P* versus median-seeding date			
−4 weeks	0.020	<0.0001	0.198
−2 weeks	0.298	<0.0001	0.128
+2 weeks	0.002	<0.0001	<0.0001
+4 weeks	<0.0001	<0.0001	<0.0001
	Jay, FL		
−4 weeks	NA	3605	5006

Cover crop seeding date	Growing season		
	2003–2004	2004–2005	2005–2006
	Rye biomass (kg ha^{-1})		
	Belle Mina, AL		
−2 weeks	NA	2982	5341
Median date	NA	2559	4695
+2 weeks	NA	1687	3349
+4 weeks	NA	1545	2706
SE	253		
Dunnett's *P* versus median-seeding date			
−4 weeks	NA	0.005	0.727
−2 weeks	NA	0.480	0.142
+2 weeks	NA	0.026	<0.0001
+4 weeks	NA	0.007	<0.0001

Table 7. Rye biomass (kg ha^{-1}) by location and year as influenced by cover-crop seeding date, which were based on the 30-year average day of first frost at each location. Further seeding dates were either 2 or 4 week prior (−) or later (+) than that date. Data are averaged over termination dates.

Delaying cereal rye planting 4 weeks significantly lowered the rye biomass yield in all the years. Biomass production was in general less at this location in 2003/2004 and 2004/2005 growing seasons. Earlier termination of rye also significantly reduced biomass. Biomass production in all the years was increased if rye was terminated a week or 2 prior to cotton planting (**Table 7**). However, no significant differences in biomass production were observed if rye was terminated 3 or 4 weeks prior to cotton planting.

At Shorter location, all the interactions and main effects were significant for rye biomass production. Delayed seeding of rye significantly reduced dry biomass accumulation (**Table 7**). In 2004–2005, no significant differences in rye dry biomass accumulation occurred if rye was seeded on the third seeding date or later. Significant planting and termination date interaction were also observed at this location. The maximum biomass production was 8523 kg ha^{-1} in year 2006 when rye was planted 2 weeks before the 0°C temperature date and terminated a week prior to cash crop planting. The least biomass produced at Shorter was 140 kg ha^{-1} when covers were planted on the last planting date and terminated on the first planting date (data not shown).

At our southernmost location Jay, all two-way interactions and main effects were significant. Rye biomass production was better in year 2006 compared to year 2005. As observed at other two locations, delayed seeding or earlier termination reduced dry biomass accumulation by rye (data not shown). The maximum observed rye biomass at this location was 7468 kg ha^{-1} produced when rye was planted 4 weeks prior to the average 0°C temperature and terminated 2 weeks before the seeding of cotton.

3.5. Weed biomass in cotton

Dry weights of weeds were more in cotton compared to corn at all site years due to the earlier sampling time in corn when fewer summer annual weeds had emerged. The cover-crop biomass observed at each location was reflected in the subsequent results observed for weed control. The three-way interaction was not significant at any of the locations. The interaction of year with seeding and termination date was significant at all the locations except at Jay. The seeding by termination date interaction was not significant at any location.

In general, there was an increase in weed biomass in cotton with earlier termination and late planting of the rye cover crop. At Belle Mina, numerically less weed dry biomass was observed corresponding to a high rye cover-crop residue (**Table 8**).

Cover crop seeding date	**Growing season**		
	2003–2004	**2004–2005**	**2005–2006**
	Belle Mina, AL		
−4 weeks	31	133	214
−2 weeks	54	182	455
Median date	406	275	945
+2 weeks	250	297	368
+4 weeks	345	478	664
SE	102		
Dunnett's *P* versus median-seeding date			
−4 weeks	0.010	0.601	<0.0001
−2 weeks	0.017	0.865	<0.0001
+2 weeks	0.519	0.999	<0.0001
+4 weeks	0.965	0.283	0.077
	Shorter, AL		
−4 weeks	316	289	62
−2 weeks	318	381	53
Median date	470	440	58
+2 weeks	474	467	81
+4 weeks	970	378	88
SE	101		
Dunnett's *P* versus median-seeding date			
−4 weeks	0.425	0.438	1.000
−2 weeks	0.437	0.953	1.000
+2 weeks	1.000	0.997	0.998

Cover crop seeding date	Growing season		
	2003–2004	2004–2005	2005–2006
	Belle Mina, AL		
+4 weeks	<0.0001	0.944	0.996
	Jay, FL		
−4 weeks	NA	48	53
−2 weeks	NA	50	48
Median date	NA	80	88
+2 weeks	NA	53	85
+4 weeks	NA	87	65
SE	14		
Dunnett's *P* versus median-seeding date			
−4 weeks	NA	0.338	0.259
−2 weeks	NA	0.390	0.160
+2 weeks	NA	0.495	1.000
+4 weeks	NA	0.993	0.626

Table 8. Weed dry biomass (kg ha^{-1}) in cotton by location and year as influenced by cover-crop seeding date, which were based on the 30-year average day of first frost at each location. Further seeding dates were either 2 or 4 week prior (−) or later (+) than that date. Data are averaged over termination dates.

Weed biomass averaged only 31 kg ha^{-1} corresponding to rye biomass of 8878 kg ha^{-1} in plots seeded with rye 4 weeks before the average 0°C temperature in 2003. No significant differences in weed biomass production were observed in 2004 among different seeding dates. In 2005, weed biomass was maximum in plots seeded with rye on the median seeding date averaging 945 kg ha^{-1} and less in the later-seeded plots. This is likely due to less rye biomass (2479 kg ha $^{-1}$) production in these plots. No significant differences in the weed biomass production were observed among the termination dates in 2003 and 2004 (data not shown). In 2005, however, the plots terminated on the final termination date had the least weed biomass.

At Shorter, no significant differences in weed biomass production were observed among seeding dates in 2004 and 2005 (**Table 8**). The maximum observed weed biomass was 970 kg ha^{-1} corresponding to rye biomass of 1276 kg ha^{-1} in 2005, when rye was seeded 4 weeks after 0°C freeze. The effect of termination dates on weed biomass production was significant in 2003; weed biomass decreased with delay in rye cover-crop termination date (**Table 9**).

At Jay location, weed biomass production was less compared to other two locations. No differences in weed biomass production were observed among seeding dates at this location (**Table 8**). The delay in rye termination decreased weed biomass production. In 2004, however, plots terminated a week before cotton planting had more weed biomass than plots terminated 2 and 3 weeks prior to cotton planting (**Table 9**).

Cover crop seeding date	Growing season		
	2003–2004	2004–2005	2005–2006
	Belle Mina, AL		
−1 week prior	287	201	272
−2 week prior	153	150	424
−3 week prior	165	397	755
−4 week prior	265	345	665
SE	116		
Dunnett's *P* versus first termination date			
−1 week prior	0.998	0.678	0.035
−2 week prior	0.815	0.456	0.288
−3 week prior	0.858	0.975	0.890
	Shorter, AL		
−1 week prior	104	141	17
−2 week prior	341	389	74
−3 week prior	532	430	64
−4 week prior	1061	603	118
SE	24		
Dunnett's *P* versus first termination date			
−1 week prior	<0.0001	0.001	0.771
−2 week prior	<0.0001	0.228	0.973
−3 week prior	<0.0001	0.392	0.952
	Jay, FL		
−1 week prior	NA	64	20
−2 week prior	NA	51	51
−3 week prior	NA	48	83
−4 week prior	NA	91	118
SE	77		
Dunnett's *P* versus first termination date			
−1 week prior	NA	0.322	<0.0001
−2 week prior	NA	0.070	0.001
−3 week prior	NA	0.052	0.125

Table 9. Weed dry biomass (kg ha^{-1}) in cotton by location and year as influenced by cover-crop termination date, which were 4, 3, 2, and 1 week prior to cotton planting. Termination dates were based on 30-year average soil temperature. Data are averaged over seeding dates.

The decrease in dry weed biomass with corresponding increase in rye biomass is in accordance with the previous studies. Teasdale [29] concluded that weed biomass production is correlated with the cover-crop biomass. Smeda and Weller [30] also reported an increase in residual weed suppression by no-till-rye residues when the time between cover-crop desiccation and crop planting was reduced, probably due to allelopathic effects.

3.6. Cotton seed lint yield

There were differences in cotton seed lint yield among the years likely due to weather conditions but cotton lint yield was not affected by the rye cover-crop seeding and termination dates at any site year (data not shown). Cotton seed lint yield averaged 3784 kg ha^{-1} in 2003, 4269 kg ha^{-1} in 2004 to 2252 kg ha^{-1} in 2005 at Belle Mina. At Shorter, the maximum seed cotton lint yield was obtained in the year 2004 averaging 4065 kg ha^{-1}. At Jay, yield was less in 2005 but was comparable to other two locations in 2005. Thus, cover-crop biomass did not interfere with attaining yields, and it reflects current knowledge on residue management at planting.

4. Conclusions

In this study, early planting of the cover crop with its later termination for subsequent corn and cotton plantings has increased cover-crop biomass accumulation compared to the late planting and early termination of the cover crop. Increased cover-crop biomass suppressed subsequent total weed dry biomass. These findings indicate that high-residue cover crops have predictable potential for suppressing early-season weeds in corn and cotton. If farmers are utilizing glyphosate-resistant corn-cotton rotation systems, these findings hold particular importance with current glyphosate-resistant weed-control issues. Because corn and cotton yields were not negatively impacted, we can conclude that high residue obtained by planting crimson clover or rye cover crops timely and terminating either a week or 2 prior to cash crop planting is feasible. Ideal management will result in maximum cover-crop biomass production and subsequent weed suppression.

Author details

Andrew J. Price[1*], Edzard van Santen[2] and Lina Sarunaite[3]

*Address all correspondence to: andrew.price@ars.usda.gov

1 United States Department of Agriculture, Agricultural Research Service, National Soil Dynamics Laboratory, Auburn, Alabama, United States

2 Auburn University, Auburn, Alabama, United States

3 Institute of Agriculture, Lithuanian Research Center for Agriculture and Forestry, Akademija, Lithuania

References

[1] Price AJ, Balkcom KS, Culpepper SA, Kelton JA, Nichols RL, and Schomberg H. Glyphosate-resistant Palmer amaranth: a threat to conservation tillage. J Soil Water Conserv. 2011; 66: 265–275. doi:10.2489/jswc.66.4.265

[2] Culpepper AS, York AC, Kichler J, and J Smith. University of Georgia programs for controlling Palmer amaranth in 2016 cotton, University of Georgia Cooperative Extension circular 952, Athens, GA [Internet]. Available from: http://extension.uga.edu/publications/files/pdf/C%20952_7.PDF

[3] Scott RC and Smith K. Prevention and control of glyphosate-resistant pigweed in Roundup Ready™ soybean and cotton. University of Arkansas Cooperative Extension Fact Sheet FSA2152 [Internet]. Available from: http://www.uaex.edu/publications/PDF/FSA-2152.pdf 2006. [Accessed: 2015-08-01]

[4] Edmisten KL, Yelverton FH, Spears JF, Bowman DT, Bachelor JS, Koenning SR, Crozier CR, Meijer AD, and Culpepper AS. 2010 cotton information. NCSU Cooperative Extension Publication [Internet]. Available from: http://ipm.ncsu.edu/cotton/insect-corner/PDF/Cotton2010.pdf 2010. [Accessed: 2015-01-08]

[5] Sosnoskie LM and Culpepper AS. Glyphosate-resistant Palmer amaranth (*Amaranthus palmeri*) increases herbicide use, tillage, and hand-weeding in Georgia cotton. Weed Sci. 2014; 62: 393–402. doi:10.1614/WS-D-13-00077.1

[6] [UA] University of Arkansas. Herbicide resistance: A growing issue in Arkansas. University of Arkansas Cooperative Extension Publication [Internet]. Available from: https://www.uaex.edu/farm-ranch/crops-commercial-horticulture/cotton/Herbicide%20Resistance.pdf 2006. [Accessed: 2015-01-09]

[7] Norsworthy JK, Ward SM, Shaw DR, Llewellyn RS, Nichols RL, Webster TM, Bradley KW, Frisvold G, Powles SB, Burgos NR, Witt WW, and Barrett M. Reducing the risks of herbicide resistance: best management practices and recommendations. Weed Sci. 2012; 60: 31–62. doi:10.1614/WS-D-11-00155.1

[8] Aulakh JS, Price AJ, and Balkcom KS. Weed management and cotton yield under two row spacings in conventional and conservation tillage systems utilizing conventional, glufosinate-, and glyphosate-based weed management systems. Weed Technol. 2011; 25: 542–547. doi:10.1614/WT-D-10-00124.1

[9] DeVore JD, Norsworthy JK, and Brye KR. Influence of deep tillage, a rye cover crop, and various soybean production systems on Palmer amaranth emergence in soybean. Weed Technol. 2013; 27: 263–270. doi:10.1614/WT-D-12-00125.1

[10] Mirsky SB, Curran WS, Mortensen DM, Ryan MR, and Shumway DL. Timing of cover crop management effects on seed suppression in no-till planted soybean using a roller-crimper. Weed Sci. 2011; 59:380–389. doi:10.1614/WT-D-12-00078.1

[11] Price AJ, Balkcom KS, Raper RL, Monks CD, Barentine RM, and Iversen KV. Controlling glyphosate-resistant pigweed in conservation tillage cotton systems. Special Publication 09. [Internet] http://www.ars.usda.gov/SP2UserFiles/Place/60100500/csr/SpecialPubs/SP09.pdf. 2011b. [Accessed 1/8/2015]

[12] Price AJ, Reeves DW, Patterson MG, Gamble BE, Balkcom KS, Arriaga FJ, and Monks CD. Weed control in peanut in a high residue conservation-tillage system. Peanut Sci. 2007; 34: 59–64. doi:10.5772/61650

[13] Price AJ, Reeves DW, and Patterson MG. Evaluation of weed control provided by three winter cereals in conservation-tillage soybean. Renew Agr Food Syst. 2006; 21: 159–164. doi:10.1079/RAF2005135

[14] Reeves DW, Price AJ, and Patterson MG. Evaluation of three winter cereals for weed control in conservation-tillage non-transgenic cotton. Weed Technol. 2005; 19: 731–736. doi:10.1614/WT-04-245R1.1

[15] Ryan MR, Curran WS, Grantham AM, Hunsberger LK, Mirsky SB, Mortensen DA, Nord EA, and Wilson DO. Effects of seeding rate and poultry litter on weed suppression from a rolled cereal rye cover crop. Weed Sci. 2011; 59: 438–444. doi:10.1614/WS-D-10-00180.1

[16] Smith AN, Reberg-Horton SC, Place GT, Meijer AD, Arellano C, and Mueller JP. Rolled rye mulch for weed suppression in organic no-tillage soybeans. Weed Sci. 2011; 59: 224–231. doi:10.1614/WS-D-10-00112.1

[17] Teasdale JR. Contribution of cover crops to weed management in sustainable agricultural systems. J Prod Agric. 2013; 9: 475–479. doi:10.2134/jpa1996.0475

[18] Wiggins MS, McClure MA, Hayes RM, and Steckel LE. Integrating cover crops and POST herbicides for glyphosate-resistant Palmer amaranth (*Amaranthus palmeri*) control in corn. Weed Technol. 2015; 29: 412–418. doi:10.1614/WT-D-14-00145.1

[19] Norsworthy JK, McClelland M, Griffith G, Bangarwa SK, and Still J. Evaluation of cereal and Brassica cover crops in conservation-tillage, enhanced glyphosate-resistant cotton. Weed Technol. 2011; 26: 490–498. doi:10.1614/WT-D-10-00040.1

[20] Vasilakoglou I, Dhima I, Eleftherohorinos E, and Lithourgidis A. Winter cereal cover crop mulches and inter-row cultivation effects on cotton development and grass suppression. Agron J. 2006; 98: 1290–1297. doi:10.2134/agronj2006.0002

[21] Yenish JP, Worsham AD, and York AC. Cover crops for herbicide replacement in no-tillage corn (*Zea mays*). Weed Technol. 1996; 10: 815–821.

[22] Teasdale JR and Mohler CR. The quantitative relationship between weed emergence and the physical properties of mulches. Weed Sci. 2000; 48: 385–392. doi: 10.1614/0043-1745(2000)048[0385:TQRBWE]2.0.CO;2

[23] Jost P, Brown S, Culpepper S, Harris G, Kemerait B, Roberts P, Shurley D, and Williams J. Conservation tillage. In P. Jost, ed. 2004 Georgia Cotton Production Guide. University of Georgia Cooperative Extension Service, Athens, GA. 2004.

[24] McCarty WH, Blaine A, and Byrd JD. Cotton no-till production. Mississippi State University Cooperative Extension Service Publication P1695. 2003.

[25] Bauer PJ and Reeves DW. A comparison of winter cereal species and planting dates as residue cover for cotton growth with conservation tillage. Crop Sci. 1999; 39: 1824–1830. doi: 10.2135/cropsci1999.3961824x

[26] Collins G, Whitaker J, Culpepper S, Harris G, Kemerait B, Perry C, Roberts P, Shurley, D, Smith A, and Porter W. 2015 Georgia cotton production guide, University of Georgia Cooperative Extension publication CSS-15-01, Athens, GA [Internet]. Available from: http://www.ugacotton.com/vault/file/2015-UGA-Cotton-Production-Guide.pdf.2015. [Accessed: 2015-01-09]

[27] Reeves DW. Cover crops and rotations. *In* J. L. Hatfield and B. A. Stewart, eds. Advances in Soil Science: Crops Residue Management. Lewis Publishers, CRC Press Inc., Boca Raton, FL, pp. 125–172 . 1994.

[28] Ashford DL and Reeves DW. Use of a mechanical roller-crimper as an alternative kill method for cover crops. Am J Altern Agric. 2003; 18: 37–45. doi:10.1079/AJAA200232

[29] Teasdale JR. Contribution of cover crops to weed management in sustainable agricultural systems. J Prod Agric. 1996; 9: 475–479. doi:10.2134/jpa1996.0475

[30] Smeda RJ and Weller SC. Potential of rye (*Secale cereal*) for weed management in transplant tomatoes (*Lycopersicon esculentum*). Weed Sci. 1996; 44: 596–602.

Section 3

Cotton Genetics, Breeding and Biotechnology

Chapter 7

Molecular Breeding of Cotton

Yuksel Bolek, Khezir Hayat, Adem Bardak and Muhammad Tehseen Azhar

Additional information is available at the end of the chapter

http://dx.doi.org/10.5772/64593

Abstract

Molecular characterization provides comprehensive information about the extent of genetic diversity, it assists for the development of an effective, highly accurate, and rapid marker-assisted cotton breeding program. Due to one of the world's leading fiber crops, molecular studies of cotton are being explored widely by cotton researchers. Cotton provides raw material to the textile industry among other products. Limitations in conventional breeding program for genetic improvement are due to the complexity and limited knowledge on economically important traits. The use of molecular markers for the detection and exploitation of DNA polymorphism is one of the most significant developments in molecular genetics. In the present scenerio, cotton molecular breeding has become a reliable source through the study and exploitation of its genetic diversity and due to better understanding of the cotton genomes using the next-generation sequencing technologies. Cotton breeders should utilize genomics in breeding programs for effective selection of best parents for agronomic and fiber-related traits, as well as for the development of resistance against biotic and abiotic stresses. The genomic research work could be based upon genotyping using DNA markers, quantitative trait loci mapping, genome-wide associations, and next-generation sequencing. The objective of this chapter is to describe evolution as well as utilization of various molecular markers and review the contribution of marker-assisted selection (MAS) in cotton breeding.

Keywords: cotton, DNA markers, genotyping by sequencing (GBS), genome-wide association studies (GWAS), marker-assisted selection (MAS)

1. Introduction

Plant breeders select those plants, which looks phenotypically more promising due to the presence of desirable traits. Most of the traits are controlled by polygenes with complex nonallelic quantitative effects and environmental interactions. In most cases, despite the fact that biometrical genetics reveals the presence of additive or non-additive effects on loci involved in the inheritance of quantitative trait, a specific locus may not be detected [1]. Tightly linked loci with desired trait can support plant breeding program by rapid introgression of quantitative trait loci (QTL) using associated molecular markers [2]. Genomic region having genes of interest for a particular trait is designated as QTL (Quantitative Trait Loc). QTL analysis involves partioning of genetic variation in single component. So, DNA-based molecular markers provide a tool to plant breeders for the selection of desirable plants based on genotype instead of phenotype.

The expression of gene(s) individually their interaction with the climatic factors and agronomic measures can determine the cultivar adaptability [3]. Selection of new plant varieties with the desirable traits under given environmental conditions and cultural practices is the fundamental basis of plant breeding [4], genetic variability produced in germplasm as a result of selection, which alter the inheritance pattern of the traits, is quite useful to screen and select the cultivars for required traits. New cultivars have been developed by exploiting genotypes with enormous variation [5]. Rapid changes are needed in agricultural production, and biologically diverse as well as low-input novel farming systems must be developed and employed. There is also a need for new crop varieties that are (1) fitting-in to global climate change in the present era, (2) adapted to biodiverse farming systems, and finally (3) giving more products to farmers and eventually to consumers.

Cotton (*Gossypium* spp.) is one of the most intensively cultivated species grown in more than 80 countries in varying climatic conditions [6]. Globally, cotton is the ultimate source of fiber for industry and provides oil to diet [7]. Being utmost fiber manufacturing crop and the third contributor to oilseed production; China, India and USA are top contributors for fiber [8]. *Gossypium* genus is divided into eight genomes (A-G and K) and comprised of 45 diploids and five allotetraploid species which are found in the arid and semiarid regions of Africa, Central and South America, Galapagos, Indian subcontinent, Australia, Arabia, and Hawaii [9–11].

At the beginning of the 20th century, scientists discovered that Mendelian factors controlling inheritance are organized in linear order on chromosomes. It was shown that genes could be inherited individually or in combination with other genes. The individual fragments flanking within a defined interval are known as molecular DNA markers [12]. Precise DNA portion with a known position on the chromosome [13], or a measurable trait that is associated with variation in DNA sequence [14, 15] or a difference may act as a genetic marker if it identifies characteristics of an individual.

Markers are broadly divided into three classes: (1) morphological markers, which themselves have phenotypic traits meaning the morphological and physiological features of plants are used to understand the genetic variation. Although morphological features may be indicative of the phenotype, they are also highly affected by environmental factors and growth practices; (2) biochemical markers, including isozymes, which involve allelic variants of proteins/ enzymes; (3) molecular markers, manifest mutations in heredity material such as DNAs and RNAs [16–19].

Polymorphism of molecular markers shows differentiation of homozygotes and heterozygotes [20]. Thottappilly et al. [21] refer to molecular markers as naturally occurring polymorphism, which include the proteins and nucleic acids that indicate certain differences. The use of molecular markers in plant breeding is called marker-assisted selection, often referred as MAS or marker-assisted breeding (MAB) (**Figure 1**) [4, 22].

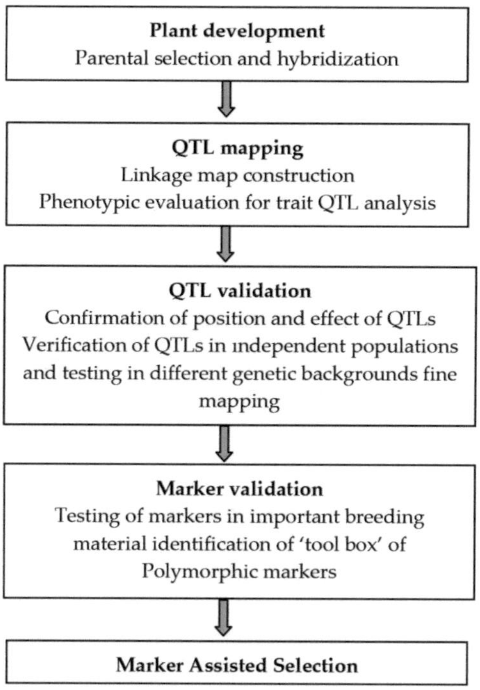

Figure 1. Marker-assisted scheme [4].

In traditional plant breeding, traits are selected depending on the phenotype, which is highly affected by the climatic factors. This approach makes the breeding a slow, expensive, and challenging process [23–25]. Practical advantages of using genetic markers, potential values of linkage maps, and exploiting for direct selection in plant breeding were begun to be studied about the 1930s [26]. Molecular markers are essential for mapping the genes of interest, MAS/ MAB, and cloning of genes using mapping-based cloning strategies [27]. In addition, the use of molecular markers includes gene introgression through backcrossing, germplasm characterization, and phylogenetic analysis [28]. It has been observed that MAS is more efficient than conventional breeding techniques [4, 29, 30]. Selection based on genotypic structure through employment of molecular markers in the field crops [31] has laid the foundation of MAS [32,

33]. Many biological and medical science applications and studies, including genetic diversity, molecular tagging of economic traits, and procurement of heritable diseases have successfully utilized molecular markers [2, 34–37]. Thus far, molecular markers have been exploited in rice [38], wheat [39], maize [40, 41], and barley [42, 43]. However, MAS has achieved the desired goals in cotton with limited success due to a genetic bottleneck through historic domestication and limited polymorphism in cultivar germplasm [44–47].

About 145 morphological markers are reported in cotton so far, but they have low utility in variety development because of incapability to assemble diverse markers in a genotype [48]. Isozymes produced through allelic variants are considered more authentic but not widely used due to their differential expression in different growth stages. For improving productivity and other key quantitative traits, cotton genetic markers have more value than morphological or isozyme markers [48]. DNA markers have become handy and effective tools for plant breeders because their expression is not necessary for their detection [49]. In order to enhance the benefits through molecular markers, vast developments have been made in 'omics', which, in turn, allowed the use of these markers in diverse ways for genetic studies instead of using them solely for phylogenetic studies [50]. Obtaining pure DNA plays a major role for the development of molecular markers in cotton [51–53]; genetic analysis has many drawbacks due to the presence of phenolic compounds, which affect quality of DNA and protein during tissues grinding [51].

Polygenic traits are mostly affected by the climatic conditions and show discrete variability after hybridization. Recombination frequency allows investigators to differentiate genes on linkage map by relative distance between a generation and their parents. The main hindrance for QTL mapping of agronomic traits is related to a large number of genes involved in phenotypic expression and their interaction with the environment [54]. As number of genes affects the trait phenotypically, it is desired that more loci should be evaluated for QTL determination, and the screening of individuals should be done at multiple locations/environments to maximize the use of QTLs. MAB uses QTLs to pyramid favorable alleles and break linkage groups for tagging QTLs of interest [55–57]. In recent years, conventional plant breeders started to use MAS for the identification of traits with high heritability such as disease resistance, as well as the yield of major field crops [57]. However, yield-related components have low heritability, which is a major challenge for the utilization of MAS [56, 58]. MAS is being employed for the identification of transgressive segregants. Transgressive segregation is the production of plants in F_2 generation that are superior to both parents for one or more traits. Transgressive breeding aims at improving yield or contributing to yield-related traits through transgressive segregation [59–61]. Several QTLs have been identified for seed cotton yield, fiber quality, plant architecture, resistance to diseases such as bacterial blight and *Verticillium* wilt [57], resistance to pests like root knot nematode, and flowering date [62] as well as for abiotic stresses (drought, salt tolerance) [55, 63].

There is a gap between discovery of useful genes and QTLs, and their utilization in breeding programs. To date, few examples are reported [55, 63] for the successful release of genotypes developed by MAS, and they have shown significant contribution to yield improvement. High-throughput, high-density genome-profiling tools enable the rapid and low-cost of crop genome in a precise and high-resolution manner. Identification of molecular variants in DNA sequence opens opportunities for plant scientists [55]. The potential exists in plant breeding for efficient use of next-generation sequencing (NGS) that also has revolutionized the plant genomics [55]. Markers can be analyzed across the genomes simply and accurately, with high-throughput. Increased number of next generation sequencing allows conducting genome-wide association studies (GWAS) [63]. It is thanks to the developments in knowledge of useful genetic diversity and QTLs, advances in sequencing, genotyping, and bioinformatics approaches that rapid, high-throughput molecular marker discovery methods have been enabled.

Day-by-day developments of new, specific markers, and trait determination tools makes molecular markers important in understanding the genomic variability and diversity within and among species. In this chapter, we discuss about the applications and types of molecular markers, next-generation sequencing, and role of molecular breeding in development of plants with improved economical traits in cotton.

2. Breeding for polygenic traits

Economically important traits such as nutritive value, earliness, agronomic traits, resistance etc. can be improved through MAS [64, 65]. Polygenic mapping allows breeders to estimate and assess the hereditary pattern of the traits governed by many genes found throughout genome; Ultimately it leads to efficient utilization of these traits for molecular breeding. Highly saturated genetic maps in a high population index permits to observe the impact of many regions of genomes on a single trait value. Paterson [66] revealed that sharing of homologues during crossing over is the basis of QTLs. The regions of the genomes connected to the traits of economic value are QTLs [67]. Association of a marker's genotypic value to a phenotype is the basis of QTL mapping. Recombination frequency is used to evaluate the relative distance among markers in the linkage map. It is assumed that markers at or lower recombination ratio of 50% are considered as unlinked found either on homologues or alternative loci while the markers which are tightly connected will be transferred to offspring more often than the unlinked markers [67].

Reinisch et al. [68] developed the pioneer genetic map of cotton during 1994. Although large number linkage maps have been constructed since then due to abundance of several DNA markers, it is still needed to determine reliable QTLs from breeding perspective. Yu et al. [69] screened genotypes by simple sequence repeats (SSRs) to map loci connected to fiber quality and lint yield in a backcross inbred line and developed a pioneer genetic map using BIL within allotetraploid cultivated cotton species. Map consisted of 392 highly cosegregated loci covering 2895 cM length and having mean interlocus distance 7.4 cM. As a whole, 39 QTLs were directly connected to yield components and 28 were associated to fiber quality.

Altaf et al. [70] explored F_2 population developed from three different species of *Gossypium* for identification of evolutionary relationship among these species by linkage map. Eleven linkage groups were constructed having 521.7 cM map size in cotton genome and relative distance of

16.8 cM was found among markers through screening randomly amplified polymorphic DNAs (RAPDs) and amplified fragment length polymorphisms (AFLPs). Jiang et al. [71] utilized F_2 population developed from *G. hirsutum* × *G. barbadense*, and produced a restriction fragment length polymorphism (RFLP) genetic map having 3767 cM length; 27 linkage groups with distance of 14.4 cM among loci.

Shappley et al. [72] used $F_{2:3}$ families derived from HS-46 and MARCABUCAAG-1-8896 genotypes and constructed genetic map by using 120 RFLPs which spanned to 865 cM and arranged in 31 linkage groups. Fifty one linked groups were developed through a map constructed with RFLP and RAPD markers [73] spanning to 6663 cM including 332 AFLPs, 91 RAPDs and three morphological markers. Khan et al. [74] studied comparison for ploidy level to diploid ancestors and tetraploid cotton with RAPD markers. 119 $F_{2:3}$ families developed from MD5678ne × Prema and utilized RFLPs for genetic map. Seventeen linkage panels were distributed on 700.7 cM map having mean distance of 7–8 cM among the markers [75].

RFLP, AFLP, and SSRs were screened in a backcrossed breeding population derived from crosses of [(*G. hirsutum* cv. Guazunchoz × *G. barbadense* cv. VH8-4602) × *G. hirsutum* cv. Guazunchoz] [76]. Linkage map covered 4400 cM of genome and consist of 888 loci arranged on 26 and 11, long- and short-linkage groups, respectively. EST-SSRs from *G. arboreum* were used for linkage map construction in backcross inbred line [(TM1 × Hai7124) × TM1] [77]. Map spans to 5644.3 cM with mean interlocus distance of 9.0 cM. As a whole, 111 loci were detected with these 99 EST-SSRs incorporated into backbone map including 511 SSR loci. These EST-SSRs will be useful in MAS for improving fiber quality.

Mei et al. [78] developed interspecific population among *G. hirsutum* L. cv. Acala-44 and *G. barbadense* L. cv. Pima S-7 and published genetic map, which covers 3287 cM of the genome. They used AFLPs, RFLPs, and SSRs and have; identified total 392 loci being 333, 12, and 47 markers, respectively. They were able to identify high repetitive DNA and heterochromatin in D-genome and relative distance among mapped loci in A-genomes that were also compared to homologous in D-genome [79].

Two hundred and thirty-three linked loci were mapped in backcross population of [*G. hirsutum* cv. Guazunchoz × *G. barbadense* VH8-4602) × *G. hirsutum* cv. Guazunchoz] by using 204 SSR markers, which produced 261 polymorphic bands [80]. Linkage map was published by adding 233 loci to already developed map [76] covering 5519 cM genome and having mean inter-related marker distance of 4.8 cM and consisting of 1160 loci. Nugyun et al. [80] applied STS markers for developing linkage maps that will fasten the genomics era by using diploid and tetraploid (AtDt) genomes. The genetic map consists of 2584 loci having İnter-locus marker distance of 1.72 cM and 763 loci intervals depending on 2007 probes from allotetraploid genome while 763 loci at relative marker distance of 1.96 cM intervals identified by 662 probes in D-genome. All desired homologous chromosome pairs were observed owing to locus repetition. Moreover, number of chromosomal variations including number of inversions and reciprocal translocations were observed.

Wang et al. [81] applied microsatellites for identifying QTLs related to fiber quality in RIL population. The genetic map was published with two common QTLs for lint percentage and fiber length. The results were in accordance to earlier studies and can be utilized in marker-assisted breeding. Lin et al. [82], screened SRAP, SSR, and RAPDs, have constructed linkage map, and a mean relevant distance was 9.08 cM among markers and total length of the map was 5141.8 cM. Park et al. [83] published the pioneer linkage map by applying EST-SSRs in RIL population derived from (*G. hirsutum* TM1 × *G. barbadense* Pima) for fiber. The linkage having about 27% genome coverage, covering 1277 cM genome and having 193 loci of those 121 newly mapped for fiber traits.

Researchers [84, 85] have used SSRs and AFLPs for determining oligonucleotides that is a good source for pyramiding of genes for marker-assisted selection. The mapping population developed by crossing parents having diversity for drought. Highly favorable environment was used; dryland and irrigated regimes for screening of genotypes. Quantitative trait loci mapped on different loci including one QTL (BNL1693) for seed cotton production on chromosomes 1 and 15 and two additional QTLs (BNL1153 and BNL2884) on chromosome 6. Moreover, chromosomes 6, 14, and 25 having BNL2884, BNL3259, and BNL1153 marker-associated QTLs found for osmotic pressure for drought in highly uniform lines. Researchers also revealed that NAU2715 and NAU2954 can be used as marker for relative water contents while relative water contents with NAU2954 will contribute a lot to drought tolerance in cotton.

SSRs were analyzed for establishing genetic diversity and QTLs [86]. F_2 population of crosses (7235 × TM 1), (HS 427-10 × TM-1), and (PD 6992 × SM 3) utilized for assigning QTLs for fiber traits in the three different linkage maps which span to 666.7, 557.8, and 588 cM, respectively, with number of mapped loci with difference of 86, 56, and 73 [86].

He et al. [87] screened RAPDs, Retrotransposon-microsatellite amplified polymorphism (REMAP), SSRs, and sequence-related amplified polymorphisms in hybrids of *G. hirsutum* L. cv. Handan 208 and *G. barbadense* L. cv. Pima 90 for construction of linkage map. As a whole, 1029 loci were mapped on 26 chromosomes; map spans to 5472.3 cM with mean İnter-locus distance of 5.32 cM. Saleem et al. [85] determined two QTLs related to drought tolerance in F_2 progeny developed from diverse parents by applying SSRs and EST-SSRs. The progeny screened with parents for osmotic pressure using hydroponic culture.

Abdurakhmonov et al. [88] revealed that chromosomes 12, 18, 23, and 26 having QTLs controlling lint percentage by applying SSRs and EST-SSRs in a RIL population. Four QTLs for lint index, eight for seed index, 11 for lint yield, four for seed cotton yield, nine for number of seeds per boll, three for fiber strength, five for fiber length, and eight for fiber fineness were determined in F_2 population (*G. hirsutum* L. cv. Handan 208 × *G. barbadense* L. cv. Pima 90) [87].

SSRs were used to screen F_2 progeny for nematode resistance [89], and researchers identified gene "GB713" that control resistance, and could be used for *reniform* nematode resistance. They found two QTLs located on chromosome 21 having 168.6 cM on the genetic map while other QTL was located on chromosome 18. Morphological traits of RIL populations developed by hybridization of *G. hirsutum* and *G. barbadense* [90]. QTLs governing the plant architecture including plant height, number of primary and secondary branches were screened. Researchers found that angle of branch, angle of fruits, plant height, leaf size, main fruiting, etc. were governed by a single QTL. Infestation of disease is a severe problem in cotton, e.g., *Xanthomonas oxysporum* [91], root knot nematode [89, 92–94], *Verticillium* [57], and cotton leaf curl disease (CLCuD) [95, 96] that warn the cotton scientist to find natural resistance sources and their urgent exploitation by using MAS.

3. DNA makers in cotton

Several types of molecular markers are available for characterization of germplasm of crop plants (**Table 1**). The amount of variation prevailing in the germplasm helps to maintain genetic conservation [98]. Availability of vast genomic database provides opportunity to develop enormous markers for detection of genetic variation [99, 100]. According to Weising et al. [101], these molecular markers must be (1) highly polymorphic, (2) codominant, (3) evenly distributed in a genome, (4) without pleiotropic effects, (5) easy to handle and fast assayed, (6) low cost and reproducible.

The cost of production of a marker is directly related to marker technique in use, polymorphic nature, and efficiency [102]. Polymorphic markers are divided into three types: (1) hybridization-based, (2) polymerase chain reaction (PCR) based, and (3) DNA sequence based markers [103].

3.1. Hybridization-based markers

Hybridization is occurred to the fragments of genomic DNAs produced by restriction endonucleases with various lengths among individuals. These types of markers are called "hybridization-based markers."

3.1.1. Restriction fragment length polymorphism

Restriction fragment length polymorphism (RFLP) is a type of hybridization-based marker in plant genome and initially used for detection of polymorphism in a DNA sequence for gene mapping during the 1975s [31]. Nucleotide sequences of 4, 5, 6, or 8 bp, called restriction sites, are recognized by restriction endonucleases [104]. Digestion of DNA with restriction enzymes results in fragments whose number and size can vary among individuals, populations, and even within species.

Many scientists developed genetic mapping during the 1975s populations of cottons that were analyzed by using RFLP. Domestication of *G. hirsutum* was investigated with RFLPs [105]; they have revealed that Yucatan is the wild ancestor of upland cotton. Wright et al. [106] used RFLP for MAS and evaluated resistance allele for bacterial blight resistance. Hybridization carried out with probes for microsatellite sequences to yield a variable number of tandem repeats (VNTR) and allow oligonucleotide fingerprinting [107]. Joint map was constructed by using $F_{2:3}$ populations derived from different intra-hirsutum accessions [108]. Two hundred and eighty-four polymorphic markers and 49 linked pairs were observed on the map. The genetic map spanned to 1502.6 cM having 5.3 cM distance between markers. RFLPs have played a significant part for omics studies [109]. Low level of polymorphism, costly chemicals, and more time for analysis limit RFLP use in MAS [104].

S.N.	Feature	RFLP	RAPD	AFLP	SSRs	SNPs
1	DNA require (µg)	10	0.02	0.5–1.0	0.05	0.05
2	PCR based	No	Yes	Yes	Yes	Yes
3	DNA quality	High	High	Moderate	Moderate	High
4	No of polymorphic loci analyzed	1–3	1.50–50	20–100	1–3	1
5	Type of polymorphism	Single base change, insertion deletion	Single base change, insertion deletion	Single base change, insertion deletion	Change in repeat length	Single base change, insertion deletion
6	Dominance	Codominant	Dominant	Dominant/ codominant	Codominant	Codominant
7	Reproducibility	High	Unreliable	High	High	High
8	Ease of use and development	Not easy	Easy	Easy	Easy	Easy
9	Automation	Low	Moderate	Moderate	High	High
10	Cost per analysis	High	Low	Moderate	Low	Low
11	Developmental cost	Low	Low	Moderate	High	High
12	Need for sequence data	Yes	No	No	Yes	Yes
13	Accuracy	Very high	Very low	Medium	High	Very high
14	Radioactivity detection	Usually yes	No	No	No	Yes
15	Genomic abundance	High	Very high	Very high	Medium	Medium
16	Part of genome surveyed	Low copy coding regions	Whole genome	Whole genome	Whole genome	Whole genome
17	Level of polymorphism	Low	Low to moderate	Low to moderate	High	High
18	Inheritance	Codominant	Dominant	Dominant	Codominant	Codominant
19	Detection of alleles	Yes	No	No	Yes	Yes
20	Utility for genetic mapping	Species specific	Cross specific	Cross specific	Species specific	Species specific
21	Utility in marker-assisted selection	Moderate	Low to moderate	Low to moderate	High	Low to moderate
22	Cost and labor involved in generation	High	Low moderate	Low moderate	High	High

Table 1. Salient features of various molecular markers [97].

Ulloa et al. [110] published genetic maps by using intraspecific populations developed from parents having diverse genetic background. Fifteen linkage groups were used for designating the chromosomes. Earlier mapped data was used for construction of map by observing the deficiency analysis of the probes. QTLs were determined for fiber and yield traits by using this map. As a whole 63 QTLs were found in A subgenome at five different loci and 29 QTLs observed at 3-loci of D-subgenome. First genetic map spans to 117 cM produced 26 QTLs with 54 RFLPs while second map produced 19 QTLs with 27 RFLPs, and spanned to 77.6 cM. It was revealed that these maps will serve as map-based cloning for fiber quality.

3.2. PCR-based markers

PCR-based markers, i.e., RAPD [111–113], AFLP [114-116], microsatellites (SSRs) [117-119], and inter-simple sequence repeats (ISSRs) [120-121] represent major class of markers in cotton genomics due to their high utility and exploitation. Below are the major advantages of PCR techniques as compared to hybridization-based methods: (1) low amount of DNA used for genotyping; (2) capacity to amplify fragments from frozen cells; (3) high polymorphism that enables to generate many genetic markers within a short time; and (4) ability to screen many genes simultaneously either for direct collection of data or provide opportunity to collect information prior to submit for nucleotide sequencing [109].

The comparison of different aspects of generally used molecular markers is given in (**Table 1**) and brief description of these three classes of molecular markers is described below with reference to cotton genetics.

3.2.1. Amplified fragment length polymorphism

Amplified fragment length polymorphism (AFLP) relies on the restricted sequences and PCR amplification. Initially, genomic DNA is digested by a restriction enzyme and resulting fragments are ligated with adapters to both ends. Then, the adapter and restriction site sequences are selectively amplified; only the fragments whose ends are complementary to 3′ ends of selective primers are amplified resulting in small sequences. Finally, a gel is run for the separation of amplified fragments and it is visualized by fluorescence [34]. The focal point of this methodology relies on the magnification of endonuclease restricted fragments through PCR.

The important advantages of using of AFLP markers is that they exist in large numbers in genomes, they have a great reproducibility due to high PCR annealing temperatures, and less cost per marker basis [104]. In addition to reliability and reproducibility [116], there is no need of DNA sequence for analysis. In contrast to RFLPs and microsatellites, enormous polymorphic loci can be investigated by having single oligonucleotide pair running a single gel through AFLPs [122]. For digestion; partially degraded DNA and good quality DNA can be utilized, but care should be taken that isolated genomic DNA should be free of chemicals that interferes with polymerase chain reaction.

Lacape et al. [97] initially developed RILs population by introgression of Guazuncho 2 (*G. hirsutum*) and VH8-4602 (*G. barbadense*), and constructed a genetic map with 800 markers

(AFLP, RFLP, and SSR) loci. AFLPs and RAPDs were used for development of linkage map in cotton [123]. Three hundred and seven SSR markers and 72 AFLP oligonucleotides were used for the development of genetic map in F_2 population which derived from intra-hirsutum hybridization. The map consisted of 27 linkage groups and it has 21, 72 cM distance between the markers [114]. Map saturation in various genotypes of cottons was analyzed [115].

AFLPs were screened in a backcross population developed from intra-hirsutum cultivars for agronomic traits and fiber quality enhancement [124]. They found 50 AFLPs associated with the fiber quality traits and few for other; further evaluated that E1M1-106, E1M4-153; E1M3-168, E6M3-266 for lint yield and lint percentage, respectively can be used in future for MAS [124]. AFLPs were used for introgression among *G. hirsutum* and *G. tomentosum* being close relative to Upland cotton [125]. Through analysis, species-specific [11, 16] AFLP markers were selected from *G. hirsutum* and *G. tomentosum*, respectively for assessing *G. hirsutum* relatedness. These species-specific AFLP markers would be useful for detecting gene flow between *G. hirsutum* and *G. tomentosum*.

Jixang et al. [124] revealed genetic diversity in a germplasm by using AFLPs. A range of 0.1–0.34 estimates of genetic diversity were found among the genotypes, and showed that genotypes having significant variation in the gene stock include AU 5367, Acala 1517-99, and LA 05307025.

3.2.2. Random amplified polymorphic DNA

Randomly amplified polymorphic DNA (RAPD) relies on use of short and random primers to amplify random portions of genome [126]. Such markers have found to be widespread in population genetic studies whose characterizations of genetic diversity and divergence within and among populations are based on assumptions of Hardy-Weinberg equilibrium and selective neutrality of the markers is employed [127]. Ultimate success of RAPDs is shown in the increase of molecular markers which require small amount of DNA and no need for sequencing, except of having all prerequisites for PCR conditions [126]. DNA fragments having sequence of about 10 bp are amplified with artificial primers by using PCR [128]. RAPDs are being used vigorously for profiling of genotype of important field crops, also for mapping for certain traits in addition to biotic and abiotic stresses. For such studies, RAPD primers show polymorphism and should be free from palindromic sequences and should have minimum 40% GC contents in the fragments [113].

Many scientists have explored RAPDs in cotton for studying different aspects like phylogenetic studies, genetic diversity, and CLCuV disease screening [111, 112, 128]. R-6592 and UBC607500 [113, 129] male sterility and fertility restorer traits can be improved by using RAPDs. Lan et al. [130] applied RAPDs for mapping fertility genes that is of immense value in cotton and tagged fertility restorer gene *R-6592* which may be utilized for productivity enhancement. Lan et al. [130] conducted phylogenetic studies in cotton and argued that this procedure is helpful and reliable for introgression of desirable traits. RAPDs were used in cotton for comparing cotton cultivars resistance to jassids, mites, and aphids [131]. DNA finger printing, mapping and genetic diversity has been studied in cotton through RAPDs [132–134].

Noormohammadi et al. [135] screened F_2 population of Upland cotton and Opal variety by using 10 homo-primers and seven hetero-primers out of 26 RAPDs and found 261 reproducible bands, with an average of 4.18 [261 bands/17 primers = 15 bands/primer] bands per primer and 22% polymorphism for analyzing genetic resemblance in agronomic traits with 45 (Upland) and 80% (Opal) polymorphism, respectively. By applying agarose gel, multilocus genotyping can be carried out by staining with ethidium bromide and this facility is available in every lab working on molecular breeding [136].

RAPDs are often laboratory dependent and require immense care to design protocols for getting polymorphism. Several factors have been reported to influence the reproducibility of RAPD results such as quantity of template DNA, buffers of polymerase, concentration of magnesium chloride, primer to template ratio, annealing temperature, type or source of DNA polymerase, and brand of thermal cycler [137]. RAPDs also fail to discriminate between homozygotes and heterozygotes and complication of expressing Mendelian ratio of loci [138].

3.2.3. Intersimple sequence repeat

Modifications of microsatellites, which utilize microsatellites-complementary primers, overcome the need for flanking fragment information [139]. Polymorphism is revealed among simple sequence repeat (SSR) markers by using primer (16–25 bp) adjacent to a single SSR and annealing occur at either ends [139]. ISSR utilizes microsatellites as oligonucleotides in a PCR reaction to amplify inter simple sequence repeats for desired DNA. ISSRs utilize SSRs repeats dinucleotide, trinucleotide, and tetranucleotide as oligonucleotide [140]. Usually, ISSR primers have substantial fragments contrary to RAPD primers, enabling elevated annealing temperature, which produce highly polymorphic bands as compared to RAPDs [120, 141]. The amplified products can be separated by agarose and polyacrylamide gel due to longer length ranged from 200 to 2000 bp [139].

ISSR markers have been vastly used in cotton improvement, phylogenetic study and for mapping of germplasm [120, 121]. Parkihya et al. [142] studied genetic diversity among cotton genotypes by using nine ISSR oligonucleotides and detected 86 bands of which 54 bands exhibited polymorphism of 62.79% having mean of six bands per primer. The PIC ranged from 0.8616 to 0.9090 and genetic similarity ranged from 0.60 to 0.917. Phylogenetic relation was revealed in 21 cotton genotypes by using 12 intersimple sequence repeat primers and observed 49.6% reproducibility [143].

Genetic diversity was studied in cotton with 10 ISSR and showed 88.5% polymorphism [144]. Liu and Wendel [145] showed that ISSR can be designed with low cost. Genetic diversity observed in genepool comprised of wild species and elite lines through SSRs and ISSR [146]. They observed 173 alleles having mean 3.93 alleles per locus by analyzing 39 SSRs and 5 ISSR markers which produced 89.6% reproducible bands. Among genotypes variation ranged from 0.04 to 0.58 while in diploid and tetraploid species it was 0.23–0.57%. Similar to RAPD, there may be some fragments with the same mobility originate from non-homologous regions [120].

3.2.4. *Sequence characterized amplified region*

RAPDs have more demerits of polymorphism as compared to other PCR-based markers which are used for analyzing a large number of individuals with low cost. This problem was overcome by using sequence characterized amplified region. PCR assay uses couple of distinct oligonucleotides for DNA sequence at a specific locus [147]; oligonucleotides might be having a high-copy, dispersed fragment within polymorphic loci. After sequencing the two ends of the two reproducible DNA fragments, one can develop two SCAR markers. SCAR 431_{1920} can be used in MAS program for screening genotypes with fiber strength. By using SCAR, codominance is produced [148].

These markers have been used in genetic analysis and used for molecular breeding [149, 150]. Extended sequence specificity of primers in SCARs results in higher reproducibility than RAPDs [151]. SCAR is widely used among researchers for mapping studies within closely related species [152]. SCARs are more authentic for MAS after conversion of DNA markers. SCAR markers are cost effective and highly polymorphic which make them suitable to be used for evaluating large number of mapping populations in cotton [152]. QTLs for leaf traits were observed [153].

3.2.5. *Sequence-tagged site*

Oslen et al. [154] developed sequence tag sites (STS) through observing impact of the PCR on human genome research, and argued that single-copy DNA sequences of known map location could serve as markers for genetic and physical mapping of genes along the chromosome. STS marker allows the utilization of PCR with specific primers which produces one oligonucleotide connected to the trait of interest. In order to utilize STS for molecular breeding, RFLP, AFLP, and RAPDs are usually converted into STS [155]. Thus, in a broad sense, STS include the markers such as microsatellites (SSRs), SCARs, and ISSRs mentioned above. Backcross breeding population was developed [(B416R × Ark8518) × Ark8518] and used for identification of STS markers related to fertility [155]. Tetraploid and diploid species were involved and artificial hybrids created by colchiploidy.

RAPDs such as UBC1471400, UBC607500, UBC979700, and UBC169800 loci were associated to productivity restoration, and it was verified that UBC607500 is having enormous value for pyramiding genes to be used in molecular breeding [129]. Linkage maps were developed by using STS for diploid and tetraploid (A_tD_t) *Gossypium* genomes [156]. Genetic map composed of 763 loci at 1.96 cM (approximately 500 kb) intervals detected by 662 probes (D), and 2584 loci at 1.72 cM (approximately 600 kb) intervals based on 2007 probes (A_tD_t).

Several cotton breeders have used STS markers for identification of male restorer parental lines for hybrid cotton [129] who mapped cotton genotypes by using backcross inbred lines (BILs) and RIL populations with informative primers, and detected 21 and 7 polymorphic STS markers in BILs and RIL populations, respectively. Twelve STS markers were mapped in BIL population, and four of them were located along with resistance gene analog-amplified fragment length polymorphism (RGA-AFLP) markers on the same chromosome. Importantly, two were mapped on chromosome c 4, flanking two main-effect QTLs, which were previously detected. These STS markers should be useful for high-throughput genotyping, gene mapping, and MAS for disease resistance including *Verticillium* wilt resistance in cotton.

3.2.6. Simple sequence repeats

Tandem repeats composed of several to over hundred repeats of one to four nucleotide motifs are found in all eukaryotic genomes. These repeats are designated as $(AAAC)_n$, here "*n*" represents number of tandem repeats. The flanking sequences of simple sequence repeats (SSRs) are used for the development of oligonucleotides [118]. Tandem repeats induce variability, which evolve polymorphism of different size due to slipped strand arise because of mispairing occurs during DNA replication [118], variation in size of PCR amplification/ products induce polymorphism which can be separated by electrophoresis.

Kinship studies are conducted by employing SSR markers assess the extent of variation [119]. Vos et al. [157] used agarose and polyacrylamide gel for the identification of SSRs having codominance nature like AFLP. Akkaya et al. [158] stated that genetic mapping is on fast track due to the use of SSRs in self-pollinated crops where these markers are of great interest for breeders [159, 160]. SSRs are mostly codominant, and are indeed excellent for studying of population genetics and mapping [161–163]. The use of fluorescent primers in combination with automatic capillary or gel-based DNA sequencers has got its way in most advanced laboratories, and SSRs are also shown to be excellent markers for fluorescent techniques, multiplexing and high-throughput analysis.

Derived from trispecies hybridization that can be segregated for natural leaf defoliation trait. This RIL population screened with microsatellite markers, JESPR-13, JESPR-153, and JESPR178 tandem repeats were found to be highly associated to leaf defoliation trait value [162]. It was found that JESPR178 is closely linked to this trait in cotton. It has an immense importance that gene pyramiding can be accomplished for molecular breeding [164]. QTLs were tagged using SSRs in the nematode resistance RIL population developed via introgression from *G. barbadense* [165]. In that study, a single marker analysis identified four major QTLs located on chromosomes 3, 4, 11, and 17 were identified to account for 8.0–12.3% of the phenotypic variance.

Fiber length was increased up to 12–20% in cotton by using microsatellites in a population derived from interspecific hybridization and loci were discovered for marker-assisted selection [166]. Twenty-three chromosomes were analyzed by SSRs and found on an average relative distance of 4.9 cM [167]. Researchers [168–170] have utilized SSR markers for studying genetic diversity in cotton and observed limited genetic variations. Reddy et al. [171] used SSR-enriched genomic libraries and identified 300 SSR markers. Multinational Seed Company has reported more than 1200 SSRs [172].

Abdurakhmonov et al. [173] conducted genome-wide association mapping based on linkage disequilibrium (LD), scanning Upland germplasm consisting of 334 *G. hirsutum* accessions collected from Uzbek, Latin American, and Australian ecotypes. Screening under different climates and by using mixed linear model involving population kinship and population structure 12–22 SSR markers were associated with fiber length, fiber strength, fiber fineness and six other fiber quality traits. Mei et al. [78] have reported 145 SSR polymorphic markers for yield and yield components in cotton by screening germplasm of 358 upland cotton varieties. Cao et al. [174] assessed genetic stock fiber quality and reported 97 polymorphic SSR markers by using LD.

Bolek et al. [57] used SSR markers for verticilium resistance in cotton by using F_2 population; 255 SSRs were screened over bulks constituted by 10 resistant, and 10 susceptible progenies. QTLs were tagged by using 60 polymorphic markers. Genetic map produced 11 linkage groups having 15.17 cM inter-locus distance and spanning 531 cM.

Backcross inbred lines used [175] for observing the genetic variation of 446 SSR markers having relative mean distance of 10 cM interspecific linkage map and also detected 58 QTLs related to fiber quality and yield components. By using SSRs, genetic markers associated to cotton earliness were determined in progeny developed from intra-hirsutum hybrids [117], and these markers correspond to bud to flower duration and flower to boll period.

Earliness in cotton can be induced by the introgression of QTLS located near to the SSR markers such as BNL1044, DPL0209, NAU1004a, NAU 5046, NAU6078, and TMB0481 [117]. F_2 progeny was developed within *G. hirsutum* for utilizing gene pyramiding in marker-assisted breeding to enhance fiber quality and agronomic traits of economical value by using SSRs, SRAPs, EST-SSRs, and SSCP-SNPs [176]. Economically valuable traits were evaluated through construction of linkage map, segregation pattern observed among the traits and 33 QTLs were identified [176].

Textile industry entirely depends upon fiber with good quality. Marker-assisted selection allows developing a cultivar having good fiber quality. There are many SSRs which can be used for fostering the breeding program; for example, lint percentage can be approved by using TMB0471 and MGHES-31, TMB0366, BNL3590, BNL1395, BNL1672, BNL1694, JESPER101, JESPR204, NAU3308, BNL1672, NAU3308; NAU4024 [168, 177–180]. Genetic base can be broadened for span length by using BNL 1395, DC40182, NAU2980, BNL2752, NAU2985, NAU1167, NAU1200, NAU2277 [50, 123, 177, 179]. BNL1122, BNL1317, BNL3145, BNL1521, CIR307, CGR6164, CGR6683, GH454, BNL3463, JESPER153, DC40182, NAU 1037, SHIN-0463, TEMB1618, NAU3736, NAU445, NAU780, NAU1102, NAU1197, NAU1322, NAU1369, JESPR218, TMD05 can be applied for fiber strength enhancement [52, 92, 173, 174, 176, 181–188].

3.2.7. *Single nucleotide polymorphism*

Single nucleotide polymorphisms (SNPs) manifest alteration in single base. SNPs are the most frequent occurring variability in the individuals which is found in each 1000 bases [189]. These are changes in bases from transitions (C/T or G/A) to transversions (C/G, A/T, C/A, or T/G) while insertions and deletions also induce SNPs which show single base changes. SNPs show useful allelic variations and have been markers of choice in various genetic studies [190]. Rapid progress in high-through put sequencing has allowed discovering SNPs in complex genomes with economic value by using genotyping by sequencing [191]. Frelichowski et al. [167] revealed that reproducibility is a major hindrance for using large number of markers developed in *G. arboreum, G. raimondii* and *G. hirsutum* [192]. In combination with genome and expressed sequence tags (ESTs) in model plant species [193], the efficiency of Sanger sequencing has been improved to accelerate the identification of variations at single base pair resolution [194].

Genotyping in plant sciences is progressing rapidly because SNPs for observing variation in a specific locus are utilized. Moreover, availability of enormous SNPs due to insertions-deletions and whole genome genomic studies is laying the corner stone for next generation sequencing [195]. Developed genomic databases and SNPs information allow evolving SNPs to an influential research for related relatives. Owing to most common type of DNA polymorphism, SNPs are also flexible in the selection of SNP variants at target loci, and they provide the option to choose from a large number of genome-wide loci when selecting sets of informative markers for specific germplasm pools [196]. Breeding programs comprised of genomic estimated breeding values are highly favored for whole genome techniques additional to targeted loci [197–199].

Economically important traits from breeding perspective are also investigated through genome-wide sequencing [200], saturated mapping of polygenic traits [201], and by using LD-mapping [202]. An et al. [203] studied the expression of R2R3-MYB transcription factors where few are expressed during fiber initiation and elongation. They observed phylogenetic relation among R2R3-MYB genes and published a map by using SNPs in Upland cotton. QTLs were mapped in population derived from intra-hirsutum and interspecific (*G. hirsutum* × *G. barbadense*) [204]. Researchers [204] have collected all published QTL data. QTLs were identified for seed, yield and fiber quality by using two populations through meta-analysis. QTLs connected to biotic and abiotic stressed were also detected. However, the development of high-throughput genotyping platforms for large numbers (thousands to millions) of SNPs has proved to be relatively time-consuming and costly.

Deynze et al. [205] reported more than 200 loci in *G. hirsutum* breeding germplasm, which were genetically mapped on mapping population derived from TM-1 and 3-79. Genepool comprised of 24-accessions derived from 8-parental lines of mapping populations of six cotton species and16 promising cotton strains used for genotyping. As a whole more than 1000 SNPs were polymorphic among G. *hirsutum* and G. barbadense were developed from 270 loci and 290 indels from 92 loci. [205]. Roche 454 pyrosequencing platform in four allotetraploid cottons using reduced representation library (RRL) have helped to map a large number of SNPs [206]. The conversion rate of SNPs using KASPar assay was about 35.8%. Three hundred and sixty-seven SNP markers were used for linkage map construction, which spanned to 1688 cM. High-resolution maps can be formed rapidly by utilizing parallel sequencing methods to determine the reads in resequencing. Pacific Biosciences technologies used for long reads [207] while Illumina and Ion Torrent are applied in sequencing for getting short reads [196].

4. Mapping populations

The group of plants, which is used for screening of molecular markers and segregated for the trait of interest, is designated as "mapping population." From commercial point of view, such populations are developed from within species and can be also developed between different species for creating desirable variation. Polymorphism is compulsory in the progenitors for required trait [208]. The exchange of chromosome fragments during crossing over produces recombination, which provides the basis for developing linkage maps [59]. Populations are required for creating genetic maps in order to locate the quantitative trait loci from economical point of view.

Mapping populations can be exemplified by F_2, backcross, recombinant inbred lines (RILs), doubled haploid lines (DHL), F_2-derived F_3 (F_2:F_3) populations, and near-isogenic lines (NILs). F_1 is produced by selfing two parents, having extreme properties for trait of interest that show a significant polymorphism for whichever type of loci are scored. Mostly, this population is used for genetic mapping as it requires less time for development. However, there are some drawbacks for this population, most important of which is the fact that it is not stable. Qualitative and quantitative traits in cotton have been mapped by using F_2 [70, 74, 81, 86].

Backcross (BC) population is developed by crossing a genotype with an elite cultivar, which is deficient for a single gene or QTL [67]. A concept of BC population was developed in 1922 and widely applied in plant breeding programs till 1960 [209]. Backcross population has been used for linkage mapping in cotton for improving various traits [129, 155–156].

Near isogenic lines(NILs) can be developed either by using selfing until purity is Achieved; for all traits with wide variation of the trait of interest among NILs or by hybridizing the donor parent to the F_1 plants and choosing the desired trait [63]. NILs are of high importance for genetic studies as they are stable like RILs. Researchers [210] used NILs for observing QTLs related to yield and drought related traits. They evaluated that NILs can be used for evaluating drought and can be used for MAS. Essenberg et al. [116] developed NILs in cotton and mapped bacterial blight resistance. They revealed that lines having Acala-44 in their parentage are showing dominance to bacterial blight.

Recombinant inbred lines (RIL) are stable and are developed by using single seed descent method from first filial generation. It continues until homozygosity is obtained in the individuals. RILs are permanent and can be screened at multiple locations for desired traits. Each strain is homozygous and stable in the RIL population. Each cycle of selfing results in enhanced recombination frequency and these populations are highly suitable for saturated mapping [129]. Moreover, for genetic mapping in cotton this population has been utilized for various traits including nematode resistance [165], fiber quality improvement [166], and verticilium resistance [175]. One of the drawbacks of this population is long duration for development in which segregation bias can occur due to removal of some genotypes after selfing. Another disadvantage of using these populations is that major QTLs are having a masking effect, and multiple QTLs are having epistatic effects.

Nested association mapping (NAM) [188] is designed for precise identification of QTLs [177]. Economically valued traits related to yield and subsequently to textile sector can be efficiently studied through developing new populations like NAM. NAM populations potentially address the limitations of conventional mapping populations

5. Some applications of markers in breeding schemes

5.1. Marker-assisted backcrossing

The simplest, most widely used, and the most efficient form of MAS is MAB. In this form, two parents are used for the development; one is "donor parent" having trait of interest for transferring the targeted gene/loci and the other is "recipient parent" which is lacking gene. Parents are hybridized and F_1 is developed. Marker-assisted backcrossing relies upon the presence of a molecular marker associated with the trait, instead of targeting the expression of phenotypic value in traditional breeding. F_1 is planted for confirming the marker loci at initial stages of development, and pure F_1 is hybridized to recurrent parent. Markers are evaluated among individuals at the initial development stages of BCF_1 and hybridized to recurrent parent having alternative alleles. BC_1 individuals show segregation frequency of F1 population gametes as two genotypes are involved in this population. Highly efficient map is constructed by using this population in contrast to F_2 population. This population is mostly used for overcoming hybrid in viability and hybrid breakdown in interspecific crosses [129]. This process is continued until three to four filial generation for stabilizing the marker and its associated trait of interest. MAB population has been utilized for observing traits of interest through quantitative trait loci [115].

5.2. Pedigree selection

Breeding techniques within the two cultivated tetraploid species rely on crossing and selection of traits using pedigree and recurrent selection methods. Promising genotypes having desirable traits can be developed using MAS and can be combined into a pedigree-based selection. Mostly, the efficiency of MAS was investigated using two populations from pedigree selection, and modified backcrossing pyramiding has been developed [211]. The selection efficiency for the fiber strength was greatly increased when QTLfs-1 was selected simultaneously with two molecular markers with known genetic distance [211].

5.3. Marker-assisted recurrent selection (MARS)

Molecular markers should be applied for plant improvement in conjunction with the latest breeding methodologies. Marker-assisted recurrent selection offers an opportunity to get maximum output from a recurrent selection [212]; and it is used for introgression of multiple genes.

Quantitative traits can be enhanced efficiently by using MARS, which allows selfing and genotyping within same cropping season in one cycle of selection. The increase in genetic gain was doubled from MARS in some populations as compared to phenotypic selection [213]. In cotton, resistance to American bollworm was achieved by using marker-assisted recurrent selection; they revealed highly significant differences in individuals studied by MARS for this insect resistance [214].

6. Gene pyramiding for MAS

Gene pyramiding has been widely used for combining number of genes especially disease resistance genes for specific races of a pathogen. Vertical resistance for different strains of pathogens is done by involving multiple strains. It is also done by "molecular breeding" because breeding for resistance is extremely difficult to achieve using conventional methods. Gutiérrez et al. [215] have used this technique for nematode resistance in cotton while [155] they applied sequence tag sites and screened STS markers associated with fertility restoring genes in cotton.

7. Next-generation sequencing (NGS)

SNP genotyping with latest high-throughput sequencing has the potential to speed up the breeding programs [216]. New DNA sequencing technologies have made it possible for the breeders and investigators to perform a genome analysis not only more rapidly but also less expensively [179]. High-throughput bioinformatics assist to identify large number of nucleotides per run [217]. Researchers have developed a lot of NGS methods with success in diverse platforms, which include Roche 454 FLX Titanium [218–220], Illumina MiSeq and HiSeq2500 [221], Ion Torrent PGM [222]. Genomic research contributes immensely to plant and animal sciences thanks to the advances in sequencing techniques [180, 221, 223–228]. The ultimate aim of all these techniques is to discover an authentic marker that could be used for sequencing in MAS with economical benefits [229–230].

Polyploidy is the main hindrance for isolation of useful SNPs in cotton because it produces homeologous and paralogous sequence variants which are combined together in allelic variations among cultivars [231–232]. Two cultivated tetraploids species were screened for the development of genomic SNPs through NGS by using reduced representation library obtained from Roche 454 pyrosequencing [206]. Competitive allele-specific PCR (KASPar) showed 35.8% validity of SNPs and developed the genetic map of *G. hirsutm* via 367 SNP markers which spanned to 1688 cM.

Gore et al. [233] developed a linkage map in a RIL population derived from intra-hirsutum cv. TM-1, and NM24016. The genetic map covered about 50% of the *G. hirsutum* genome which consisted of 429 SSRs and 412 SNPs. They also tagged 10 QTLs related to fiber quality, which provided a unique resource for mapping. Before Affymetrix became commercially available, Gene Chip cotton genome array consisting of 239,777 probe sets that represent 21,485 cotton transcripts has been developed [234, 235]. Sequences from Genome database, dbEST and

RefSeq were used for the development of Chip which promises to be an excellent source for genomics.

8. Genotyping by sequencing

In agricultural sciences, the discovery of reliable and true SNPs is compulsory for knowing about the utilization and importance of particular sequences. Molecular breeding tools can be applied to explore germplasm without available genomic data through genotyping by sequencing (GBS) methodology. GBS permits researchers to analyze complex genomes of polyploid species efficiently at low cost and it has been widely used due to the latest developments in high-throughput sequencing [191]. Reduced representative libraries are developed by using endonucleases [55, 178, 236]. Single nucleotide polymorphism is discovered for genomic studies [237]. Genomic techniques; genome-wide association study (GWAS), genomic diversity, genetic linkage analysis, molecular marker discovery offer to screen genotypes upon genotypic basis for traits of interest through GBS. Genotyping and reproducibility of markers are performed in a single step through GBS and SNPs are developed [238].

GBS-based sequencing data are used for developing genetic map and tagging markers with quantitative traits in populations derived from different ways, i.e., filial generations, RILs, etc. and germplasm collections [218]. GBS approach has been used efficiently for genetic analysis and marker development of rapeseed, lupin, lettuce, switchgrass, soybean, maize, and cotton [38, 219, 222–224, 233, 239].

The merits of GBS over existing marker development methodologies include availability of large number of markers, fast screening of populations composed of more number of individuals, diverse genotyping systems to tackle multiple traits, and more precise SNPs discovery and validity due to availability of high-throughput sequencing data [216]. Recently, GBS approach has been used to identify SNPs in the collections of RILs of wheat and to map various traits useful for breeding programs [55]. It is needed that efforts should be made to develop strategies for getting the benefits of NGS and advanced genotyping from breeder perspectives [196]. GBS protocol of Poland et al. [236] likely is needed to maximize the cost-effective concurrent discovery and genotyping of SNPs within cotton populations.

Although very efficient and productive in terms of achieving the desired goals, there are some drawbacks in GBS as well. GBS has incapability to assign true alleles of each locus in polyploids as compared to other techniques. As exemplified, Huang et al. [178] used RILs and biparental populations for assessing the utility of GBS in hexaploid oat. They observed that data analysis algorithm factors involved in SNP discovery, developed GBS derived loci description by forming two bioinformatics workflow. Its genetic map spans to 45,117 loci, which will be a source of further genetic studies [178].

Islam et al. [240] used GBS with two different approaches in cultivated cotton germplasm consisting of 11 diverse cultivars and their random-mated RILs. Authors have discovered a large set of polymorphic SNPs with broad applicability. They identified 4441 and 1176 polymorphic SNPs with minor allele frequency of ≥0.1. The utility of developed SNP markers were confirmed using SNPs in 154 Upland cotton accessions with high genetic diversity.

9. Association mapping

Genome-wide association study is used for developing highly saturated maps in cotton germplasm [241]. This technique allows detecting association among various markers and traits through assessing of the genetic diversity of required traits [242]. Linkage disequilibrium-based mapping (LD-mapping) is the advanced tool to study complex traits governed by many genes. LD-mapping has been successfully used in self-pollinated plants [243]. Microsatellites were screened in germplasm consisting of varieties at different locations to tag yield and fiber quality QTLs [202]. QTLs mapped for yield and fiber quality traits will serve as a reliable source to determine the diversity within the species and will contribute a lot in MAS [202]. In contrast to biparental populations, association mapping fosters molecular breeding because a vast genetic diversity is present in germplasms due to diverse sources [173]. Several protocols have been developed including complexity reduction of polymorphic sequences (CRoPS) [244], restriction site associated DNA (RAD) [216], GBS [195], and sequence-based genotyping (SBG) [245, 246] for genome analysis. Of all protocols, LD-mapping is on the top thanks to innovations done for high resolution. Association mapping is an authentic way for molecular tagging as it allows the screening of quantitative traits of value in a precise way [247]. Genome-wide association makes it possible to detect association among various markers and traits.

Abdurakhmonov et al. [46] used LD-mapping in a germplasm collection, which included photoperiodic lines. Simple sequence repeats were used for assessing the extent of LD in cotton and the major fiber quality QTLs were tagged using mixed linear model.

Nested association mapping is also being used for identification of suitable SSRs in a NAM population derived from 20 diverse genotypes of *G. hirsutum* with Namangan-77. SSR marker screening for development of highly saturated map through NAM $F_{2:3}$ populations for traits of immense value in cotton is underway [188].

10. Public data resources

Sequenced genomic information allows breeders to analyze the genetic variation [248]. Major databases, which serve as a foundation, include CottonGen [58], Comparative Evolutionary Genomics of Cotton [249], National Center for Biotechnology Information [250] for Express sequence tags resource, TropGENE Database [251], the Cotton Diversity Database [252] and BACMan resources at Plant Genome Mapping Laboratory [253]. These resources provide genomic and heredity data of the cotton germplasm, QTLs tagged to loci and highly saturated linkage maps.

11. Targeting-induced local lesions in genomes (TILLINGS)

Phenotypic variation in plant genomes is produced by variation in DNA bases, which can be induced naturally and/or using different chemicals [254]. The targeting-induced local lesions in genomes (TILLING) technique allows determining an allelic variation precisely in a single-base pair for the targeted gene. Chemical treatments have been applied to generate SNP mutations. Point mutations, which are useful from breeder's perspective, can be detected by TILLING and ECOTILLING techniques [255]. The mutagens used for induction of point mutation are highly selective and optimal concentration can spontaneously produce single base alternations at a high frequency in TILLING.

Knock-out population is developed by treating the seed with chemicals, inducing change in DNA sequence [256]. Auld et al. [257] used TILLING in *G. arboreum* and demonstrated the applicability of this technique in cotton. The ultimate success to produce large number of sequence variations of target genome depends upon duration of application, relative capability of ethyl methane sulfonate (EMS), and γ-rays [53]. Aslam et al. [53] screened three *Gossypium* sp. (*G. hirsutum, G. barbadense* and *G. arboreum*) and constructed a kill curve. They observed the impact of different mutagens (EMS and γ-rays) consisting of eight different concentrations of EMS (0.1–0.8%) and two levels of γ-rays (100–800 Gy). The genotypes of each species were evaluated with morphological parameters emergence and plant height, and yield traits (number of bolls per plant, boll weight, lint yield and lint percentage). For reverse and forward genetics point of view, viable accessions were selected from mutagenized genotypes. They revealed that EMS showed significantly high mutation rate than γ-rays.

There are many software tools which help to observe the bases variation; for instance, the method that determines whether a change occurs in an amino acid hampering codon is named conservation-based SIFT (sorting intolerant from tolerant) [258]. Taylor [259] described that any alternation of a gene can be detected by PARSESNP (for Project Aligned Related Sequences and Evaluate SNPs [260]; graphs show the changes in sequence by using precise co-segregating information, positioning of coding/and noncoding regions and reference DNA sequence.

12. Conclusions

Developing reliable markers, which will work in different populations and utilized in the breeding to enhance selection efficiency, is a very important step for breeding. Markers should allow desired genotype selection because of their tight linkage to the trait of interest. On the other hand, emerging technologies like high-throughput marker systems and marker-based selection methodologies have been developed, and are currently being used efficiently in cotton breeding. It is also promising that some economically important traits like fiber quality, yield, *Verticillium* wilt resistance, cotton leaf curl virus, drought tolerance, nematode resistance can be enhanced by using MAS. Genetic diversity can also be evaluated by using DNA markers before starting breeding program. Tremendous efforts have been carried for studying genetic diversity from genotypic and phenotypic aspects in germplasm accessions of cotton. Many

QTLs related to economical traits have been discovered. It is an emerging concern that efforts should be made for the utilization of molecular breeding methodologies to enhance cotton productivity, which can be enhanced through the recent developments in NGS. Moreover, highly saturated maps are useful for determining genetic manipulations from heredity perspectives, and SNPs are the best for this purpose. These markers along with QTLs provide innovative tools in the cotton genomics era.

Author details

Yuksel Bolek[1], Khezir Hayat[1], Adem Bardak[1*] and Muhammad Tehseen Azhar[2]

*Address all correspondence to: adembardak@ksu.edu.tr

1 Faculty of Agriculture, Agricultural Biotechnology Department, Kahramanmaras Sutcu Imam University, Kahramanmaras, Turkey

2 Department of Plant Breeding and Genetics, University of Agriculture, Faisalabad, Pakistan

References

[1] Edwards MD, Stuber CW, Wendel JF. Molecular-marker-facilitated investigations of quantitative-trait loci in maize. I. Numbers, genomic distribution and types of gene action. Genetics, 1987; 116: 113–125. PMCID: 1203110.

[2] Van Esbroeck GA, Bowman DT, Calhoun DS, May OL. Changes in the genetic diversity of cotton in the U.S. from 1970 to 1995. Crop Science, 1998; 38: 33–37. DOI: 10.2135/cropsci1998.0011183X003800010006x.

[3] Collins NC, Tardieu F, Tuberosa R. Quantitative trait loci and crop performance under abiotic stress: where do we stand? Plant Physiology, 2008; 147: 469–486. DOI: www.plantphysiology.org/cgi/doi/10.1104/pp.108.118117.

[4] Collard CYB, Mackill JD. Marker-assisted selection. An approach for precision plant breeding in the twenty-first century. Philosophical Transactions of the Royal Society B: Biological Sciences, 2008; 363: 557–572. DOI: 10.1098/rstb.2007.2170.

[5] Budak H, Bolek Y, Dokuyucu T, Akkaya VA. Potential uses of molecular markers in crop improvement. KSÜ Fen ve Mühendislik Dergisi. 2004; 7: 75–79.

[6] Kalivas A, Xanthopoulos F, Kehagia O, Tsaftaris AS. Agronomic characterization, genetic diversity and association analysis of cotton cultivars using simple sequence

repeat molecular markers. Genetics and Molecular Research, 2011; 10: 208–217. DOI: 10.4238/vol10-1gmr998.

[7] Zhang Y, Lin Z, Li W, Tu L, Nie Y, Zhang X. Studies of new EST-SSRs derived from *Gossypium barbadense*. Chinese Science Bulletin, 2007; 51, 2522–2531. DOI: 10.1007/s11434-007-0399-2.

[8] Available from: http://www.textileworld.com/textile-world/fiber-world/2015/10/icac-stable-world-cotton-trade-expected-in-2015-16/ [18-03-2016].

[9] Fryxell PA. A revised taxonomic interpretation of *Gossypium* L. (*Malvaceae*), Rheedea, 1992; 2: 108–165.

[10] Beasley JO. The production of polyploids in *Gossypium*. Journal of Heredity, 1940; 31: 39–48.

[11] Endrizzi J. Turcotte EL, Kohel RJ. Genetics, cytology and evolution of *Gossypium*. Advances in Genetics, 1985; 23: 271–375.

[12] Ortiz R. Biotechnology with horticultural and agronomic crops in Africa. Acta Horticulture. 2004; 642: 4356.

[13] Kumar LS. DNA markers in plant improvement: an overview. Biotechnology Advances, 1999; 17: 143–182. DOI: 10.1016/S0734-9750(98)00018-4.

[14] King RC, Stansfield WD. A Dictionary of Genetics. 4th ed. New York: Oxford University Press; 1990. p. 188.

[15] Schulmann AH. Molecular markers to assess genetic diversity. Euphytica, 2007; 158: 313–321. DOI: 10.1007/s10681-006-9282-5.

[16] Joshi C, Nguyen H. RAPD (random amplified polymorphic DNA) analysis based inter varietal genetic relationships among hexaploid wheats. Plant Science, 1993; 93: 95–103. .DOI: 10.1016/0168-9452(93)90038-2.

[17] Winter P, Kahl G. Molecular marker technologies for plant improvement. World Journal of Microbiology & Biotechnology, 1995; 11: 438–448. DOI: 10.1007/BF00364619.

[18] Jones CJ, Edwaeds KJ, Castaglione S, Winfield MO, Sela F, Van De Weil C, Bredemeijer G, Vosman B, Matthes M, Daly A, Brettschneider R, Bettni P, Buitti M, Maestri E, Malcevschi A, Marmiroli N, Aert R, Volckaert G, Rueda J, Linacero R, Vazquetz A, Karp A. Reproducibility testing of RAPD, AFLP and SSR markers in plants by a network of European laboratories. Molecular Breeding. 1997; 3: 381–390. DOI: 10.1023/A:1009612517139.

[19] Gupta PK, Balyan HS, Sharma PC, Ramesh B. Microsatellites in plants: a new class of molecular markers. Current Science, 1996; 70: 45–53.

[20] Roychowdhury R, Taoutaou A, Hakeem KR, Gawwad MRA, Tah J. Molecular marker-assisted technologies for crop improvement. In: Roychowdhury R, editor. Crop

Improvement in the Era of Climate Change. International Publishing House, India DOI: 10.13140/RG.2.1.2822.2560.

[21] Thottappilly G, Magonouna HD, Omitogun OG. The use of DNA markers for rapid improvement of crops in Africa. African Crop Science Journal. 2000; 8: 99–108.

[22] Aken JV. Marker-Assisted Selection: A Noninvasive Biotechnology Alternative to Genetic Engineering of Plant Varieties. AZ Amsterdam, The Netherlands: Greenpeace International Ottho Heldringstraat; 2009.

[23] Mohan M, Nair S, Bhagwat A, Krishna TG, Yano M, Bhatia CR, Sasaki T. Genome mapping, molecular markers and marker-assisted selection in crop plants. Molecular Breeding, 2012; *3*: 87–103. DOI: 10.1023/A:1009651919792.

[24] Francia E, Tacconi G, Crosatti C, Barabaschi D, Bulgarelli D, Dall AE, Vale G. Marker-assisted selection in crop plants. Plant Cell and Tissue Organ Culture, 2005; 82: 317–342. DOI: 10.1007/s11240-005-2387-z.

[25] Brumlop, Sarah, Finckh MR. Applications and potentials of marker-assisted selection (MAS) in plant breeding. Federal Agency for Nature Conservation Konstantinstrasse Bonn, Germany Bundesamt für Naturschutz (BfN); 2010. p. 31. URL: http://www.bfn.de.

[26] Crouch JH, Ortiz R. Applied genomics in the improvement of crops grown in Africa. African Journal of Biotechnology, 2004; 3: 489–496. DOI: 10.5897/AJB2004.000-2099.

[27] Hayashi K, Yoshida H, Ashikawa I. Development of PCR-based SNP markers for rice blast resistance genes at the Piz locus. Theoretical and Applied Genetics, 2004; 108: 1212–1280. DOI: 10.1007/s00122-003-1553-0.

[28] Jain SM, Brar DS, Ahloowalia BS. Molecular Techniques in Crop Improvement. 2nd ed. Dordrecht, The Netherlands: Kluwer Academic Publishers: 2002. p. 772.

[29] Kumpatla SP, Buyyarapu R, Abdurakhmonov IY, Mammadov JA. In: Ibrokhim IY, editor. Genomics-Assisted Plant Breeding in the 21st Century: Technological Advances and Progress. Croatia: In Tech. Plant Breeding; 2012;.

[30] Gupta PK, Kumar J, Mir RR, Kumar A. Marker-assisted selection as a component of conventional plant breeding. Plant Breeding Reviews, 2010; 33, 145–217.

[31] Helentjaris T, Slocum M, Wright S, Schaefer A, Nienhuis J. Construction of genetic linkage maps in maize and tomato using restriction fragment length polymorphisms. Theoretical and Applied Genetics, 1986; 61: 650–658. DOI: http://dx.doi.org/10.1155/2014/607091.

[32] Welsh J, McClelland M. Fingerprinting genomes using PCR with arbitrary primers. Nucleic Acids Research, 1990; 18: 7213–7218.

[33] Vos P, Hogers R, Bleeker M, Reijans M, Van DLT, Hornes M et al. AFLP: a new technique for DNA fingerprinting. Nucleic Acids Research, 1995; 23: 4407–4414.

[34] Semagn K, Bjornstad A, Ndjiondjop MN. An overview of molecular marker methods for plants. African Journal of Biotechnology, 2006; 5, 2540–256.

[35] Lam HM, Xu X, Liu X, Chen W, Yang G, Wong FL, et al. Resequencing of 31 wild and cultivated soybean genomes identifies patterns of genetic diversity and selection. Nature Genetics, 2010; 42: 1053–1059. DOI:10.1038/ng.715.

[36] Singh H, Deshmukh RK, Singh A, Singh AK, Gaikwad K. Highly variable SSR markers suitable for rice genotyping using agarose gels. Molecular Breeding, 2010; 25: 359–364. DOI: 10.1007/s11032-009-9328.

[37] Sonah H, Deshmukh RK, Singh VP, Gupta DK, Singh NK, Sharma TR. Genomic resources in horticultural crops: status, utility and challenges. Biotechnology Advances, 2011; 29, 199–209. DOI: 10.1016/j.biotechadv.2010.11.002.

[38] Conaway C, Cartinhour S, Ayres N, McClung AM, Lai XH, Marchetti MA, Park WD. PCR based markers linked to blast resistance genes in rice. In: Proceedings of the 27th Rice Technical Working Group Meeting, Reno-Sparks, NV, USA, 1–4 March 1998. p. 77.

[39] Koebner RMD, Summers RW. 21st century wheat breeding: plot selection or plate detection? Trends in Biotechnology, 2003; 21: 59–63. DOI: 10.1016/S0167-7799(02)00036-7.

[40] Stuber CW, Polacco M, Senior ML. Synergy of empirical breeding, marker-assisted selection, and genomics to increase crop yield potential. Crop Science, 1999; 39: 1571–1583. DOI: 10.2135/cropsci1999.3961571x.

[41] Tuberosa R, Salvi S, Sanguineti MC, Maccaferri M, Giuliani S, Landi P. Searching for QTLs controlling root traits in maize: a critical appraisal. Plant and Soil, 2003; 255: 35–54. DOI: 10.1023/A:1026146615248.

[42] Thomas W. Prospects for molecular breeding of barley. Annals of Applied Biology, 2003; 142: 1–12. DOI: 10.1111/j.1744-7348.2003.tb00223.x.

[43] Williams KJ. The molecular genetics of disease resistance in barley. Australian Journal of Agricultural Research 2003; 54: 1065–1079. DOI: 10.1071/AR02219. 0004-9409/03/111065.

[44] Iqbal MJ, Reddy OUK, El-Zik KM, Pepper AE. A genetic bottleneck in the evolution under domestication of upland cotton *Gossypium hirsutum* L. examined using DNA fingerprinting. Theoretical and Applied Genetics, 2001; 103: 547–554. DOI: 10.1007/PL00002908.

[45] Rahman M, Asif M, Ullah I, Malik KA, Zafar Y. Overview of cotton genomic studies in Pakistan. Plant & Animal Genome Conference XIII. San Diego, 2005, CA, USA.

[46] Abdurakhmonov IY, Kohel RJ, Yu JZ, Pepper AE, Abdullaev AA, Kushanov FN, Salakhutdinov IB, Buriev ZT, Saha S, Scheffler BE, Jenkins JN, Abdukarimov A.

Molecular diversity and association mapping of fibre quality traits in exotic *G. hirsutum* L. germplasm. Genomics, 2008; 92: 478–487. DOI: 10.1016/j.ygeno.2008.07.013.

[47] Zehr UB, editor, Cotton, Biotechnology in Agriculture and Forestry. Heidelberg: Springer-Verlag; 2012. DOI: 10.1007/978-3-642-04796-1_5.

[48] Percy RG, Kohel RJ. Qualitative genetics. In: Smith CW, Cothren JT, editors. Cotton. Origin, History, Technology, and Production. New York: John Wiley & Sons; 1999. p. 319–360.

[49] Arshad M, Sajjad H. Molecular marker technology for cotton plant improvement. ICAC, 2002; March 8–13.

[50] Joshi SP, Prabhakar K, Ranjekar PK, Gupta VS. Molecular markers in plant genome analysis. http/www.ias.ac.in/currsci/jul25/articles 15.htm; 2011. p. 1–19.

[51] Saha S, Karaca M, Jenkins JN, Zipf AE, Reddy UK, Kantey RV. Simple sequence repeats as useful resources to study transcribed genes of cotton. Euphytica, 2003; 130: 355–364. 51. DOI: 10.1023/A:1023077209170.

[52] Sun FD, Zhang JH, Wang SF, Gong WK, Shi YZ, Liu AY, Li JW, Gong JW, Shang HH, Yuan YL. QTL mapping for fiber quality traits across multiple generations and environments in upland cotton. Molecular Breeding, 2012; 30: 569–582. DOI: 10.1007/s11032-011-9645-z.

[53] Aslam U, Khan AA, Cheema HMN, F. Imtiaz, Malik W. Kill curve analysis and response of ethyl methanesulfonate and γ-rays in diploid and tetraploid cotton. International Journal of Agricultural and Biological Engineering, 2013; 15: 11–18. DOI: 12–724/2013/15–1–11–18.

[54] Lee M. DNA markers and plant breeding programs. Advances in Agronomy, 1995; 55: 265–344. DOI: 10.1016/s0065-2113(08)60542-8.

[55] Elshire RJ, Glaubitz JC, Sun Q, Poland JA, Kawamoto K, Buckler ES, Mitchell SE. A robust, simple genotyping-by-sequencing (GBS) approach for high diversity species. PLoS One 2011; 6: e19379. DOI: 10.1371/journal.pone.0019379.

[56] Ribaut JM, Hoisington D. Marker-assisted selection: new tools and strategies. Trends in Plant Science, 1998; 3: 236–238.

[57] Bolek Y, El-Zik KM, Pepper AE, Bell AA, Magill CW, Thaxton PM, Reddy OK. Mapping of *Verticillium* wilt resistance genes in cotton. Plant Science, 2005; 168: 1581–1590. DOI: 10.1016/j.plantsci.2005.02.008.

[58] CottonGeN [internet]. 2016. Available from: https://www.cottongen.org. [Accessed 2016-03-08]

[59] Tanksley SD, Young ND, Paterson AH, Bonierbale MW. RFLP mapping in plant breeding: new tools for an old science. Biotechnology, 1989; 7: 257–264. DOI: 10.1038/nbt0389-257.

[60] Paterson AH. Molecular Dissection of Complex Traits. CRC Press (Taylor & Francis Group) UK; 1997. ISBN 9780849376863. CAT# 7686.

[61] Abdurakhmonov IY, Buriev ZT, Shermatov SE, et al. Marker-assisted selection for complex fiber traits in cotton. 5th World Cotton Research Conference, Special session of ICGI, Mumbai, India; 2011, 7–12 November 2011.

[62] Voss-Fels K, Snowdon RJ. Understanding and utilizing crop genome diversity via high-resolution genotyping. Plant Biotechnology, Journal, 2015. DOI: 10.1111/pbi.12456.

[63] Wang S, Chen† J, Zhang W, Hu Y, Chang L, Fang L, Wang Q, Lv F, Wu H, Si H, et al. Sequence-based ultra-dense genetic and physical maps reveal structural variations of allopolyploid cotton genomes. Genome Biology, 2015; 16: 108. DOI: 10.1186/s13059-015-0678-1.

[64] Qin H, Chen M, Yi X, Bie S, Zhang C, Zhang Y, Lan J, Meng Y, Yuan Y, Jiao C. Identification of associated SSR markers for yield component and fiber quality traits based on frame map and upland cotton collections. PLoS One, 2015; 10: e0118073. DOI: 10.1371/journal.pone.0118073.

[65] Thornsberry JM, Goodman MM, Doebley J, Kresovich S, Nielsen D, Buckler ES. Dwarf8 polymorphisms associate with variation in flowering time. Nature Genetics, 2001; 28: 286–289. DOI: 10.1038/90135.

[66] Paterson, AH. Making genetic maps. In: Genome Mapping in Plants (Biotechnology Intelligence Unit). San Diego, CA: Academic Press; 1996. p. 23–39.

[67] Collard BCY, Jahufer MZZ, Brouwer JB, Pang ECK. An introduction to markers, quantitative trait loci (QTL) mapping and marker-assisted selection for crop improvement: the basic concepts. Euphytica, 2005; 142: 169–196. DOI: 10.1007/s10681-005-1681-5.

[68] Reinisch AJ, Dong JM, Brubaker CL, Stelly DM, Wendel JF, Paterson AH. A detailed RFLP map of cotton, *Gossypium hirsutum* × *Gossypium barbadense*: chromosome organization and evolution in a disomic polyploid genome. Genetics, 1994; 138: 829–847. PMCID: PMC1206231.

[69] Yu J, Zhang K, Li S, Yu S, Zhai M, Wu X, Li S, et al. Mapping quantitative trait loci for lint yield and fiber quality across environments in a *Gossypium hirsutum* × *Gossypium barbadense* backcross inbred line population. Theoretical and Applied Genetics, 2013; 126: 275–287. DOI: 10.1007/s00122-012-1980-x.

[70] Altaf J, Stewart McD, Wajahatullah MK, Zhang J. Molecular and morphological genetics of a trispecies F_2 population of cotton. Proceedings of the Beltwide Cotton Conference, 1997; 1: 448–452, National Cotton Council, Memphis, TN.

[71] Jiang CX, Wright RJ, El-Zik KM, Paterson AH. Polyploid formation created unique avenues for response to selection in *Gossypium* (cotton). Proceedings of the National

Academy of Sciences of the United States of America, 1998; 95: 4419–4424. DOI: 10.1073/pnas.95.8.4419.

[72] Shappley ZW, Jenkins JN, Meredith WR, McCarty JC. 1998. An RFLP linkage map of upland cotton (*Gossypium hirsutum* L.). Theoretical and Applied Genetics, 97: 756–761. DOI: 10.1007/s001220050952.

[73] Khan MA, Zhang J, Stewart MCDJ. Integrated molecular map based on a trispecific F_2 population on cotton. In: Herber DJ, Richter DA, editors. Proceedings of Beltwide Cotton Improvement Conference; 1998, San Diego, CA. p. 491–492.

[74] Khan MA, Stewart JMCD, Zhang J, Myers GO, Cantrell RG. Addition of new markers to trispecific cotton map. In: Proceedings of Beltwide Cotton Conference; 1999. p. 439.

[75] Ulloa M, Meredith WR. Genetic linkage map and QTL analysis of agronomic and fiber quality traits in an intraspecific population. Journal Cotton Science, 2000; 4: 161–170.

[76] Lacape JM, Nguyen TB, Thibivilliers S, Bojinov B, Courtois B, Cantrell RG, Burr B, Hau B. A combined RFLP-SSR-AFLP map of tetraploid cotton based on a *Gossypium hirsutum* × *Gossypium barbadense* backcross population. Genome, 2003; 46: 612–626. DOI: 10.1139/g03-050.

[77] Han Z, Guo W, Song X, Zhang T Genetic mapping of EST derived microsatellites from the diploid *Gossypium arboreum* in allotetraploid cotton. Molecular Genetics and Genomics, 2004; 272: 308–327. DOI: 10.1007/s00438-004-1059-8.

[78] Mei M, Syed NH, Gao W, Thaxton PM, Smith CW, Stelly DM, Chen ZJ. Genetic mapping and QTL analysis of fiber related traits in cotton. Theoretical and Applied Genetics, 2004; 108: 280–291. DOI: 10.1007/s00122-003-1433-7.

[79] Liu S, Saha S, Stelly D, Burr B, Cantrell RG. Chromosomal assignment of microsatellite loci in cotton. Journal of Heredity, 2000; 91: 326-332. DOI: 10.1093/jhered/91.4.326.

[80] Nguyen TB, Giband M, Brottier P, Risterucci AM, Lascape JM. Wide coverage of the tetraploid cotton genome using newly developed microsatellite markers. Theoretical and Applied Genetics, 2004; 109: 167–175. DOI: 10.1007/s00122-004-1612-1.

[81] Wang FR, Gong YC, Zhang CY, Liu GD, et al. Genetic effects of introgression genomic components from Sea Island cotton (*Gossypium barbadense* L.) on fiber related traits in upland cotton (*G. hirsutum* L.). Euphytica, 2011; 181: 41–53. DOI: 10.1007/s10681-011-0378-1.

[82] Lin Z, He D, Zhang X, Nie Y, Guo X, Feng C, Stewart JMCD. Linkage map construction and mapping QTL to cotton fibre quality using SRAP, SSR and RAPD. Plant Breeding, 2005; 124: 180–187. DOI: 10.1111/j.1439-0523.2004.01039.x.

[83] Park YH, Alabady MS, Ulloa M, Sickler B, Wilkins TA, Yu J, Stelly D, Kohel RJ, El-Shiny OM, Cantrell RG. Genetic mapping of new cotton fibre loci using EST-derived micro-

satellites in an interspecific recombinant inbred (RIL) cotton population. Molecular Genetics and Genomics, 2005; 274: 428–441. DOI: 10.1007/s00438-005-0037-0.

[84] Babar M, Saranga Y, Iqbal Z, Arif M, Zafar Y, Lubbers E, Chee P. Identification of QTLs and impact of selection from various environments (dry vs irrigated) on the genetic relationships among the selected cotton lines from F6 population using a phylogenetic approach. African Journal of Biotechnology, 2009; 8: 4802–4810. DOI: 10.4314/ajb.v8i19.65170.

[85] Saleem MA, Malik TA., Shakeel A, Ashraf M. QTL mapping for some important drought tolerant traits in upland cotton. The Journal of Animal & Plant Science, 2015; 25: 502–509.

[86] Shen X, Guo W, Zhu X, Yuan Y, Yu JZ, Kohel RJ, Zhang T. Molecular mapping of QTLs for qualities in three diverse lines in upland cotton using SSR markers. Molecular Breeding, 2005; 15: 169–181. DOI: 10.1007/s11032-004-4731-0.

[87] He DH, Lin ZX, Zhang XL, Nie YC, Guo XP, Zhang YX, Li W. QTL mapping for economic traits based on a dense genetic map of cotton with PCR-based markers using the interspecific cross of *Gossypium hirsutum* vs *Gossypium barbadense*. Euphytica, 2007; 153: 181–197. DOI: 10.1007/s10681-006-9254-9.

[88] Abdurakhmonov IY, Buriev ZT, Saha S, Pepper AE, Musaev JA, Almatov A, Shermatov, SE, Kushanov FN, Mavlonov GT, Reddy, UK, Yu JZ, Jenkins, JN, Kohel RJ, Abdukarimov A. Microsatellite markers associated with lint percentage trait in cotton, *Gossypium hirsutum*. Euphytica, 2007; 156: 141–156. DOI: 10.1007/s10681-007-9361-2.

[89] Ynturi P, Jenkins JN, McCarty JC, Gutierrez OA, Saha S. Association of root-knot nematode resistance genes with simple sequence repeat markers on two chromosomes in cotton. Crop Science, 2006; 46: 2670–2674. DOI: 10.2135/cropsci2006.05.0319.

[90] Song XL, Wang K, Guo WZ, Han ZG, Zhang TZ. Quantitative trait loci mapping of leaf morphological traits and chlorophyll content in cultivated tetraploid cotton. Acta Botanica Sinica, 2005; 47: 13821390. DOI: 10.1139/g04-126.

[91] Rungis D, Llewellyn D, Dennis ES, Lyon BR. Investigation of the chromosomal location of the bacterial blight resistance gene present in an Australian cotton (*Gossypium hirsutum* L.) cultivar. Australian Journal of Agricultural Research, 2005; 53: 551–560. DOI: 10.1071/ar04190.

[92] Shen XL, Van Becelaere G, Kumar P, Davis RF, May OL, Chee P. QTL mapping for resistance to root-knot nematodes in the M-120 RNR Upland cotton line (*Gossypium hirsutum* L.) of the Auburn 623 RNR source. Theoretical and Applied Genetics, 2006; 113: 1539–1549. DOI: 10.1007/s00122-006-0401-4.

[93] Wang C, Ulloa M, Roberts PA. Identification and mapping of microsatellite markers linked to a root-knot nematode resistance gene (rkn1) in Acala NemX cotton (*Gossypium*

hirsutum L.). Theoretical and Applied Genetics, 2006; 112: 770–777. DOI: 10.1007/s00122-005-0183-0.

[94] Niu C, Hinchliffe DJ, Cantrell RG, Wang CL, Roberts PA, Zhang JF. Identification of molecular markers associated with rootknot nematode resistance in upland cotton. Crop Science, 2007; 47: 951–960. DOI: 10.2135/cropsci2006.07.0499.

[95] Rahman M, Hussain D, Malik TA, Zafar Y. Genetics of resistance to cotton leaf curl disease in *Gossypium hirsutum*. Plant Pathology, 2005; 54: 764–772. DOI: 10.1111/j.1365-3059.2005.01280.x.

[96] Rahman M, Ahmed N, Asif M, Zafar Y. Identification of DNA markers linked with cotton leaf curl disease (CLCD). International Cotton Genome Initiative (ICGI) Workshop, 2006; Brasilia, Brazil. p. 77–78.

[97] Lacape JM, Jacobs J, Arioli T, Derijcker R, Forestier N, Chiron D, Llewellyn, Jean J, Thomas E, Viot C. A new interspecific, *Gossypium hirsutum* × *G. barbadense*, RIL population: towards a unified consensus linkage map of tetraploid cotton. Theoretical and Applied Genetics, 2009; 119: 281–292. DOI: 10.1007/s00122-009-1037-y.

[98] Jubrael J, Udupa S, Baum M. Assessment of AFLP-based genetic relationships among date palm (*Phoenix Dactylifera* L.) varieties of Iraq. Journal of the American Society for Horticultural Science, 2005; 130: 442–447.

[99] Andersen JR, Lubberstedt T. Functional markers in plants. Trends in Plant Science, 2003; 8: 554–560. DOI: 10.1016/j.tplants.2003.09.010.

[100] Kalia RK, Rai MK, Kalia S, Singh R, Dhawan AK. Microsatellite markers: an overview of the recent progress in plants. Euphytica, 2011; 177: 309–334. DOI: 10.1007/s10681-010-0286-9.

[101] Weising K, Nybom H, Wolff K, Kahl G. DNA fingerprinting in plants: Principles, Methods and Applications. 2nd ed. Boca Raton, FL: CRC Press, Taylor & Francis Group; 2005.

[102] Gupta P, Varshney R, Sharma P, Ramesh B. Molecular markers and their applications in wheat breeding. Plant Breeding, 1999; 118: 369–390. DOI: 10.1046/j.1439-0523.1999.00401.x.

[103] Kumar P, Gupta VK, Misra AK, Modi DR, Pandey BK. Potential of molecular markers in plant biotechnology. Plant Omics Journal, 2009; 2: 141–162.

[104] Liu ZJ, Cordes JF. DNA marker technologies and their applications in aquaculture genetics. Aquaculture, 2004; 238: 1–37. DOI:10.1016/j.aquaculture.2004.05.027.

[105] Brubaker CL, Wendel JF. Reevaluating the origin of domesticated cotton (*Gossypium hirsutum*; Malvaceae) using nuclear restriction fragment length polymorphisms (RFLPs). American Journal of Botany, 1994; 81: 1309–1326. DOI: 10.2307/2445407.

[106] Wright RJ, Thaxton PM, El-Zik KM, Paterson AH. D-subgenome bias of Xcm resistance genes in tetraploid *Gossypium* (cotton) suggests that polyploid formation has created novel avenues for evolution. Genetics, 1998; 149: 1987–1996. PMID: 9691052.

[107] Karp A, Edwards KJ. DNA markers: a global overview. In: Caetano Anolles G, Gresshoff PM, editors. DNA Markers: Protocols, Applications, and Overviews. Wiley-Liss, Inc. USA; 1997. 364 p.

[108] Ulloa M, Meredith JWR, Shappley ZW, Kahler AL. RFLP genetic linkage maps from four $F_{2.3}$ populations and a joinmap of *Gossypium hirsutum* L. Theoretical and Applied Genetics, 2002; 104: 200–208. http://naldc.nal.usda.gov/download/12760/PDF.

[109] Caeteno-Annolas. MAAP: a versatile and universal tool for genome analysis. Plant Molecular Biology, 1994; 25: 1011–1026.

[110] Ulloa M, Saha S, Jenkins JN, Meredith WRJ, JC Mccarty JR, Stelly DM. Chromosomal assignment of RFLP linkage groups harboring important QTLs on an intraspecific cotton (*Gossypium hirsutum* L.) joinmap. Journal of Heredity, 2005; 96: 132–144. DOI: 10.1093/jhered/esi020.

[111] Khan SA, Hussain D, Askari E, Stewart JMcD, Malik KA. Zafar Y. Molecular phylogeny of *Gossypium* species by DNA fingerprinting. Theoretical and Applied Genetics, 2000; 101: 931–938. DOI: 10.1007/s001220051564.

[112] Rahman M, Hussain D, Zafar Y. Estimation of genetic divergence among elite cotton (*Gossypium hirsutum* L.) cultivars/genotypes by DNA fingerprinting technology. Crop Science, 2002; 42: 2137–2144. DOI: 10.2135/cropsci2002.2137.

[113] Preetha S, Raveendren TS. Molecular marker technology in cotton. Biotechnology and Molecular Biology Review, 2008; 3: 32–45.

[114] Bardak A. Mapping of genes related to fiber and fuzz formation in cotton (*G. hirsutum* L.) genome and QTL analysis. Ph.D. Thesis. Department of Field Crops, March 2012. p. 141.

[115] Badigannavar A, Myers GO, Jones DC. Molecular diversity revealed by AFLP markers in upland cotton genotypes. Journal of Crop Improvement, 2012; 26: 627–640. DOI: 10.1080/15427528.2012.664614.

[116] Essenberg M, Bayles MB, Samad RA, Hall JA, Brinkerhoff LA, Verhalen MA. Four near-isogenic lines of cotton with different genes for bacterial blight resistance. Phytopathology, 2002; 92: 1323–1328. DOI: 10.1094/PHYTO.2002.92.12.1323.

[117] Li C, Wang X, Dong N, Zhao H, Xia Z, Wang R, Converse RL. Wang Q. QTL analysis for early-maturing traits in cotton using two upland cotton (*Gossypium hirsutum* L.) crosses. Breeding Science, 2013; 63: 154–163. DOI: 10.1270/jsbbs.63.154.

[118] Xiao J, Wu K, Fang DD, Stelly DM, Yu J, Cantrell RG. New SSR markers for use in cotton (*Gossypium* spp.) improvement. Journal of Cotton Science, 2009; 13: 75–157.

[119] Qureshi SN, Saha S, Kantety RV, Jenkins JN, Saha S. Molecular biology and physiology: EST-SSR: a new class of genetic markers in cotton. Journal of Cotton Science, 2004; 8: 112–123.

[120] Reddy MP, Sarla N, Siddiq EA. Inter simple sequence repeat (ISSR) polymorphism and its application in plant breeding. Euphytica, 2002; 128: 9–17. DOI: 10.1023/A: 1020691618797.

[121] Bornet B, Muller C, Paulus F, Branchard ML. Highly informative nature of inter simple sequence repeat (ISSR) sequences amplified using tri and tetra-nucleotide primers from DNA of cauliflower (*Brassica oleracea* var. botrytis L.). Genome, 2002; 45: 890–896. DOI: 10.1139/g02-061.

[122] Russell JR, Fuller JD, Macaulay M, Hatz BG, Jahoor A, et al. Direct comparison of levels of genetic variation among barley accessions detected by RFLPs, AFLPs, SSRs and RAPDs. Theoretical and Applied Genetics, 1997; 95: 714–722. DOI: 10.1007/ s001220050617.

[123] Altaf MK, Stewart JM, Wajahatullah MK, Zhang JF. Molecular and morphological genetics of a trispecies F_2 population of cotton. In: Dugger P, Richter DA, editors. Proceedings of the Beltwide Cotton Production Research Conferences. National Cotton Council of America, Memphis, TN. Animal Genome VI, January 18–22; 1998. San Diego, California, USA; 1997. p. 448–452.

[124] Wu J, Jenkins JN, McCarty JC, Zhong M. AFLP marker associations with agronomic and fiber traits in cotton. Euphytica, 2007; 153: 153–163. DOI: 10.1007/s10681-006-9250-0.

[125] Hawkins J, Pleasants, Wendel JF. Identification of AFLP markers that discriminate between cultivated cotton and the Hawaiian island endemic, *Gossypium tomentosum* Nuttall ex Seeman. Genetic Resources and Crop Evolution, 2005; 52: 1069–1078. DOI: 10.1007/s10722-004-6115-z.

[126] Bardakci F. Random amplified polymorphic DNA (RAPD) markers. Turkish Journal of Biology, 2001; *25*: 185–196.

[127] Lee SW, Thomas F, Ledig, Johnson DR. Genetic variation at allozyme and RAPD markers in *Pinus longaeva* (Pinaceae) of the White Mountains, California. American Journal of Botany, 2002; 89: 566–577. PMID: 21665657.

[128] Khanam S, Sham A, Bennetzen JL, Aly MAM. Analysis of molecular marker-based characterization and genetic variation in date palm (*Phoenix dactylifera* L.). AJCS, 2012; 6: 1236–1244.

[129] Tian J, Deng Z, Zhang K, Yu H, Jiang X, Li C. Genetic Analyses of Wheat and Molecular Marker-Assisted Breeding, Volume 1, © Science Press, Beijing and Springer Science+Business Media Dordrecht; 2015. DOI: 10.1007/978-94-017-7390-4_2.

[130] Lan TH, Cook CG, Paterson AH. Identification of a RAPD marker linked to male fertility restoration gene in cotton (*Gossypium hirsutum* L.). Journal of Agricultural Genomics, 1999; 1: 1–5.

[131] Geng CD, Gong ZZ, Huang JQ, Zhang ZC. Identification of difference between cotton cultivars (*G. hirsutum*) using the RAPD method. Jiangsu Journal of Agricultural Science, 1995; 11: 21–24.

[132] Zahra N, Shojaei-Jesvaghani F, Sheidai M, Farahani F, Omran A, Inter simple sequence repeats (ISSR) and random amplified polymorphic DNA (RAPD) analyses of genetic diversity in Mehr cotton cultivar and its crossing progenies. African Journal of Biotechnology, 2011; 10: 11839–11847. DOI: 10.1371/journal.pbio.0030038.

[133] Farzaneh T, et al. Cytogenetic and RAPD analysis of cotton cultivars and their F_1 progenies. Caryologia, 2010; 63: 73–81. DOI: 10.1080/00087114.2010.10589710.

[134] Noormohammadi Z, Shojaei-Jeshvaghani F, Sheidai M, Farahani F, et al. ISSR and RAPD analysis of genetic diversity in Mehr cotton cultivar and its crossing progenies. African Journal of Biotechnology, 2011; 10: 11839–11847. DOI: 10.5897/AJB11.1377.

[135] Noormohammadi Z, Farahani Y, Sheidai HAM, Ghasemzadeh-Baraki S, Alishah O. Genetic diversity analysis in Opal cotton hybrids based on SSR, ISSR, and RAPD markers. Genetics and Molecular Research, 2013; 12: 256–269. DOI: 10.4238/2013.January.30.12.

[136] Ulloa M, Abdurakhmonov IY, Claudia PM, Percy R, Stewart McDJ. Genetic diversity and population structure of cotton (*Gossypium* spp.) of the New World assessed by SSR markers. Botany, 2013; 91: 251–259. DOI: 10.1139/cjb-2012-0192.

[137] Wolff K, Schoen ED, Peters-Van RJ. Optimizing the generation of random amplified polymorphic DNA in chrysanthemum. Theoretical and Applied Genetics, 1993; 86: 1033–1037. DOI: 10.1007/BF00211058.

[138] Liu ZJ, Cordes JF. DNA marker technologies and their applications in aquaculture genetics. Aquaculture, 2004. DOI:10.1016/j.aquaculture.2004.05.027

[139] Singh PK, Sharma H, Srivastava N, Bhagyawant SS. Analysis of genetic diversity among wild and cultivated chickpea genotypes employing ISSR and RAPD markers. American Journal of Plant Sciences, 2014; 5: 676–682. DOI: http://dx.doi.org/10.4236/ajps.2014.55082.

[140] Mishra KK, Fougat RS, Ballani A, Thakur Vinita, Yachana J. Madhumat B. Potential and application of molecular markers techniques for plant genome analysis. International Journal of Pure & Applied Bioscience, 2014; 2: 169–188.

[141] Bornet B, Branchard M. Non-anchored inter simple sequence repeat (ISSR) markers: reproducible and specific tools for genome fingerprinting. Plant Molecular Biology Reporter, 2001; 19: 209–215. DOI: 10.1007/BF02772892.

[142] Parkhyia S, Gohel K, Mehta DDR. Genetic diversity analysis of cotton (*G. hirsutum* L.) genotypes using ISSR markers. IJAPSA, 2014; 1: 7–19.

[143] Gupta M, Chyi YS, Romero-Severson J, Owen JL. Amplification of DNA markers from evolutionarily diverse genomes using single primers of simple sequence repeats. Theoretical and Applied Genetics, 1994; 89: 998–1006. DOI: 10.1007/BF00224530.

[144] Tsumura Y, Ohba K, Strauss SH. Diversity and inheritance of inter-simple sequence repeat polymorphisms in Douglas fir (*Pseudotsuga menziesii*) and sugi (*Cryptomeria japonica*). Theoretical and Applied Genetics, 1996; 92: 40–45. DOI: 10.1007/BF00222949.

[145] Liu B, Wendel JF. Intersimple sequence repeat (ISSR) polymorphisms as a genetic marker system in cotton. Molecular Ecology Notes, 2001; 1: 205–208. DOI: 10.1046/j. 1471-8278.2001.00073.x.

[146] Wang G, Mahalingan R, Knap HT. (C-A) and (GA) anchored simple sequence repeats (ASSRs) generated polymorphism in soybean, *Glycine max* (L.) Merr. Theoretical and Applied Genetics, 1998; 96: 1086–1096. DOI: 10.1007/s001220050843.

[147] Paran I, Michelmore RW. Development of reliable PCR based markers linked to downy mildew resistance genes in lettuce. Theoretical and Applied Genetics, 1993; 85: 985–993. DOI: 10.1007/BF00215038.

[148] Dnyaneshwar W, Preeti C, Joshi K, Patwardhan B. Development and application of RAPD-SCAR marker for identification of *Phyllanthus emblica* Linn. Biological and Pharmaceutical Bulletin, 2006; 2911: 2313–2316. DOI: 10.1248/bpb.29.2313.

[149] Li SF, Tang SJ, Cai, WQ. RAPD-SCAR markers for genetically improved NEW GIFT Nile Tilapia (*Oreochrmis niloticus niloticus* L.) and their application in strain identification. Zoological Research, 2010; 31: 147–153. DOI: 10.3724/SP.J.1141.2010.02147.

[150] Rajesh MK, Jerard BA, Preethi P, Thomas RJ, Fayas TP, Rachana KE, Karun A. Development of a RAPD-derived SCAR marker associated with tall-type palm trait in coconut. Scientia Horticulturae, 2013; 150: 312–316. DOI: 10.1016/j.scienta.2012.11.023.

[151] Kumla S, Doolgindachbaporn S, Sudmoon R, Sattayasai N. Genetic variation, population structure and identification of yellow catfish, *Mystus nemurus* (C&V) in Thailand using RAPD, ISSR and SCAR marker. Molecular Biology Reports, 2012; *39*: 5201–5210. DOI: 10.1007/s11033-011-1317-x.

[152] Guo W, Zhang T, Shen X, Yu ZJ, Kohel RJ. Development of SCAR marker linked to a major QTL for high fiber strength and its usage in molecular-marker-assisted selection in Upland cotton. Crop Science, 2003; 43: 2252–2256. DOI: 10.2135/cropsci2003.2252.

[153] Jiang C, Wright RJ, Woo SS, DelMonte TA, Paterson AH. QTL analysis of leaf morphology in tetraploid *Gossypium* (cotton). Theoretical and Applied Genetics, 2000; 100: 409–418.

[154] Olsen M, Hood L, Cantor C, Botstein D. A common language for physical mapping of the human genome. Science, 1989; 245: 1434–1435. DOI: 10.1126/science.2781285.

[155] Feng CD, Stewart JMc, Zhang JF. STS markers linked to the Rf 1 fertility restorer gene of cotton. Theoretical and Applied Genetics, 2005; 110: 237–243. DOI: 10.1007/s00122-004-1817-3.

[156] Rong J, Abbey C, Bowers JE, Brubaker CL, Chang C, Chee PW, Delmonte TA, Ding X, Garza JJ, Marler BS, et al. A 3347-locus genetic recombination map of sequence tagged sites reveals features of genome organization, transmission and evolution of cotton (*Gossypium*). Genetics, 2004; 166: 389–417. DOI: 10.1534/genetics.166.1.389.

[157] Vos P, Hogers R, Bleeker M, Reijans M, Lee van de T, Hornes M, Frijters A, Pot J, Peleman J, Kuiper M, Zabeau M. AFLP: a new technique for DNA fingerprinting. Nucleic Acids Research, 1995; 23: 4407–4414. PMCID: PMC307397.

[158] Akkaya MS, Bhagwat AA, Cregan PB. Length polymorphisms of simple sequence repeat DNA in soybean. Genetics, 1992; 132: 1131–1139. PMCID: PMC1205234.

[159] Roder MS, Korzun V, Wendehake K, Plaschke J, Tixier MH, Leroy P, Ganal MW. A microsatellite map of wheat. Genetics, 1998; 149: 2007–2023. PMCID: PMC1460256.

[160] Gupta PK, Varshney RK. The development and use of microsatellite markers for genetic analysis and plant breeding with emphasis on bread wheat. Euphytica, 2000; 113: 163–185. DOI: 10.1023/A:1003910819967.

[161] Jarne P, Lagoda PJL. Microsatellites, from molecules to populations and back. Trends in Ecology & Evolution, 1996; 11: 424–429. DOI: 10.1016/0169-5347(96)10049-5.

[162] Abdurakhmonov IY, Abdullaev AA, Saha S, Buriev ZT, Arslanov D, Kuryazov Z, Mavlonov GT, Rizaeva SM, Reddy UK, Jenkins JN, Abdullaev A, Abdukarimov A. Simple sequence repeat marker associated with a natural leaf defoliation trait in tetraploid cotton. Journal of Heredity, 2005; 96: 644–653. DOI: 10.1093/jhered/esi097.

[163] Bardak A, Bolek Y. Genetic diversity of diploid and tetraploid cottons determined by SSR and ISSR markers. Turkish Journal of Field Crops, 2012; 17: 139–144.

[164] Abdurakhmonov IY, Buriev ZT, Shermatov SE, Kushanov FN, Makamov A, Shopulatov U, Turaev O, Norov T, Akhmedov C, Mirzaakhmedov M, Abdukarimov A. Utilization of natural diversity in Upland cotton (*G. hirsutum*) germplasm collection for pyramiding genes via marker-assisted selection program. In: 5th Meeting of the Asian Cotton Research and Development Network. February 23–25, 2011.

[165] Chee P, Draye X, Jiang CX, Decanini L, Delmonte TA, Bredhauer R, Smith CW, Paterson AH. Molecular dissection of interspecific variation between *Gossypium hirsutum* and *Gossypium barbadense* (cotton) by a backcross-self approach. I. Fiber elongation. Theoretical and Applied Genetics, 2005; 111: 757–763. DOI: 10.1007/s00122-005-2063-z.

[166] Mumtaz H. Identification of structural and functional genomic markers for fiber quality traits in cotton using interspecific population (*G. hirsutum* × *G. barbadense*). MPhil Thesis; 2007; QA University, Islamabad, Pakistan,

[167] Frelichowski JM, Palmer MB, Main D, Tomkins JP, Cantrell RG, Stelly DM, et al. Cotton genome mapping with new microsatellites from Acala 'Maxa' BAC-ends. Molecular Genetics and Genomics, 2006; 275: 479–491. DOI: 10.1007/s00438006-0106-z.

[168] Abdalla M, Reddy OUK, Ei-Zik KM, Pepper AE. Genetic diversity and relationships of diploid and tetraploid cotton. Theoretical and Applied Genetics, 2001; 6: 222–229. DOI: 10.1007/s001220051639.

[169] Van EGA, Bowman DT, Calhoun DS, May OL. Changes in the genetic diversity of cotton in the USA from 1970 to 1995. Crop Science, 1998; 38: 33–37. DOI: 10.2135/cropsci1998.0011183X003800010006x.

[170] Sapkal DR, Sutar SR, Thakre PB, Patil BR, Paterson AH, Waghmare VN. Genetic diversity analysis of maintainer and restorer accessions in upland cotton (*Gossypium hirsutum* L.). Journal of Plant Biochemistry and Biotechnology, 2011; 20: 20–28. DOI: 10.1007/s13562-010-0020-7.

[171] Reddy OUK, Pepper AE, Abdurakhmonov I, Saha S, Jenkins JN, Brooks T, Bolek Y, El-Zik KM. New dinucleotide and trinucleotide microsatellite marker resources for cotton genome research. The Journal of Cotton Science, 2001; 5: 103–113.

[172] Kumpatla SP, Horne EC, Shah MR, Gupta M, Thompson SA. Development of SSR markers: towards genetic mapping in cotton (*Gossypium hirsutum* L.). In: 3rd International Cotton Genome Initiative Workshop, Nanjing, China. Cotton Science, 2002; 14: 28.

[173] Abdurakhmonov IY, Saha S, Jenkins JN, Buriev ZT, Shermatov SE, et al. Linkage disequilibrium based association mapping of fiber quality traits in *G. hirsutum* L. variety germplasm. Genetica, 2009; 136: 401–417. DOI: 10.1007/s10709-008-9337-8.

[174] Cao Z., Wang P., Zhu X., et al. SSR marker-assisted improvement of fiber qualities in *Gossypium hirsutum* using *Gossypium barbadense* introgression. Theoretical and Applied Genetics, 2014; 14: 587–594. DOI: 10.1007/s00122-013-2241-3.

[175] Nie X, Tu J, Wang B, Zhou X, Lin Z. A BIL population derived from *G. hirsutum* and *G. barbadense* provides a resource for cotton genetics and breeding. PLoS One, 2015; 10: e0141064. DOI: 10.1371/journal.pone.0141064.

[176] Wang XQ, Yu Y, Sang J, Wu QZ, Zhang XL, Lin ZX. Intraspecific linkage map construction and QTL mapping of yield and fiber quality of *Gossypium babrdense*. Australian Journal of Crop Science, 2013; 7: 1252–1261.

[177] Pathak D, Bhatia D. Development of advanced mapping populations in cotton. ICAC 2015; XXXIII.

[178] Huang YF, Poland JA, Wight CP, Jackson EW, Tinker NA. Using genotyping-by-sequencing (GBS) for genomic discovery in cultivated oat. PLoS One, 2014; 9: e102448. DOI: 10.1371/journal.pone.0102448.

[179] Bolukbasi MF, Mizrak A, Ozdener GB, Madlener S, Strobel T, Erkan EP, Fan JB, Breakefield XO, Saydam O. miR-1289 and "Zipcode"-like sequence enrich mRNAs in microvesicles. Molecular Therapy — Nucleic Acids, 2012; 1: e10. DOI: 10.1038/mtna.2011.2.

[180] Bolger ME, Weisshaar B, Scholz U, Stein N, Usadel B, Mayer KF. Plant genome sequencing—applications for crop improvement. Current Opinion in Biotechnology, 2014; 26: 31–37. DOI: 10.1016/j.copbio.2013.08.019.

[181] Qin YS, Liu RZ, Mei HX, Zhang TZ, Guo WZ. QTL mapping for yield traits in upland cotton (*Gossypium hirsutum* L.). Acta Ecologica Sinica, 2009; 35: 1812–1821. DOI: 10.3724/SP.J.1006.2009.01812.

[182] Li FG, Fan GY, Lu CR, Xiao GH, Zou CS, Kohel RJ, et al. Genome sequence of cultivated Upland cotton (*Gossypium hirsutum* TM-1). Nature Biotechnology, 2015; 33: 524–530. DOI: 10.1038/nbt.3208.

[183] Chen H, Qian N, Guo WZ, Song QP, Li BC, Deng FJ, Dong CG, Zhang TZ. Using three overlapped RILs to dissect genetically clustered QTL for fiber strength on Chro. D8 in Upland cotton. Theoretical and Applied Genetics, 2009; 119: 605–612. DOI: 10.1007/s00122-009-1070-x.

[184] Zhang K, Zhang J, Ma J, Tang SY, Liu DJ, Teng ZH, et al. Genetic mapping and quantitative trait locus analysis of fiber quality traits using a three-parent composite population in upland cotton (*Gossypium hirsutum* L.). Molecular Breeding, 2012; 29: 335–348. DOI: 10.1007/s11032-011-9549-y.

[185] Liang QZ, Cheng HU, Hua H, Li , Zhao H, Ping JH. Construction of a linkage map and QTL mapping for fiber quality traits in upland cotton (*Gossypium hirsutum* L.). Plant Genetics, 2013; 58: 3233-3243. DOI: 10.1007/s11434-013-5807-1.

[186] Islam MS, Zeng LH, Delhom CD, Song HL, Kim HJ, Li P, et al. Identification of cotton fiber quality quantitative trait loci using intraspecific crosses derived from two near-isogenic lines differing in fiber bundle strength. Molecular Breeding, 2014; 34: 373–384. DOI: 10.1007/s11032-014-0040-4.

[187] Islam MS, Linghe Z, Thyssen GN, Christopher D, Delhom H, Jin K, Ping L, D. Fang. Mapping by sequencing in cotton (*Gossypium hirsutum*) line MD52ne identified candidate genes for fiber strength and its related quality attributes. Theoretical and Applied Genetics, DOI: 10.1007/s00122-016-2684-4.

[188] Abdurakhmonov IY, Shapulatov UM, Shermatov SE, Buriev ZT, Abdullaev AA, Kushanov FN, Egamberdiev SS, Salahutdinov IB, Ubaydullaeva HA, Makamov AH, Darmanov MM, Ayubov MS, Norov TM, Tulanov AA, Mavlonov GT, Abdukarimov

A. Achievements and perspectives of cotton "omics" in Uzbekistan. In: Proceedings of the International Cotton conference Bremen, 19–21 March 2014, Bremen, Germany.

[189] Collin FS, Brooks LD, Charkravarti AA. DNA polymorphism discovery resource for research on human genetic variation. Genome Research, 1998; 8: 1229–1231. DOI: 10.1101/gr.8.12.1229.

[190] Rafalski JA. Applications of single nucleotide polymorphisms in crop genetics. Current Opinion in Plant Biology, 2002; 5: 94-100. DOI: 10.1016/S1369-5266(02)00240-6.

[191] Zhu YL, Song QJ, Hyten DL, Tassell VCP, Matukumalli LK, Grimm DR, Hyatt SM, Fickus EW, Young ND, Cregan PB. Single-nucleotide polymorphism in soybean. Genetics, 2003; 163: 1123–1134. PMCID: PMC1462490.

[192] Krawczak M. Informativity assessment for biallelic single nucleotide polymorphisms. Electrophoresis, 1999; 20: 1676–1681. DOI: 10.1002/(SICI)1522-2683(19990101)20:8<1676::AID-ELPS1676>3.0.CO;2-D.

[193] Zhu W, Schlueter SD, Brendel V. Refined annotation of the Arabidopsis genome by complete expressed sequence tag mapping. Plant Physiology, 2003; 132: 469–484. DOI: 10.1104/pp.102.018101.

[194] Wang DG, Fan JB, Siao CJ, Berno A, Young P, Sapolsky R, Ghandour G, Perkins N, Winchester E, Spencer J, et al. Large-scale identification, mapping, and genotyping of single-nucleotide polymorphisms in the human genome. Science, 1998; 280: 1077–1082. DOI: 10.1126/science.280.5366.1077.

[195] He J, Zhao X, Laroche A, Lu ZX, Liu H, Li Z. Genotyping by-sequencing (GBS), an ultimate marker-assisted selection (MAS) tool to accelerate plant breeding. Front. Plant Science, 2014; 5: 484. DOI: 10.3389/fpls.2014.004.

[196] Thomson MJ, Zhao K, Wright M, McNally KL, Rey J, Tung CW, Reynolds A, Scheffler B, Eizenga G, McClung A, Kim H, Ismail AM, de Ocampo M, Mojica C, Reveche MY, Dilla-Ermita CJ, Mauleon R, Leung H, Bustamante C, McCouch SR. High-throughput single nucleotide polymorphism genotyping for breeding applications in rice using the BeadXpress platform. Molecular Breeding, 2012; 29: 875–886. DOI: 10.1007/s11032-011-9663-x.

[197] Heffner EL. Sorrells, ME, Jannink JL. Genomic selection for crop improvement. Crop Science, 2009; 49: 1–12. DOI: 10.2135/cropsci2008.08.0512.

[198] Bernardo R. Genomewide selection with minimal crossing in self-pollinated crops. Crop Science, 2010; 50: 624–627. DOI: 10.2135/cropsci2009.05.0250.

[199] Jannink JL, Lorenz AJ, Iwata H. Genomic selection in plant breeding: from theory to practice. Briefings in Functional Genomics, 2010; 9: 166–177. DOI: 10.1093/bfgp/elq00.

[200] Nicolae DL, et al. Trait-associated SNPs are more likely to be eQTLs: annotation to enhance discovery from GWAS. PLoS Genetics, 2010; 6, e1000888. DOI: 10.1371/journal.pgen.1000888.

[201] Zhang ZS, Hu MC, Zhang J, Liu DJ. Construction of a comprehensive PCR-based marker linkage map and QTL mapping for fiber quality traits in upland cotton (*Gossypium hirsutum* L.). Molecular BreedIng, 2009; 24: 49–61. DOI: 10.1007/s11032-009-9271-1.

[202] Mei HX, Zhu XF, Zhang TZ. Favorable QTL alleles for yield and its components identified by association mapping in Chinese upland cotton cultivars. PLoS One, 2013; 8: e82193. DOI: 10.1371/journal.pone.0082193 PMID: 24386089.

[203] An C, Saha S, Jenkins JN, Ma DP, Scheffler BE, et al. Cotton (*Gossypium* spp.) R2R3-MYB transcription factors SNP identification, phylogenomic characterization, chromosome localization, and linkage mapping. Theoretical and Applied Genetics, 2008; 116: 1015–1026. DOI: 10.1007/s00122-008-0732-4.

[204] Said JI, Song M, Wang H, Lin Z, Zhang X, Fang DD, Zhang J. A comparative meta-analysis of QTL between intraspecific *Gossypium hirsutum* and interspecific *G. hirsutum* × *G. barbadense* population. Molecular Genetics and Genomics, 2015; 290: 1003–1025. DOI 10.1007/s00438-014-0963-9.

[205] Deynze V, Stoffel K, Lee M, Wilkins TA, Kozik A, Cantrell RG, Yu JZ, Kohel RJ, Stelly DM. Sampling nucleotide diversity in cotton. BMC Plant Biology, 2009; 9: 125. DOI: 10.1186/1471-2229-9-125.

[206] Byers RL, Harker DB, Yourstone SM, Maughan PJ, Udall JA. Development and mapping of SNP assays in allotetraploid cotton. Theoretical and Applied Genetics, 2012; 124: 1201–1214. DOI: 10.1007/s00122-0111780-8.

[207] Pacific Biosciences [Internet]. 2016. Available from: http//www.pacificbiosciences.com.

[208] Datta D, Gupta S, Chaturvedi SK, Nadarajan N. Molecular Markers in Crop Improvement. Kanpur: Indian Institute of Pulses Research; 2011.

[209] Stoskopf NC, Tomes DT, Christie BR. Plant Breeding: Theory and Practice. San Francisco, CA, Oxford: Westview Press Inc.; 1993

[210] Levi A, Paterson AH, Barak V, Yakir D, Wang B, Chee W, Saranga Y. Field evaluation of cotton near-isogenic lines introgressed with QTLs for productivity and drought related traits. Molecular Breeding, 2009; 23: 179–195. DOI: 10.1007/s11032-008-9224-0.

[211] Guo WZ, Zhang TZ, Ding YZ, Zhu YC, Shen XL, Zhu XF. Molecular marker-assisted selection and pyramiding of two QTLs for fiber strength in upland cotton. Acta Genitica Sinica, 2005; 32: 1275–1285.

[212] Jiang GL, Dong Y, Shi J, Ward RW. QTL analysis of resistance to *Fusarium* head blight in the novel wheat germplasm CJ9306. II. Resistance to deoxylevinaeol accumulation

and grain yield loss. Theoretical and Applied Genetics, 2007; 115: 1043–1052. DOI: 10.1007/s00122-007-0630-1.

[213] Ethington SR, Crosbie TM, Edwards MD, Reiter RS, Bull JK. Molecular markers in commercial breeding program. Crop Science, 2007; 47: S154–S163. DOI: 10.2135/cropsci2007.04.0015IPBS.

[214] Yi C, Guo W, Zhu X, Min L, Zhang T. Pyramiding breeding by marker-assisted recurrent selection in upland cotton II. Selection effects on resistance to *Helicoverpa armigera*. Scientia Agricultura Sinica, 2004; 37: 801–807.

[215] Gutiérrez, Osman A, et al. Identification of QTL regions and SSR markers associated with resistance to *reniform* nematode in *Gossypium barbadense* L. accession GB713. Theoretical and Applied Genetics, 2011; 122: 271–280. DOI: 10.1007/s00122-010-1442-2.

[216] Baird NA, Etter PD, Atwood TS, Currey MC, Shiver AL, Lewis ZA, Selker EU, Cresko WA, Johnson EA. Rapid SNP discovery and genetic mapping using sequenced RAD markers. PLoS One, 2008; 3: e3376. DOI: 10.1371/journal.pone.0003376.

[217] Shendure J, Hanli J. Next-generation DNA sequencing. Nature Biotechnology, 2008; 26, 1135–1145. DOI: 10.1038/nbt1486

[218] Deschamps S, Llaca V, Gregory DM, Bus, et al. Genotyping-by-sequencing in plants. Biology, 2012; 1: 460–483. DOI: 10.3390/biology1030460.

[219] Quail MA, Smith M, Coupland P, Otto TD, Harris SR, Connor, et al. A tale of three next generation sequencing platforms: comparison of Ion Torrent, Pacific Biosciences and Illumina MiSeq sequencers. BMC Genomics, 2012; 13: 341. DOI: 1471-2164/13/341.

[220] Thudi M, Li Y, Jackson SA, May GD, Varshney RK. Current state-of-art of sequencing technologies for plant genomics research. Briefings in Functional Genomics, 2012; 11: 3–11. DOI: 10.1093/bfgp/elr045.

[221] Bentley DR, et al. Accurate whole human genome sequencing using reversible terminator chemistry. Nature, 2008; 456: 53–59. DOI: 10.1038/nature07517.

[222] Rothberg JM, Hinz W, Rearick TM, Schultz J, Mileski W, Davey M, Leamon JH, Johnson K, Milgrew MJ, Edwards M, Hoon J, Simons JF, Marran D, Myers JW, Davidson JF, Branting A, Nobile JR, Puc BP, Light D, Clark TA, Huber M, Branciforte JT, Stoner IB, Cawley SE, Lyons M, Fu Y, Homer N, Sedova M, Miao X, Reed B, Sabina J, Feierstein E, Schorn M, Alanjary M, Dimalanta E, Dressman D, Kasinskas R, Sokolsky T, Fidanza JA, Namsaraev E, McKernan KJ, Williams AJ, Roth GT, Bustillo J. An integrated semiconductor device enabling non-optical genome sequencing. Nature, 2011; 475: 348. DOI: 10.1038/nature10242.

[223] Schuster SC. Next-generation sequencing transforms today's biology. Nature Methods, 2008; 5: 16–18. DOI: 10.1038/nmeth1156.

[224] Rounsley S, Marri PR, He Yu, Sisneros R, Goicoechea N, Lee JL, Angelova SJ, Kudrna A, Luo D, Affourtit M, Desany J, Knight B, Niazi J, Egholm F, Wing RA. De novo next

generation sequencing of plant genomes. Rice, 2009; 2: 35–43. DOI: 10.1007/s12284-009-9025-z.

[225] Morrell PL, Buckler ES, Ross-Ibarra J. Crop genomics: advances and applications. Nature Reviews Genetics, 2012; 13: 85–96. DOI: 10.1038/nrg3097.

[226] Paterson AH, Bowers JE, Bruggmann R, Dubchak I, Grimwood J, Gundlach H, Haberer G, Hellsten U, Mitros T, Poliakov A, et al. The Sorghum bicolor genome and the diversification of grasses. Nature, 547: 2009; 551–556. DOI: 10.1038/nature07723.

[227] Huang X, Lu T, Han B. Re-sequencing rice genomes: an emerging new era of rice genomics. Trends Genetics, 2013; 29: 225–232. DOI: 10.1016/j.tig.2012.12.001.

[228] Li JY, Wang J, Zeigler RS. The 3000 rice genomes project: new opportunities and challenges for future rice research. Giga Science, 2014; 3: 1–3. DOI: 10.1186/2047-217X-3-8.

[229] Mardis ER. Next-Generation DNA sequencing methods. Annual Review of Genomics and Human Genetics, 2008; 9: 387–402. DOI: 10.1146/annurev.genom.9.081307.164359.

[230] Gupta PK, Rustgi S, Mir RR. Array-based high-throughput DNA markers for crop improvement. Heredity, 2008; 101: 5–18. DOI: 10.1038/hdy.2008.3.

[231] Paterson et al. Repeated polyploidization of *Gossypium* genomes and the evolution of spinnable cotton fibres. Nature, 2012; 492: 423—427. DOI: 10.1038/nature11798.

[232] Chen X, Li X, Zhang B, Xu J, Wu Z, Wang B, et al. Detection and genotyping of restriction fragment associated polymorphisms in polyploid crops with a pseudo-reference sequence: a case study in allotetraploid *Brassica napus*. BMC Genomics, 2013; 14: 346. DOI: 10.1186/1471-2164- 14-346.

[233] Gore MA, Fang DD, Poland JA, Zhang J, Percy RG, Cantrell RG, Lipka AE. Linkage map construction and quantitative trait locus analysis of agronomic and fiber quality traits in cotton. The Plant Genome, 2014; 7. DOI: 10.3835/plantgenome2013.07.00.

[234] Affymetrix [Internet]. 2016. Available from: http://www.affymetrix.com/products services/arrays/specific/cotton.affx. [Accessed 2016-03-25]

[235] Malik W, Ashraf J, Iqbal ZM, Khan AA, Qayyum A, Abid MA, Noor E, Ahmad MA, Abbasi GH. Molecular markers and cotton genetic improvement: current status and future prospects. The Scientific World Journal, 2014; http://www.hindawi.com/journals/tswj/2014/607091.

[236] Poland J, Endelman J, Dawson J, Rutkoski J, Wu S, Manes Y, Dreisigackere S, Crossae J, Sánchez-Villedae H, Sorrells M, Jannink JL. Genomic selection in wheat breeding using genotyping-by-sequencing. Plant Genome, 2012; 5: 103–113. DOI: 10.3835/plantgenome2012.06.0006.

[237] Poland JA, Rife TW. Genotyping-by-sequencing for plant breeding and genetics. Plant Genome, 2012; 5: 92–102. DOI: 10.3835/plantgenome2012.05.0005.

[238] Narum SR, Buerkle CA, Davey JW, Miller MR, Hohenlohe PA. Genotyping-by-sequencing in ecological and conservation genomics. Molecular Ecology, 2013; 22: 2841–2847. DOI: 10.1111/mec.12350.

[239] Beissinger TM, Hirsch CN, Sekhon RS, Foerster JM, Johnson JM, Muttoni G, Vaillancourt B, Buell CR, Kaeppler SM, De Leon N. Marker density and read depth for genotyping populations using genotyping-by-sequencing. Genetics, 2013; 193: 1073–1081. DOI: 10.1534/genetics.112.147710.

[240] Islam MS, Thyssen GN, Jenkins JN, Fang DD. Detection, validation, and application of genotyping-by-sequencing based single nucleotide polymorphisms in upland cotton. Plant Genome, 2015; DOI: 10.3835/plantgenome2014.3807.0034.

[241] Mather DE, Tinker NA, Laberge DE, Edney M, Jones BL, Rossnagel BG, Legge WG, Briggs KG, Irvine RB, Falk DE, Kasha KJ. Regions of the genome that affect grain and malt quality in a North American two row barley cross. Crop Science, 1997; 37: 544–554. DOI: 10.2135/cropsci1997.0011183X003700020039x.

[242] Abdurakhmonov YI, Abdukarimov A. Application of association mapping to understanding the genetic diversity of plant germplasm resources. International Journal of Plant Genomics, 2008. Article ID 574927, DOI: 10.1155/2008/574927.

[243] Kraakman ATW, Niks RE, Van den Berg PMMM, Stam P, Van Eeuwijk FA. Linkage disequilibrium mapping of yield and yield stability in modern spring barley cultivars. Genetics, 2004; 168: 435–446. DOI: 10.1534/genetics.104.026831.

[244] Mammadov W, Chen R, Ren, et al. Development of highly polymorphic SNP markers from the complexity reduced portion of maize (*Zea mays* L.) genome for use in marker-assisted breeding. Theoretical and Applied Genetics, 2010; 121: 577–588. DOI: 10.1007/s00122-010-1331-8.

[245] Truong HT, Ramos AM, Yalcin F, De Ruiter M, Van der Poel HJ, Huvenaars KH, Hogers RCJ, Van Encke-vort LJG, Janssen A, Van Orsouw NJ, Van Eijk MJ. Sequence- based genotyping for marker discovery and co-dominant scoring in germplasm and populations. PLoS One 2012; 7: e37565. DOI: 10.1371/journal.pone.0037565.

[246] Van Poecke RM, Maccaferri M, Tang J, Truong HT, Janssen A, Van Orsouw NJ, et al. Sequence-based SNP genotyping in durum wheat. Plant Biotechnology Journal 2013; 11: 809–817. DOI: 10.1111/pbi.12072.

[247] Abdurakhmonov IY, Abdukarimov A. Application of association mapping to understanding the genetic diversity of plant germplasm resources. International Journal of Plant Genomics, 2008. Article ID: 574927, DOI: 10.1155/2008/574927.

[248] Boopathi MN, Thiyagu K, Urbi B, Santhoshkumar M, Gopikrishnan A, Aravind S, Swapnashri G, Ravikesavan R. Marker-assisted breeding as next-generation strategy for genetic improvement of productivity and quality: can it be realized in cotton? International Journal of Plant Genomics, 2011; 2011: 670104. DOI: 10.1155/2011/670104.

[249] Comparative Evolutionary Genomics of Cotton [Internet]. 2016. Available from: http://cottonevolution.info. [Accessed 2016-03-25].

[250] National Center for Biotechnology Information [Internet]. 2016. Available from: http://www.ncbi.nlm.nih.gov. [Accessed 2016-03-25].

[251] TropGENE Database [Internet]. 2016. Available from: http://tropgenedb.cirad.fr. [Accessed 2016-03-25].

[252] The Plant Genome Mapping Laboratory [Internet]. 2016. Available from: http://www.plantgenome.uga.edu/. [Accessed 2016-03-25].

[253] BACMan resources at Plant Genome Mapping Laboratory [Internet]. 2016. Available from: http://www.plantgenome.uga.edu. [Accessed 2016-03-25].

[254] Till BJ, Comai L, Henikoff S, TILLING and ECOTILLING for crop improvement. Genomics-assisted crop improvement. Genomics Approaches and Platforms, 20071: 333–349.

[255] Simsek O, Kacar YA. Discovery of mutations with TILLING and ECOTILLING in plant genomes. Scientific Research and Essays, 2010; 5: 3799–3802. http://www.academicjournals.org/SRE.

[256] Mehboob R, Shaheen T, Iqbal M, Ashraf, et al. Cotton genetic resources. A review. Agronomy for Sustainable Development, Springer Verlag/EDP Sciences/INRA, 2012; 32: 419–432. DOI: 10.1007/s13593-011-0051-z.

[257] Auld D, Light GG, Fokar M, Bechere E, Allen RD. Mutagenesis system for genetic analysis of *Gossypium*. In: Paterson AH, editor. Genetics and genomics of cotton. vol. 3. Springer Inteurnational Publishing, NY, USA.; 2009. p. 209–226. DOI: 10.1007/978-0-387-70810-2_9.

[258] Ng PC, Henikoff S. SIFT: predicting amino acid changes that affect protein function. Nucleic Acids Research, 2003; 31: 3812–3814. DOI: 10.1093/nar/gkg509.

[259] Taylor NE, Greene EA. PARSESNP: a tool for the analysis of nucleotide polymorphisms. Nucleic Acids Research, 2003; 31: 3808–3811. DOI: 10.1093/nar/gkg574.

[260] Project Aligned Related Sequences and Evaluate SNPs [Internet]. 2016. Available from: http://www.proweb.org/parsesnp. [Accessed 2016-03-25].

Chapter 8

The Utilization of Translocation Lines and Microsatellite Markers for the Identification of Unknown Cotton Monosomic Lines

Marina F. Sanamyan, Abdusalom K. Makamov,
Shukhrat U. Bobokhujaev, Dilshod E. Usmonov,
Zabardas T. Buriev, Sukumar Saha and
David M. Stelly

Additional information is available at the end of the chapter

http://dx.doi.org/10.5772/64558

Abstract

Simple sequence repeats (SSR) have been applied as useful markers for understanding cotton genetics. In the last decade, chromosome-deficient stocks of *Gossypium hirsutum* L. were used in the development of chromosome substitution lines for *G. barbadense* L., *G. tomentosum* Nuttall et Seemann, and *G. mustelinum* Watt chromosomes or chromosome segments. Several DNA markers have already been assigned to the individual chromosomes of *G. hirsutum*. We created new cotton monosomic lines in Uzbekistan after irradiation of seeds by thermal neutrons or pollen gamma-irradiation to complement other global efforts in the development of cotton chromosome substitution lines. The primary objective of this chapter is to report the use of chromosome-specific SSR markers and a well-defined tester set of cotton translocation lines from the Cotton Cytogenetic Collection at Texas A&M AgriLife Research to confirm chromosome specificity of monosomic lines in Uzbekistan cytogenetic collection of cotton. Our results have assigned several different monosomic lines to the chromosomes 2, 4, 6, and telosome 11 A_t-subgenome and chromosomes 18 and 20 or 22 D_t-subgenome. These lines will be very useful in molecular mapping, the creation of substitution lines, and cotton breeding.

Keywords: cotton (*Gossypium hirsutum* L.), chromosome, identification, monosome, molecular markers

1. Introduction

Monosomic plants can be used for the synthesis of the chromosome substitution (CS-B) lines [1]. Such substitution lines are a useful means of interspecific introgression and for studying economically important genes. In upland cotton (*Gossypium hirsutum* L.), Kohel et al. [2] studied multiple traits of disomic substitution lines that contained chromosomes 6 or 17 of *G. barbadense* (L.).

About 10 years ago, replacement and additional *G. barbadense* chromosome substitution lines became available. These were developed similarly by hybridization of the same *G. barbadense* donor line to quasi-isogenic *G. hirsutum* hypoaneuploids, followed by iterative modified backcrossing and then inbreeding. Each resultant CS-B line was expected to be substituted for one chromosome or segment and to be largely though not necessarily completely devoid of unrelated *G. barbadense* segments [3, 4]. The results revealed information on the association of specific chromosomes with genes for agronomic and fiber traits. More recently, substitution lines were created for *G. tomentosum* [5] and *G. mustelinum* [6], as well as for additional chromosomes of *G. barbadense* [7]. Saha et al. subsequently used the CS-B lines to identify chromosomal locations of important traits and beneficial genes and interactions [3, 8, 9].

Simple sequence repeats (SSR) of cotton have been applied widely as molecular markers for genetics, mapping, trait analysis, and germplasm diversity analysis and comparisons of specific individuals, lines, and populations. Several SSR markers associated with lint percentage have been located to chromosomes 12, 18, 23, and 26 using deletion analysis in aneuploid chromosome substitution lines. SSRs were used to analyze the genetic identities of specific hypoaneuploid interspecific F_1 hybrids and disomic chromosome substitution intermediates genotypes, using the principles of deletion molecular analysis [10, 11]. Recent reports extended the systematic characterizations of additional hypoaneuploid chromosome substitution F_1 hybrids and many chromosome substitution lines using chromosome-specific SSR-markers [6, 7].

A Cotton Cytogenetic Collection of Uzbekistan now includes 95 primary monosomics derived from the highly inbred *G. hirsutum* line "L-458" by irradiation of the seeds with thermal neutrons and pollen with gamma-rays [12]. The chromosome identities of these monosomic lines of the Uzbek Collection need to be determined to optimize the efficiency of collection maintenance and its use in breeding-related research, for example, development of chromosome substitution lines.

The primary objective of this chapter is to report the use of chromosome-specific SSR markers and a well-defined tester set of translocation lines of the USA collection to confirm chromosome specificity of monosomic lines in Uzbekistan collection.

2. Materials and methods

2.1. Plant material

Monosomic lines of the Uzbek Cytogenetic collection were developed in a common genetic background of the highly inbred line *G. hirsutum* line L-458, which was created through multiple generations of self-pollination (F_{20}) of cultivar 108-F [13, 14]. Because all of the 95 primary monosomics were isolated from a common genetic background, some differences observed among them can be attributed to the differences in their monosomic state [15]. Irradiation of seeds by thermal neutrons or pollen gamma-irradiation gave rise to most (76) of the monosomics. Other monosomic plants were detected among progenies of desynaptic plants (17) and translocation heterozygote plants (2). The primary monosomics were numbered according to their order of detection (Mo1-Mo95).

The *G. barbadense* line 3-79 is nonphotoperiod sensitive and is highly homozygous as it is originated as a doubled haploid [16]. It has been used extensively as parent in genetic studies, genomics [17], and as a donor parent for the substituted chromosome (CS) or chromosome segments from *G. barbadense* in our study. The overall method of the CS line development was discussed in previous reports [4, 18].

A well-defined tester set of translocation lines of Cytogenetic Collection of the USA was kindly provided by Prof. D.M. Stelly through a USDA-Uzbekistan cotton germplasm exchange program. All plant materials were vegetatively maintained in the greenhouse of National University of Uzbekistan.

2.2. Cytological analyses

For studies of meiotic chromosome pairing at metaphase-I (MI) and sporad normality floral buds were collected in the morning, and after the removal of calyx and corolla, fixed in a solution of 96% alcohol and acetic acid (7:3). Buds were kept at room temperature for 3 days then immersed in fresh fixative and stored at 4°C. For cytological preparations, buds were rinsed in tap water before being examined for meiotic MI chromosome configurations in the microsporocytes, commonly known as "pollen mother cells" (PMCs) using the iron acetocarmine squash technique. Analyses of hybrid plant chromosomes were carried out on the basis of MI configurations. The development of F_1 hybrid plant PMCs was assessed based on the cytological features observed at the tetrad stage. The meiotic index was calculated as the percentage of sporads that were normal tetrads. Pollen viability was estimated as percentage of mature pollen grains stainable in acetocarmine. All cytological observations were made using Biomed (Leica, Heerbrugg, Switzerland) and Axioskop A1 (Carl Zeiss, Germany) microscopes.

2.3. Identification of hybrid F_1 monosomic translocation heterozygotes

Monosomes were chromosomally identified using translocation tests. For this purpose, the monosomic ($2n = 51$) lines from Uzbek Cytogenetic Collection were crossed as seed parent with translocation lines ($2n = 52$) of the tester set from USA Cotton Cytogenetic Collection provided by Texas A&M AgriLife Research. Floral buds of F_1 hybrid progeny were analyzed to identify individuals that were monosomic ($2n = 51$) and also heterozygous for the respective translocation, that is, monosomic translocation heterozygotes. To reveal "critical configurations" and detect common chromosomes among the chromosomes involved in interchanges with monosomes, the meiotic MI configurations were analyzed in heterozygotes of monosomic translocations heterozygous F_1 hybrids. Progeny modally forming 23II + IV + I were interpreted as indicating independence between chromosomes affected by monosomy and the translocation, whereas progeny modally forming 24II + III were interpreted as evidence of association between the monosome and one of the two translocation chromosomes. It was generally presumed that parent and progeny monosomic conditions were similar, that is, no monosomic "shift" occurred.

2.4. DNA extraction and genotyping

Genomic DNAs were extracted from young leaf samples of cytogenetically identified F_1 monosomic cotton hybrids using CTAB method [18]. Extracted genomic DNAs were checked in 0.9% agarose electrophoresis, and DNA concentrations were diluted to a working concentration of 15 μl based on Hind III-digested λ-phage DNA 25 ng/μl. PCR amplification carried out in a 10 μl volume reaction mix containing 1.0 μl 10× PCR buffer, (with 25 mM Mg Cl2), 0.2 μl BSA, 0.08 μl dNTPs (25mM), 0.2 μl primer pairs, 0.1 μl Taq-polymerase, and 2 μl DNA template. PCR runs were conducted with an initial denaturation of DNA at 94°C for 2 min, followed by 35 cycles of 94°C (step 1) for 20 sec, 55°C (step 2) for 30 sec, and 72°C (step 3) for 50 sec. After 35 cycles, the extension temperature of 72°C was held for 7 min. The PCR products were visualized in 3.5% high-resolution agarose gel, stained with ethidium bromide and photodocumented using an Alpha Imager (Innotech Inc., USA) gel documentation system.

Chromosome-specific SSR primer pairs were collected according to recently published genetic mapping papers [11, 19–27]. For each chromosome, we chose four loci that were polymorphic between L-458 (*G. hirsutum*) and 3-79 (*G. barbadense*). Documented electrophoregram results for SSRs were scored as "a/b/h" where "a" locus similar to recipient L-458, "b" locus similar to donor line 3-79 and "h" genotype similar to normal F_1 hybrid. To identify the chromosome deficient from a given F_1 monosomic cotton hybrid, the SSRs of that chromosome were expected to exhibit "b" genotype, that is, to lack of the *G. hirsutum* (maternal) allele and to possess only the *G. barbadense* (paternal) allele [10].

3. Results

3.1. Cytogenetic characteristics of the aneuploid hybrid F_1 plants

We crossed 46 monosomic and two monotelodisomic lines of *G. hirsutum* from Uzbek cytogenetic collection of cotton and a *G. barbadense* doubled haploid line Pima 3-79. Among resulting progeny, the aneuploid hybrid F_1 plants were detected in 37 interspecific F_1 progeny families based on hybrid phenotypes and meiotic metaphase-I configuration analyses. In five of the aneuploid hybrid F_1 families, three hybrid monosomic plants were detected in each progeny, in 11 aneuploid hybrid F_1 families two hybrid monosomic were isolated, and in the remaining 21 hybrid families, one aneuploid hybrid F_1 plant was detected. These results showed differences in the ease monosomic detection in various hybrid backgrounds and/or differences in maternal transmission rates for various monosomes. Deficiencies for one chromosome arm occurred in the progenies of two monotelodisomic hybrid F_1 plants.

Hybrid F_1 plants had intermediate phenotypes, including strong effects on plant shape and size; clustering (flower positions and density); number, sizes and shapes of leaves, bracts, and stipules; sizes and number bract teeth; coloration; number and sizes of external nectarines; and boll shape. Additional phenotypic effects by monosomy were super-imposed on these general phenotypic effects of interspecific hybridity.

Meiotic metaphase-I analysis of 56 monosomic hybrid F_1 plants revealed that 46 plants exhibited modal chromosome pairing of 25 bivalents and one univalent. Seven monosomic hybrid F_1 plants were characterized with the presence of additional univalents and their average univalent frequencies per cell among them ranged from 1.06 ± 0.06 in Mo67xPima 3-79 to 1.22 ± 0.15 in Mo11xPima 3-79. Three univalents were observed in some PMCs of the seven monosomic hybrid F_1 plants from Mo7, Mo11, Mo27, Mo67, Mo72, Mo75 and Mo89. Three monosomic hybrid F_1 plants from families Mo17xPima 3-79 formed three univalents in many PMCs, and they accordingly exhibited relatively high average univalent frequencies per cell, which ranged from 1.24 ± 0.13 to 1.45 ± 0.15. The similarity of relative univalent sizes across the affected cells (24 II + 3 I) suggested that the extra pair of univalents in all of these cells arose from the same pair of chromosomes. A similar effect was noted in the parental monosomic plant in selfed Mo17 progenies, and could indicate that Mo17 is affected by more than simple monosomy. The three monosomic hybrid F_1 plants (Mo17xPima 3-79) also seemed to differ in their morphology, which suggests the possibility that one or more of them arose following a univalent shifts due to irregular chromosome disjunction in meiosis of the maternal Mo17 parent.

Meiotic products were characterized by examining sporads in most of the monosomic hybrid families, looking for example for the frequency of normal tetrad conformation. Meiotic index, originally proposed by Love [28] for evaluation of meiosis in wheat, reports the normal tetrad percentage and is an indicator of meiotic stability. Most of monosomic hybrid F_1 plants had a higher meiotic index (more than 90%) than that of the control hybrid F_1 plants (L-458xPima 3-79—89.25 ± 0.58%), which indicated that their univalent chromosome underwent regular disjunction. However, the meiotic index values of four of the monosomic hybrid F_1 plants (Mo48xPima 3-79, Mo59xPima 3-79, Mo62xPima 3-79, Mo92xPima 3-79) were characterized ranging from 89.78 ± 0.50% to 85.96 ± 1.29%. Two monosomic hybrid F_1 plants showed an increase of percentage of tetrads with micronuclei to 4.41 ± 0.45% (Mo59xPima 3-79) and 4.53 ± 0.37% (Mo92xPima 3-79) in comparison with control hybrid F_1 plants (L-458xPima 3-79—1.02 ± 0.06%), which demonstrated disturbances in monosome disjunction and formation of imbalanced gametes.

Pollen viability after acetocarmine staining was studied in monosomic hybrid families. Pollen viability was high in most monosomic hybrid F_1 plants. However, nine monosomic hybrid F_1 plants had reduced pollen viability and showed early haplo-deficient microspore abortion prior to mature pollen stage. Two monosomic hybrid F_1 plants had small reductions in pollen viability (up to 20%), four monosomic hybrid F_1 plants had more reductions in pollen viability (up to 30%), and three monosomic hybrid F_1 plants had reductions in semisterile pollen (up to 50%). Thus, some of monosomic hybrid F_1 plants had decreased meiotic index and decreased pollen viability.

3.2. Molecular marker analysis

For molecular analysis of the monosomic hybrid F_1 plants, the principles of deletion molecular analysis were used [10, 11]. Considering that many DNA markers have already been assigned to the individual chromosomes of *G. hirsutum* L., we aimed to utilize chromosome-specific SSR markers to identify and reconfirm the chromosome specificity identities of monosomic lines of our collection, based on SSR content monosomic substitution F_1 hybrids created by crossing with the doubled haploid *G. barbadense* L. line 3-79. Detection and genotyping of SSR markers were straightforward and in a manner described in previous reports that utilized a PCR amplification of chromosome-specific markers in the genomic DNAs of hybrid plants. To localize SSR loci to chromosomes, we screened monosomic hybrid F_1 plants for the L-458 allele using labeled and/or unlabeled primers. For SSR loci located at sites other than the chromatin deficient segment, the L-458 marker would be present and F_1 hybrids would exhibit heterozygous phenotype. In comparison, if an SSR locus was on the segment deficient from the hypoaneuploid hybrid F_1 plant, the electropherogram would lack the L-458 allele and exhibit hemizygous pattern for the donor allele from *G. barbadense* Pima 3-79.

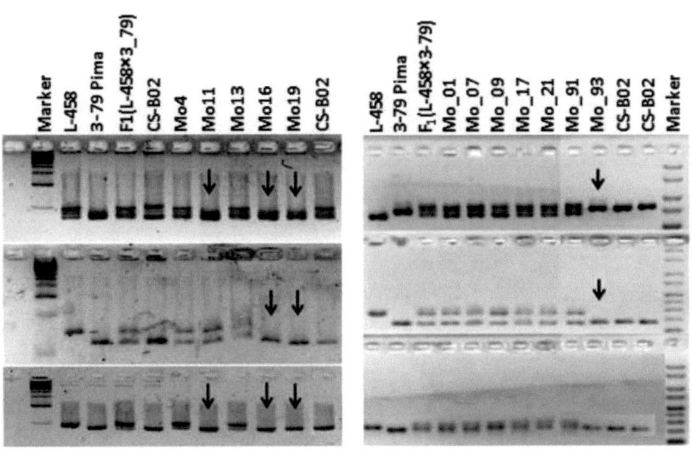

Figure 1. Chromosome identification of monosomic interspecific F_1 hybrids, monosomic *G. hirsutum* × *G. barbadense*. SSR primer pairs specific for chromosome 2 A_t-subgenome: (a) BNL3590; (b) BNL3971; (c) Gh198; (d) BNL1434; (e) BNL3971; and (f) BNL1897.

Our results revealed that four monosomic hybrid F_1 plants (Mo11xPima 3-79, Mo16xPima 3-79, Mo19xPima 3-79, and Mo93xPima 3-79) deficient for unknown chromosome(s) showed the presence of only *G. barbadense*-specific SSR markers bands (BNL3590 and GH-198 for Mo11), (BNL3971, BNL3590, and GH-198 for Mo16 and Mo19), (BNL1434, BNL1897, and BNL3971 for Mo93), and corresponding absence of the respective L-458 allele. The results helped reveal the chromosomal identities of monosomes Mo11, Mo16, Mo19, and Mo93 based on known chromosomal locations of the respective SSR markers. Because the aforementioned SSR markers were assigned previously to chromosome 2 of the A_t-subgenome of cotton [11, 19–

http://dx.doi.org/10.5772/64558

27] the SSR-based results for Mo11, Mo16, Mo19, and Mo93 indicate that they are monosomic for cotton chromosome 2 (**Figure 1**).

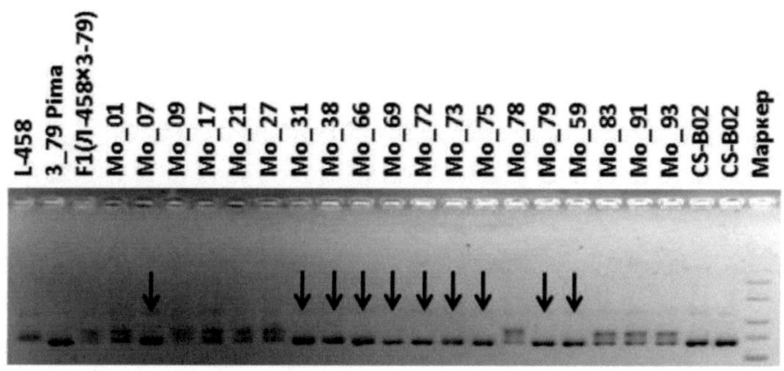

Figure 2. Chromosome identification of monosomic interspecific F_1 hybrids, monosomic *G. hirsutum* × *G. barbadense*. SSR primer pairs specific for chromosome 4 A_t-subgenome: BNL2572.

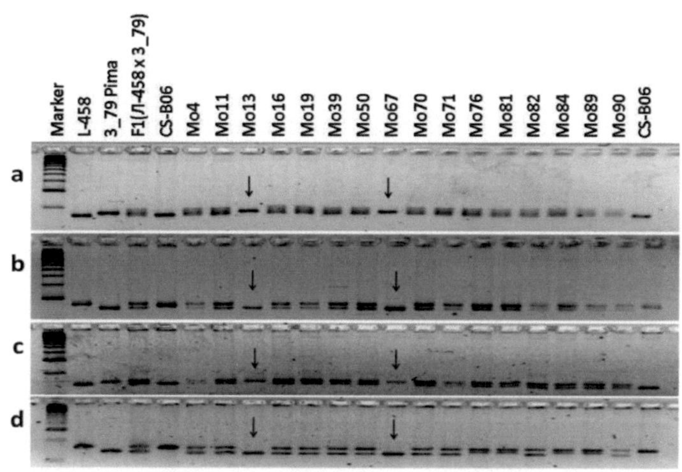

Figure 3. Chromosome identification of monosomic interspecific F_1 hybrids, monosomic *G. hirsutum* × *G. barbadense*. SSR primer pairs specific for chromosome 6 A_t-subgenome: (a) BNL2884; (b) CIR203; (c) BNL1064; and (d) Gh082.

SSR-based deficiency analysis of the six monosomic hybrid F_1 plants (Mo70xPima 3-79, Mo71xPima 3-79, Mo76xPima 3-79, Mo81xPima 3-79, Mo89xPima 3-79, and Mo90xPima 3-79), each deficient for an unknown chromosome showed the presence of only *G. barbadense*-specific SSR marker bands for BNL2572, CIR122, and GH-107, was lacking the respective L-458 alleles. Similarly, analysis of the 10 other monosomic hybrid F_1 plants (Mo7xPima 3-79, Mo31xPima 3-79, Mo38xPima 3-79, Mo59xPima 3-79, Mo66xPima 3-79, Mo69xPima 3-79, Mo72xPima 3-79, Mo73xPima 3-79, Mo75xPima 3-79, and Mo79xPima 3-79), each deficient for one unknown chromosome showed the presence of only the polymorphic *G. barbadense*-specific SSR marker bands for BNL2572, CIR122, and GH-048, was lacking the respective missing L-458 alleles.

Because all of these SSR markers previously were assigned to chromosome 4 A_t-subgenome of cotton [11, 19–27], the results indicated that the unknown monosomes Mo7, Mo31, Mo38, Mo59, Mo66, Mo69, Mo70, Mo71, Mo72, Mo73, Mo75, Mo76, Mo79, Mo81, Mo89, and Mo90 all involved monosomy for chromosome 4 of the cotton A_t-subgenome (**Figure 2**).

Further, our results revealed that two monosomic hybrid F_1 plants (Mo13xPima 3-79 and Mo67xPima 3-79), each of which deficient for unknown chromosome, showed differential presence of polymorphic *G. barbadense*-specific SSR markers BNL1064, BNL2884, BNL3650, CIR203, Gh032, Gh039, Gh082, and TMB1538 and were missing the L-458 allele. Our results indicated that the monosomic chromosome in Mo13 and Mo67 is chromosome 6 A_t-subgenome of cotton because previous assignment of these differential SSR markers has been assigned to this chromosome [11, 19–27] (**Figure 3**).

Using the similar approach, monosomic line Mo48 was assigned to the chromosome 18 of the D_t-subgenome of cotton based on polymorphism of BNL3280 marker from chromosome 18. Monosomic line Mo17 was assigned to the chromosome 20 or 22 of the D_t-subgenome using chromosome-specific SSR marker—JESPR235 genotyping experiment with monosomic F_1 substitution hybrids (Mo17x Pima 3-79) [19, 26], because of this SSR marker was assigned to these two chromosomes.

A monotelodisomic line recovered among progeny of Mo21 and was identified using the chromosome-specific SSR markers—BNL3442, Gh246, CIR212 that were polymorphic monosomic F_1 substitution hybrids (Telo21x Pima 3-79). This result suggested that monotelodisomic line Telo21 is chromosome arm 11 of the A_t-subgenome of cotton because these SSR markers are from the arm of chromosome arm 11 of cotton [11, 19–27].

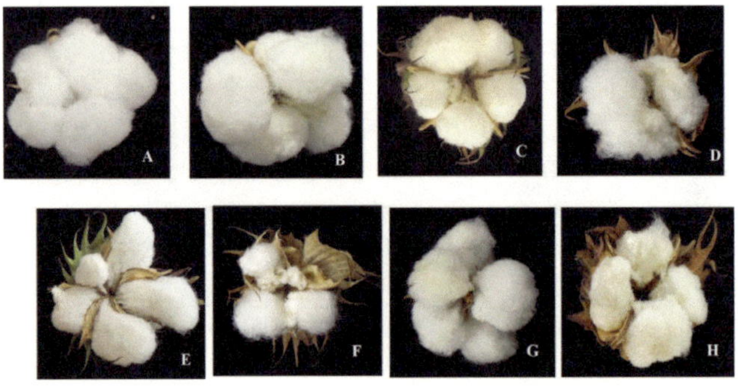

Figure 4. Examples of bolls from cotton monosomic lines with identified monosomes: (A) L-458-parental line; (B) Mo11; (C) Mo16; (D) Mo76; (E) Mo90; (F) Mo13; (G) Mo48; and (H) Mo17.

Thus, we identified chromosomes specificities for 24 monosomic and one monotelodisomic line using F_1 substitution hybrids and chromosome-specific SSR markers. Results demonstrated the differential rates of monosome occurrence and/or recovery among the cotton chromosome complement. In our Uzbekistan-based experiments, chromosome 2, 4, 6, 11, 18, and 20 or 22 were recovered as monosomic/monotelodisomic individuals. The identities of 11 additional F_1 substitution hybrids have yet to be identified, namely Mo1, Mo4, Mo9, Mo28,

http://dx.doi.org/10.5772/64558

Mo39, Mo50, Mo62, Mo82, Mo84, Mo91, and Mo92. Individual cotton chromosome deficiency had a specific influence in plant morphology and some characters such as bolls (**Figure 4**).

For instance, monosomic lines of the chromosome 2 A_t-subgenome including Mo11, Mo16, Mo19, and Mo93, all have a similar phenotypic syndrome that includes features such as dwarf plant architecture; small, narrow, and dense leaf; short sympodia and small and round bolls.

Monosomic lines of the chromosome 4 A_t-subgenome including Mo7, Mo31, Mo38, Mo59, Mo66, Mo69, Mo70, Mo71, Mo72, Mo73, Mo75, Mo76, Mo79, Mo81, Mo89, and Mo90, all have such characters as bushy plant; leaves usually with wavy margins; long peduncle and bolls; and long bolls. Monosomic lines of the chromosome 6 A_t-subgenome including Mo13 and Mo67—both have bushy plant; short sympodia; small and rounded bolls; and late flowering (**Figure 5**).

Monosomic plants deficient for a copy of chromosome 11 of the A_t-subgenome (Mo21) have dwarf plant architecture; short sympodia; small leaves; and small and defectiveed bolls with curved apical tips. Monosomic plants deficient for a copy of chromosome 18 of the D_t-subgenome (Mo48) have dwarf plant architecture, short sympodia, small leaves and bolls that are smaller and rounder. Monosomic plants deficient for a copy of chromosome 20 or 22 of the D_t-subgenome (Mo17) have dwarf plant architecture; small leaves; short sympodia; small, defective, unsymmetrical bracteoles; late flowering and set fewer seed.

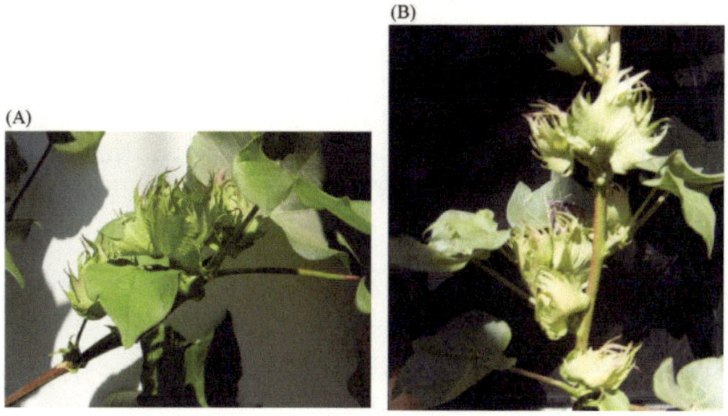

Figure 5. Some unique morphologic characters of the cotton monosomic lines with identified monosomes: (A) short sympodia on the monosomic line Mo19 (on chromosome 2) and (B) fragment of the stem of the monosomic line Mo67 (on chromosome 6).

3.3. Identification and numeration of the unknown monosomes

We have begun a new effort to identify cotton monosomic lines of the Uzbek cytogenetic cotton collection using a well-defined tester set of translocation lines of the cytogenetic collection of the USA, kindly provided by Prof. D.M. Stelly, Texas A&M University, USA, through USDA–Uzbekistan cotton germplasm exchange program. We performed numerous sexual crosses between monosomic lines of our collection and tester-translocation lines, but some monosomic lines were distinguished by low crossing characteristics and few seed set. Monosomes were identified by analyzing meiotic metaphase I configurations of monosomic translocation heterozygous F_1 hybrids. When monosome of such a hybrid involves neither of the translocated chromosomes, each metaphase I cell typically includes a quadrivalent and a monosome (23 II + 1 IV + 1 I). In contrast, when the monosome involves one of the translocated chromosomes, a trivalent typically occurs (24 II + 1 III) [29].

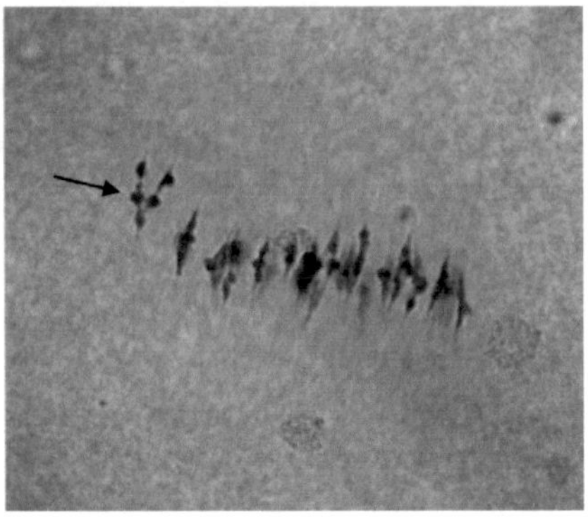

Figure 6. "Critical configuration" of the chromosomes at the meiotic metaphase I, showing 24 bivalents and 1 trivalent in cotton F_1 plant from the cross of monosomic Mo19xTT2L-6R (arrow point to the trivalent).

Cytological analyses of the two hybrid combinations involving two tester set lines (Mo19xTT6L-7L, Mo19xTT10R-11R) showed that monosome Mo19 is not chromosome 6, 7, 10, or 11 because the modal MI pairing configuration in the respective monosomic F_1 hybrids included 23 II + 1 IV + 1 I. In contrast, the tests with translocation lines TT2L-6R and TT2R-8Rb showed that the monosome Mo19 is chromosome 2, because the modal MI pairing configurations in the monosomic F_1 hybrids of Mo19xTT2L-6R and Mo19xTT2R-8Rb M I were 24 II + 1 III (**Figure 6**).

Since the monosomic line Mo19 had common chromosome 2 in the two translocation lines and it was assigned to chromosome 2 A_t-subgenome of cotton using SSR markers (BNL3971, BNL3590, and GH-198), we can now confidently tell that the monosome Mo19 from chromosome 2 A_t-subgenome (**Table 1**).

The cytological analyses of the two hybrid combinations involving two tester lines (Mo67xTT3R-5R, Mo67xTT9R-25) showed that monosome Mo67 is not chromosome 3, 5, 9, or 25 because the modal MI pairing configuration of its monosomic F_1 hybrids was 23 II + 1 IV + 1 I. The test with translocation line TT6L-7L showed, however, that the monosome Mo67 could be from chromosome 6 or 7, because in the monosomic F_1 hybrid of Mo67xTT6L-7L MI the modal MI pairing configuration was 24 II + 1 III. Molecular marker data suggested that the monosome Mo67 must be chromosome 6 of the A_t-subgenome (**Table 1**).

The cytological test of the hybrid combination involving one tester line (Mo75xTT4R-15L) showed that monosome Mo75 could be from chromosome 4 or 15, because in the monosomic F_1 hybrid of Mo75xTT4R-15L MI pairing was 24 II + 1 III. Molecular marker data suggested that the monosome Mo75 is chromosome 4 A_t-subgenome (**Table 1**; **Figure 7**).

http://dx.doi.org/10.5772/64558

Monosomic line	Origin	Year of the obtained	Chromosome		Molecular markers
			Size	Identity	
Mo11	Pollen irradiation	1991	Medium	A 2	BNL3590, GH-198
Mo16	Pollen irradiation	1991	Medium	A 2	BNL3971, BNL3590, GH198
Mo19	Pollen irradiation	1991	Large	A 2	BNL3971, BNL3590, GH198
Mo93	Pollen irradiation	2007	Medium	A 2	BNL1434, BNL1897, BNL3971
Mo7	Pollen irradiation	1990	Medium	A 4	BNL2572, CIR122, CIR048
Mo31	Pollen irradiation	1993	Medium	A 4	BNL2572, CIR122, CIR048
Mo38	Pollen irradiation	1993	Large	A 4	BNL2572, CIR122, CIR048
Mo59	Desynapsis	1996	Medium	A 4	BNL2572, CIR122, CIR048
Mo66	Pollen irradiation	1995	Medium	A 4	BNL2572, CIR122, CIR048
Mo69	Desynapsis	1997	Medium	A 4	BNL2572, CIR122, CIR048
Mo70	Desynapsis	1997	Medium	A 4	BNL2572, CIR122, GH-107
Mo71	Desynapsis	1997	Medium	A 4	BNL2572, CIR122, GH-107
Mo72	Desynapsis	1997	Medium	A 4	BNL2572, CIR122, CIR048
Mo73	Desynapsis	1997	Medium	A 4	BNL2572, CIR122, CIR048
Mo75	Pollen irradiation	1999	Medium	A 4	BNL2572, CIR122, CIR048
Mo76	Pollen irradiation	2001	Medium	A 4	BNL2572, CIR122, GH-107
Mo79	Desynapsis	2002	Small	A 4	BNL2572, CIR122, CIR048
Mo81	Pollen irradiation	2003	Medium	A 4	BNL2572, CIR122, GH-107
Mo89	Desynapsis	2003	Medium	A 4	BNL2572, CIR122, GH-107
Mo90	Pollen irradiation	2003	Small	A 4	BNL2572, CIR122, GH-107
Mo13	Pollen irradiation	1991	Large	A 6	BNL1064, BNL2884, BNL3650, CIR203, Gh032,Gh039, Gh082, TMB1538
Mo67	Translocation	1996	Large	A 6	BNL1064, BNL2884, BNL3650, CIR203, Gh032,Gh039, Gh082, TMB1538
Telo Mo21	Pollen irradiation	1991	Large	A 11	BNL3442, GH246, CIR212
Mo48	Pollen irradiation	1994	Small	D 18	BNL3280
Mo17	Pollen irradiation	1991	Medium	D 20 or 22	JESPR235

Table 1. Origin and some characters of the cotton monosomic lines of cotton *G. hirsutum* L.

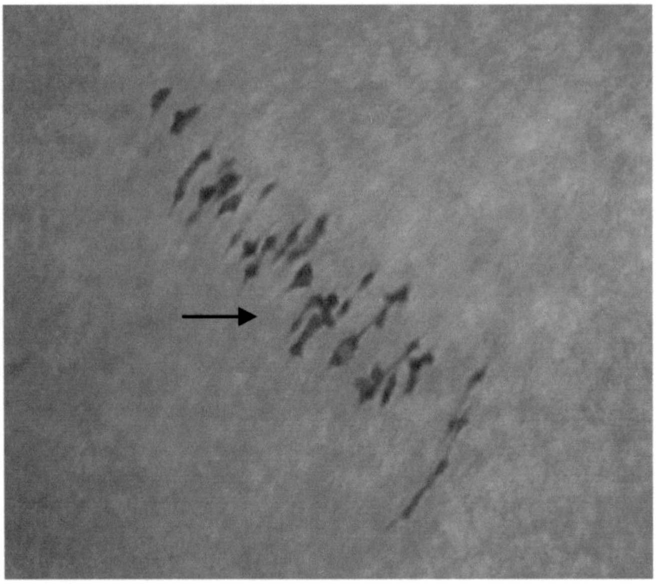

Figure 7. "Critical configuration" of the chromosomes at the meiotic metaphase I, showing 24 bivalents and 1 trivalent in cotton F_1 plant from the cross of monosomic Mo75 with TT4R-15L (arrow point to the trivalent).

Thus, out of one monotelodisomic and 24 monosomic lines identified using chromosome-specific SSR markers, three monosomes were confirmed by means of the translocation test. From 24 identified monosomic lines, four are chromosome A_t-2, 16 are chromosome A_t-4, two are chromosome A_t-6, and one each is chromosome D_t-18, chromosome D_t- 20 or 22 and telosome A_t-11.

4. Discussion

The utilization of the microsatellite markers and translocation lines for the identification of unknown cotton monosomic lines in our study provided the unified identification and numeration of the chromosomes and chromosome arm for 24 aneuploid lines of the Uzbek cytogenetic collection of cotton. On the basis of molecular-genetic and cytogenetic tests involving translocations, three of the six monosomes were designated chromosomes 2, 4, and 6 of the A_t-subgenome and two chromosomes were designated chromosomes 18 and 20 or 22 D_t-subgenome. One telosome was designated as a telosome 11 A_t-subgenome.

Twenty other monosomes were identified as duplicates of three of aforementioned monosomes (chromosomes 2, 4, and 6). Chromosome 4 of the A_t-subgenome was recovered more frequently (16 times), than chromosome 2 of the A_t-subgenome (4 times) and chromosome 6 of the A_t-subgenome (2 times) during the pollen irradiation in different doses and in progeny of the desynaptic plants (**Table 1**). The other chromosomes were recovered only once (chromosomes 18 and 20 or 22 D_t-subgenome and one telosome as a telosome 11 A_t-subgenome). These data demonstrated differences between the studied chromosomes on the response to irradiation treatments, and/or differences in their ability to survive as embryos and plants, and/or their ability to be maternally transmitted through nullisomic maternal gametes and gametophytes. It is possible that the centromeric region of the cotton chromosome 4 is more susceptible to treatments, and/or this chromosome is under less severe selection against monosomy and thus deficiencies are recovered and transmitted more frequently in the natural and irradiated populations. Identification of other monosomic lines using similar strategy is in progress in our laboratories.

According to our previous results, two monosomics lines (Mo11 and Mo19) from our collection may be involved the same monosome and were homologous because they had chromosomal associations with the same translocation line Tr16 of Uzbek cytogenetic collection [12, 15].

There are many challenges in genetic and molecular-genetic analyses of the complex genomes of cotton [5, 30–32], and the development of novel aneuploid lines for tetraploid cotton will be important to solve mapping of molecular markers in the cotton genome. Our results, which are largely based on radiation-induced aneuploidy, paralleled the findings of Endrizzi et al. [16] showed that chromosomes 4 and 6 are the two chromosomes that occur most frequently as spontaneous monosomes in natural populations of cotton. A challenge in attaining complete genome coverage, that is, monosomes for all chromosomes may be that some chromosomes may contain genes that are unique and essential to the zygote, plant, functional megaspore or megagametophyte. For these chromosomes, it may not possible to recover or sexually utilize monosomes; for others, the difficulty is likely to range from relatively easy to challenging.

5. Conclusion

The results presented in this report suggest that microsatellite markers are facile and useful tools for cytogenetic analysis of the cotton chromosome deficient plants. The utilization of the microsatellite markers for the identification of unknown cotton monosomic lines provided an opportunity to foster the identification and numeration of the chromosomes and chromosome arm for 24 aneuploid lines of the Uzbekistan cytogenetic collection of cotton. These markers can also be readily used for the development of new cotton chromosome substitution lines and germplasm introgression.

Acknowledgements

This work was partially supported by research Grants F-5-31 and KA-8009 from the Committee for Science and Technology of the Republic of Uzbekistan. We thank the administration of Center of Genomics and Bioinformatics, Academy of Science of Uzbekistan for the continued support of collaborative research and being an instrumental for the molecular experiments conducted in this study.

Author details

Marina F. Sanamyan[1*], Abdusalom K. Makamov[2], Shukhrat U. Bobokhujaev[1], Dilshod E. Usmonov[2], Zabardas T. Buriev[2], Sukumar Saha[3] and David M. Stelly[4]

*Address all correspondence to: sanam_marina@rambler.ru

1 National University of Uzbekistan, Tashkent, Uzbekistan

2 Center of Genomics and Bioinformatics, Academy of Sciences of Uzbekistan, Tashkent, Uzbekistan

3 USDA-ARS, Crop Science Research Laboratory, Mississippi State, USA

4 Department of Soil and Crop Sciences, Texas A&M University, College Station, USA

References

[1] Khush GS. Cytogenetics of aneuploids. New York and London: Academic Press; 1973. 301 p.

[2] Kohel GS. An evaluation of *Gossypium barbadense* L. chromosomes 6 and 17 in the *G. hirsutum* L. genome. Crop Science. 1977;17:404–406. DOI: 10.2135/cropsci1977.0011183X001700030016x

[3] Saha S., Wu J., Jenkins JN., McCarty JC., Gutierrez OA., Stelly DM., Percy RG., Raska DA. Effect of chromosome substitutions from *Gossypium barbadense* L. 3-79 into *G. hirsutum* L. TM-1 on agronomic and fiber traits. Journal of Cotton Science. 2004;8:162–169. DOI: 10.1007/s00122-012-1965-9

[4] Stelly DM., Saha S., Raska DA., Jenkins JN., McCarty JC., Gutierrez Jr., OA. Registration of 17 Upland (*Gossypium hirsutum*) cotton germplasm lines disomic for different *G. barbadense* chromosome or arm substitution. Crop Science. 2005;27:2663–2665. DOI: 10.2135/cropsci2004.0642

[5] Saha S., Raska DA., Stelly DM. Upland cotton (*Gossypium hirsutum* L.) × Hawaiian cotton (*G. tomentosum* Nutt. ex Seem.) F_1 hybrid hypoaneuploid chromosome substitution series. Journal of Cotton Science. 2006;10:263–272.

[6] Saha S., Raska DA., Stelly DM., Manchali S., Gutierrez OA. Hypoaneuploid chromosome substitution F_1 hybrids of *Gossypium hirsutum* L. × *G. mustelinum* Miers ex Watt. Journal of Cotton Science. 2013;17:102–114.

[7] Saha S., Stelly DM., Makamov AK., Ayubov MS., Raska D., Guitierrez OA., Manchali S., Jenkins JN., Deng D., Abdurakhmonov IY. Molecular confirmation of *Gossypium*

hirsutum chromosome substitution lines. Euphytica. 2015;205:459–473. DOI: 10.1007/s 10681-015-1407-2

[8] Saha S., Jenkins JN., Wu J., McCarty JC., Gutierrez OA., Percy RG., Roy G. Cantrell, Stelly DM. Effects of chromosome-specific introgression in upland Cotton on fiber and agronomic traits. Genetics. 2006;172:1927–1938. DOI: 10.1534/genetics.105.053371

[9] Saha S., Wu J., Jenkins JN., McCarty JC., Hayes R., Stelly DM. Genetic dissection of chromosome substitution lines of cotton to discover novel *Gossypium barbadense* L. alleles for improvement of agronomic traits. Theoretical Applied Genetics. 2010;120:1195–1205. DOI: 10.1007/s 00122-009-1247-3

[10] Liu S., Saha S., Stelly D., Burr B., Cantrel RG. The use of cotton aneuploid for the chromosomal assignment of microsatellite loci in cotton. Journal of Heredity. 2000;91:326–332.

[11] Gutierrez OA., Stelly DM., Saha S, Jenkins JN., Mc Carty JC., Raska DA., Schefler BE. Integrative placement and orientation of non-redundant SSR loci in cotton linkage group by deficiency analysis. Molecular Breeding. 2009;23:697–707. DOI: 10.1007/s11032-009-9266-y

[12] Sanamyan MF., Petlyakova J., Rakhmatullina EM., Sharipova E. Chapter 10. Cytogenetic collection of Uzbekistan. In: Abdurakhmonov IY. (Ed). World Cotton Germplasm Resources. Croatia: In Tech; 2014. pp. 247–287. DOI: 10.5772/56978

[13] Sanamyan MF., Petlyakova JE., Musaev DA. The development and cytogenetic study of monosomics of *Gossypium hirsutum* L. Biologia Plantarum. 2000;43:193–197.

[14] Sanamyan MF., Petlyakova JE., Sharipova EA., Abdurakhmonov IY. Cytogenetic characteristics of new monosomic stocks of cotton (*Gossypium hirsutum* L.). Genetics Research International. 2011;2011:1–12. DOI: 10.4061/2011/273642

[15] Sanamyan MF., Petlyakova JE., Sharipova EA., Abdurakhmonov IY. Morphological characteristics and identification of new monosomic stocks for cotton (*Gossypium hirsutum* L.). Advances in Bioscience and Biotechnology. 2010;1:372–383. DOI: 10.4236/abb.2010.15050

[16] Endrizzi JE., Turcotte EL., Kohel RJ. Genetics, cytology and evolution of Gossypium. Advances in Genetics.1985;23:271–375.

[17] Hulse-Kemp AM., Lemm J., Plieske J., et al. Development of a 63K SNP array for cotton and high-density mapping of intraspecific and interspecific populations of *Gossypium* spp. G3 Genes Genomes Genetics. 2015;5:1187–1209. DOI: 10.1534/g3.115.018416

[18] Saha S., Raska DA., Stelly DM. Chromosome substitution lines: concept, development and utilization in the genetic improvement of upland cotton. In: Abdurakhmonov IY (Ed). Plant Breeding. Croatia: In Tech; 2012. pp. 107–128. DOI: 10.5772/1389

[19] Dellaporta SJ., Wood J., Hicks JB. A plant DNA mini preparation: version II. Plant Molecular Biology Reporter. 1983;1:19–21.

[20] Guo W., Caiping C., Changbiao W., Zhiguo H., Xianliang S., Kai W., Xiaowei N., Cheng W., Keyu L., Ben S., Tianzhen, Z. A microsatellite-based, gene-rich linkage map reveals genome structure, function and evolution in *Gossypium*. Genetics. 2007;176:527–541. DOI: 10.1534/genetics.107.070375

[21] Hoffman SM., Yu JZ., Grum DS., Xiao J., Kohel RJ., Pepper AE. Identification of 700 new microsatellite loci from cotton (*G. hirsutum* L.). Journal of Cotton Science. 2007;11:208–241.

[22] Lacape J-M., Jacobs J., Arioli T., Derijcker R., Forestier-Chiron N., Llewellyn D., Jean J., Thomas E., Viot C. A new interspecific, *Gossypium hirsutum* × *G. barbadense*, RIL population: towards a unified consensus linkage map of tetraploid cotton. Theoretical Applied Genetics. 2009;119:281–292. DOI: 10.1007/s00122-009-1037-y

[23] Yu Y., Daojun Y., Shaoguang L., Ximei L., Xiaqing W., Zhongxu L., Xianlong Z. Genome structure of cotton revealed by a genome-wide SSR genetic map constructed from a BC1 population between *Gossypium hirsutum* and *G. barbadense*. BMC Genomics. 2011;12:15. DOI: 10.1186/1471-2164-12-15

[24] Yu JZ., Fang DD, Kohel RJ, Ulloa M, Hinze LL, Percy RG, Zhang J, Chee P. Scheffler BE, Jones DC. Development of a core set of SSR markers for the characterization of *Gossypium* germplasm. Euphytica. 2012a;187:203–213. DOI: 10.1007/s10681-012-0643-y

[25] Yu, JZ., Kohel RJ., Fang DD., Cho J., Van Deynze A., Ulloa M., Hoffman SM., Pepper AE., Stelly DM., Jenkins JN., Saha S., Kumpatla SP., Shah MR., Hugie WV., Percy RG. A high-density simple sequence repeat and single nucleotide polymorphism genetic map of the tetraploid cotton genome. G.3. Genes Genomes Genetics. 2012b;2:43–58. DOI: 10.1534/g3.111.001552

[26] Blenda A., Fang DD., Rami J-F., Garsmeur O., Luo F., et al. A high density consensus genetic map of tetraploid cotton that integrates multiple component maps through molecular marker redundancy check. PLoS One. 2012;7(9):e45739. DOI: 10.1371/journal.pone.0045739

[27] Zhiguo H., Changbiao W., Xianliang S., Wangzhen G., Jinying G., Chunhong LC., Tianzhen Z. Characteristics, development and mapping of *Gossypium hirsutum* derived EST-SSRs in allotetraploid cotton. Theoretical Applied Genetics. 2006;112:430–439. DOI: 10.1007/s00122-005-0142-9

[28] Love RM. Varietal differences in meiotic chromosome behavior of Brazilian wheat. Agronomy Journal. 1951;43:72–76.

[29] Endrizzi JE., Brown MS. Identification of monosomes for six chromosomes in *Gossypium hirsutum*. American Journal of Botany. 1964;51:117–120.

[30] Reinisch JA., Dong J., Brubaker CL., Stelly DM., Wendell JF., Raterson AH. A detailed RFLP map of cotton, *Cossypium hirsutum* × *Gossypium barbadense*: chromosome organi-

zation and evolution in disomic polyploid genome. Genetics. 1994;138:829–847. DOI: 10.1101/gr.3907305

[31] Han ZG., Guo WZ., Song XL., Zhang TZ. Genetic mapping of EST-derived microsatellites from the diploid *Gossypium arboreum* in allotetraploid cotton. Molecular Genetics and Genomics. 2004;272:308–327. DOI: 10.1371/journal.pone.0028676

[32] Nguyen TB., Ciband M., Brottier P., Risterucci AM., Lacape JM. Wide coverage of the tetraploid cotton genome using newly developed microsatellite markers. Theoretical Applied Genetics. 2004;109(1):167–176.

Chapter 9

Genetic Resistance to the Reniform Nematode in Cotton

Seloame T. Nyaku, Yonathan Tilahun,
Kathy Lawrence, Venkateswara R. Sripathi,
Abreeotta J. Williams and Govind C. Sharma

Additional information is available at the end of the chapter

http://dx.doi.org/10.5772/64389

Abstract

Among major nematode pests of Upland, cotton production is the reniform nematode, which is a serious threat in various cotton-producing regions. The availability of germplasm lines with tolerance or resistance to this menacing pest is a valued asset. To date, various laboratories and research institutions have collaborated to transfer the reniform nematode resistance from wild gene pools of cotton into widely cultivated Upland cotton, which have led to positive results. This chapter focuses on the current status of these introgressions and resistance mechanisms in cotton. In this overview, four major themes are being pursed: (1) tolerance mechanisms in cotton to the reniform nematode, (2) genotype evaluations, (3) introgression of reniform resistance into Upland cotton, and (4) functional analysis of reniform infection in Upland cotton. Genetic resistance in Upland cotton to the reniform nematode is the only practical solution because conventional control measures are the most cost-effective and environmentally sustainable and therefore have been and will be actively pursued. Resistance genes, if successfully introgressed into crop plants from wild relatives, should complement management of the reniform nematode with traditional methods.

Keywords: functional analysis, introgression, reniform nematode, resistance mechanisms, tolerance

1. Introduction

Cotton (*Gossypium hirsutum* L.) is one of the most important fiber crops of the world. However, in selected regions, yields are being reduced drastically by the reniform nematode, *Rotylenchulus reniformis*. This pest was reported in 1940 [1] and to date has become a significant pest of cotton in the southeastern and south-central United States [2, 3]. The estimated cotton production loss that occurred in the United States due to reniform nematode in 2005 was 115 × 106 kg (526,000 bales), conservatively worth US$1 kg^{-1} [4, 5].

The reniform nematode is a semi-endoparasite and derives its name from having a kidney-shaped body, usually of the adult female, and the males are, however, vermiform. The reniform life cycle is in four stages beginning from the egg. The first juvenile stage (J1) molts to become the second juvenile (J2) which also occurs within the egg. The J2 then hatches 1–2 weeks after eggs are laid especially when conditions are favorable [5]. Cuticles may sometimes overlay the other and are seen usually in the third- and fourth-stage juveniles, J3 and J4 [6]. Generally, after molting, there is a reduction in the body size of the reniform nematode [5]. The young adult reniform nematode females move towards the germinating host seedlings and to certain organic substances secreted by the roots [7]. Penetration by the nematode is in the elongation zone of the host plant root, proximal to the meristem. The epidermis and cortex are pierced by the vermiform young female intracellularly with the pericycle being the permanent feeding site [8, 9]. Half to two-thirds of the nematodes' body usually remains outside the root, and the nematode swells with kidney-like shape morphology.

Among the cellular changes observed after penetration of the cells by the reniform nematode include the formation of dense granular cytoplasm, hardening of cell walls through accumulation of polysaccharides, disintegration of cell walls, and enlargement of cells [10–12]. The adult female reniform nematode oviposits into a gelatinous matrix, produced by the vaginal glands, and the number of eggs within an egg mass varies, from 60 to 200 by a single adult female nematode [13]. The reniform nematode has the capability to undergo anhydrobiosis, a survival mechanism in the absence of water, making it thrive for at least 2 years in the absence of a host in dry soil [14]. The state of anhydrobiosis for the reniform nematode can last for more than 20 years in the absence of host plants [15].

Root-knot nematode (*Meloidogyne* spp.), another damaging nematode of cotton, are sedentary endoparasites that feed within the roots of host plants, resulting in drastic yield losses [16, 17]. The major observable signs on plants are the root knots that indicate colonization of roots of infected plants by these organisms. Symptoms include low yields, stunted growth, wilting, and predisposition to other pathogens. The most damaging stage is the second-stage juveniles (J2), which penetrate and invade their hosts near root tips and then migrate intercellularly toward the vascular cylinder. These nematodes puncture the cell wall continuously, and there is secretion release from the stylet into the cytoplasm, and the cytoplasm contents are ingested. The cells enlarged to form giant cells [18], and these have multiple nuclei and are very active metabolically in their functions [19]. The life cycle of *Meloidogyne* lasts for about 3 weeks, and eggs are then released into a gelatinous matrix by the adult female. During this period of feeding within the plant roots, physiological changes occur which alter gene expression mechanisms of the host [20].

2. Tolerance and resistance mechanisms of cotton to reniform nematode

Studies have shown changes in host gene expression during infection of roots by nematodes especially within the syncytium [21–23]. During the formation of syncytium, a number of changes occur within plant cells, among these are changes in cell cycle mechanisms, hormone regulation events, and cell wall architecture [24, 25]. Establishment of nematode feeding cells is through specific processes which are controlled and directed by encoded products of nematode parasitism genes found within the esophageal glands. These products are then delivered into the feeding cell through the nematode stylet [26]. Processes and events occurring at the nematode feeding sites play roles related to various degrees of susceptibility of cotton plants to the reniform nematode. Among these events are early degradation of syncytia [10], formation of wall deposits, and absence of hypertrophy in pericycle cells. These are some known mechanisms proposed for cotton resistance to reniform nematode.

Various Upland cotton varieties were planted in Unites States (US) in 2015 [27]. Among the varieties grown in United States, the largest and least acreages of cultivation were 'Deltapine' (31.2%) and 'Seed Source Genetics' (0.02%), respectively. 'Deltapine' cultivar covered about 50.1% of the acreage planted to Upland cotton in the southeastern states (Alabama, Florida, Georgia, North Carolina, South Carolina, and Virginia). Bayer CropScience ('FiberMax' and 'Stoneville') also covered significantly higher acreages (21.61 and 16.93%), respectively. An early study was conducted on susceptible (DP50-HR: 'Deltapine 50' with higher reproduction) and resistant (DP50-LR: 'Deltapine 50' with lower reproduction) genotypes, which were inoculated with 3000 reniform nematodes [28]. Roots collected 3, 6, 9, 12, and 15 days after inoculation (dai) revealed reduced reproduction in susceptible genotypes with degeneration of the syncytial cells and absence of hypertrophy within the pericycle cells.

Reniform nematodes show significant variations in populations [29–34]. Cotton genotypes will, therefore, have varying reproductive and pathogenicity responses to reniform nematode variants if present in populations. The 'LONREN 'genotypes ('LONREN-1' and 'LONREN-2' both of which are resistant to the reniform nematode) were used in association with susceptible genotypes ('FiberMax 966' and 'Deltapine 555BR') to six levels of inocula (0, 500, 1000, 5000, 10,000, or 50,000), consisting of eggs and vermiform life stages of reniform nematodes [35]. High inoculum levels (10,000 and 50,000) significantly reduced the root dry mass of 'LONREN' genotypes; however, higher levels in the susceptible genotypes rather stimulated root mass. Thus, the 'LONREN' genotypes may be involved in hypersensitive responses to nematode parasitism.

Another study was conducted on five cotton genotypes with various resistance/tolerance levels to reniform nematode isolates obtained from cotton field in Louisiana [36]. High reproduction of isolates was observed from Evan (33,793 juveniles/250 g soil) and Avoyelles (27,800 juveniles/250 g soil) genotypes. Data revealed that the *G. arboreum* ('A2-190') and 'LONREN-2' were the most resistant genotypes among the nematode isolates. However, 'TX-110' and 'BARBREN-713' both had high levels of resistance to the reniform nematodes in terms of pathogenicity. The 'LONREN-1', 'LONREN-2', and 'A2-190' genotypes showed hypersensitivity to reniform nematode invasion of roots as seen in stunted plant growth. This study therefore confirms the presence of variation in both pathogenicity and reproduction of reniform nematode isolates in cotton fields. Isolates obtained from various infested cotton fields may have various adaptive mechanisms in the soils in which they occur [37, 38]. Further, genetic variation within specific genes, for example, rRNA and ITS1 and microsatellite loci of the reniform nematode [29–31, 34, 39, 40] might influence pathogenicity and reproductive ability of nematodes. Simple sequence repeat (SSR) markers have been used to reveal the polymorphism in reniform nematode sampled from infested fields in Mississippi [40].

Exploring of host resistance to nematode parasitism is the most effective and environmentally friendly method of nematode management. Resistant cultivars pose an incompatible interaction with nematodes. A hypersensitive reaction is produced in a response to the feeding or invading nematode leading to lignification of the cells in close proximity to the reniform nematode's head, or the cells either collapse or become necrotic [41, 42]. However, in a compatible interaction, there is a formation of active syncytia with cells becoming hypertrophic, dense cytoplasm, enlarged nuclei, in most instances a partial disintegration of cell walls [29]. Application of nematicides to the resistant genotypes of cotton, for example, 'LONREN' have a positive impact on plant response and yield [43]. This hypersensitivity which is produced can be reduced in seedlings after nematicide applications. Four-resistant breeding lines from ('LONREN-1' × 'FM966') cross, a susceptible line from the 'LONREN' × 'FM966' cross, 'LONREN-1', 'BARBREN-713', and the 'DP393' (susceptible cultivar) were explored in a nematicide trial [43]. There was an increase in plant height and yield among plants to which nematicides were applied in greenhouse experiments. Furthermore, the number of reniform nematodes isolated was about 50% lower in resistant genotypes 45 days after planting (DAP). Differences were also observed among 'BARBREN-713' and 'LONREN'-derived lines in relation to reniform nematode egg number counts, with lower counts noted on 'BARBREN-713'. There was also a reduction in stunting of genotypes that received aldicarb treatment.

3. Evaluation of *G. hirsutum* genotypes to reniform nematode

Within the *Gossypium* genus, about 50 diploid and allotetraploid species are known. Two widely cultivated diploids include *Gossypium arboreum* L. and *G. herbaceum* L., and the two cultivated allotetraploids are *G. hirsutum* L. and *G. barbadense* L. [44]. There are eight diploid genome groups (A, B, C, D, E, F, G, and K) with the same chromosome number (2n = 26) [45]. Among the wild diploid species, three geographical groups are known (Australian, American, and Afro-Arabian).

Towards the end of the 1980s, some germplasm lines ('La. RN 4-4', 'La. RN 909', 'La. RN 910', and 'La. RN 1032') were developed in Louisiana State University in Baton Rouge with low-to-moderate levels of resistance to the reniform nematode [46]. These lines were from Upland cotton and were the first with some levels of resistance to the reniform nematode. Towards the latter part of 1997, the Unites States Department of Agriculture (USDA) Agricultural Research Service (ARS) scientists in Texas released four germplasm lines ('N220-1-91', 'N222-1-91', 'N320-2-91', and 'N419-1-91') with slightly higher levels resistance to the reniform nematode compared to earlier released lines [47].

Further screening of *G. hirsutum* genotypes has been conducted [46–49]. However, most of these lines have varying tolerance levels to the reniform nematode [47]. Several genotypes (*G. hirsutum* (110), *G. herbaceum* (7), *G. arboreum* (14), *G. barbadense* (6), wild *Gossypium* spp. (33), *Hibiscus* spp. (22), and other Malvaceae (7) were evaluated for their resistance against the reniform nematode, through their ability to reproduce on roots [50]. The genotypes (*G. stocksii, G. somalense,* and *G. barbadense* and 'Texas110' possessed high resistance to the reniform nematode. *Gossypium hirsutum* 893, *G. herbaceum* PI 408775, *G. arboreum* PI 41895, PI 417891, and CB 3839 also have low nematode egg productions (20%).

Resistance has also been explored in wild accessions of *G. hirsutum* and *G. barbadense* to *M. incognita* race 3 and reniform nematodes [51]. The *G. barbadense* accessions ('TX-1347' and 'TX-1348') had lower reproduction on them compared to the *G. hirsutum* accessions although were susceptible to *M. incognita* race 3. A greenhouse study was conducted on 52 cultivars of cotton to identify those with some resistance to the reniform nematode; however, all the cultivars were susceptible to this organism [48]. Among the various cultivars, those with the lowest reproductive factors (RF) were 'SG 105', 'DP 543 BGII'/'RR', 'DP 445BG'/'RR', and 'FM 989 R'. Other *G. hirsutum* lines ('MT2468 Ren1', 'MT2468 Ren2', and 'MT2468 Ren3') with resistance to the reniform nematode were released [52]. This effort was from Scientists at the USDA ARS and the Mississippi Agricultural and Forestry Experiment Station.

4. Introgression of reniform nematode resistance into Upland cotton

Researchers over the years have screened genotypes and believed to have resistance to the reniform nematode. They have proved that these genotypes are not 100% resistant to the reniform nematode [48–50]. This, therefore, has resulted in multi-institutional collaborations on the introgression of resistance into Upland cotton from close and distant relatives of *Gossypium* [53, 54]. Monosomic addition lines were developed with the aim of transferring resistance into Upland cotton from *G. longicalyx* [55]. However, after screening 12 lines that were segregating, resistance to this pest was minimal. However, there have been successful introgressions into the reniform nematode into *G. hirsutum* from *G. arboreum* [56], *G. aridum* [57], *G. barbadense* [58–60] making the introgressed lines resistant to the reniform nematode.

The introgression of the reniform nematode resistance trait of *G. longicalyx* into Upland cotton was achieved through the development of two 52-chromosome trispecies hybrids [(*G. hirsutum* × *G. longicalyx*) chromosome-doubled × *G. armourianum*] (abbreviated as HLA) and [(*G. hirsutum* × *G. herbaceum*) chromosome-doubled × *G. longicalyx*] (abbreviated as HHL) [61]. The *G. longicalyx* (F_1) had the resistance trait. In this approach, there was a need to include a genotype that could reduce ploidy characteristics existing between the 'donor' and 'recipient' genotypes. Therefore, either *G. armourianum* Kearney (D_{2-1}) or *G. herbaceum* L. (A1) were used in genetic crosses. A number of recurrent backcrossings were undertaken that produced 28 lines with reniform nematode resistance, and segregation (1:1) was observed in all the backcrosses for resistant and susceptible traits [61, 62]. This demonstrated that the trait responsible for reniform nematode resistance is single gene controlled and heritable. This effort led to the release of two *G. hirsutum* germplasm lines, 'LONREN-1' (Registration # GP-977, PI 669509) and 'LONREN-2' (Registration # GP-978, PI 669510). The release was by both USDA and Cotton Incorporated to enable cotton farmers' access to the reniform nematode-resistant germplasm with improved yields. The introgressed chromosome segments in both lines differ slightly in terms of size, with that of 'LONREN-2' much smaller than that of 'LONREN-1'. Experimental assays revealed a 95% reduction in nematode populations in growth chambers and 50–90% reductions in field trials. A disadvantage with these lines, however, is the reduced plant growth and stunting in fields with very high populations of reniform nematodes, reflecting in poor yields [63, 64]. This gene conferring high resistance to the reniform nematode has also been introgressed from the African species *G. longicalyx* (Hutch. & Lee, 2n = 2x = 26; $2F_1$) [65]. The allele conferring this resistance (*Ren*^{lon}) was linked to chromosome 11. In that study [65], two trispecies hybrids made up of *G. hirsutum* $(AD)_1$, the recipient species, *G. longicalyx* (F_1) the donor parent, and two wild diploids, *G. armourianum* (D_{2-1}) and *G. herbaceum* (A1), were used as 'bridges'.

Various screens were performed on *G. hirsutum, G. longicalyx, G. armourianum*, and HLA trispecies hybrids to identify markers that could be linked to resistance in the reniform nematode [65]. Sixty-two simple sequence repeat (SSR) markers were used in amplifying pooled DNA from *G. hirsutum* cultivars ['Auburn (Aub)-623', 'AcalaNemX', and 'Deltapine (DP)-458'] for the identification of polymorphisms on the A-sub-genome. Some primer pairs revealed polymorphisms among various groups of resistant (F_1 and HLA) and susceptible $(AD)_1$ and $(D)_{2-1}$ genotypes. These primer pairs were selected and used for screening genotypes in BC2F1 populations to identify markers associated with the reniform resistance locus *Ren*. A phenotypic marker in *G. longicalyx* could be linked with green seed fuzz (*Fzglon*) which was closely associated with the reniform nematode. This association was confirmed by screening 984 resistant and susceptible genotypes in various backcrosses.

Transfer of reniform nematode resistance into Upland cotton has also been successfully achieved through crossing the resistant *G. arboreum* (A-genome) with a D-genome species [66]. Backcrossing with Upland cotton $(AD)_1$, and screenings of the BC2F1 and the BC2F2 for resistance to reniform nematode showed plants with resistance to this pest. Another successful reniform nematode resistance introgression into *G. hirsutum* was from *G. aridum* [57]. This study involved mapping of traits from various genotypes that have been backcrossed. This included a trispecies hybrid, [*G. arboreum* × (*G. hirsutum* × *G. aridum*)], crossed with 'MD51ne' (*G. hirsutum*). One hundred and four simple sequence repeat markers were then used to identify markers linked with resistance in the reniform nematode in 50 and 26 resistant and susceptible progenies, respectively, obtained from the above crosses. Among the various markers utilized, 25 of them were resistance specific to the reniform nematode and were all localized to chromosome 21 of cotton. The locus of resistance was *Ren*^{ari} and two of these markers identified were BNL3279_132 and BNL2662_090.

Reniform nematode resistance introgression into *G. hirsutum* from *G. arboreum* accession ('A2-190') crossed with a hexaploid (AD1) × D4 bridging line (G 371) is another success story [56]. The progenies were tetraploid triple-species hybrids. They were progressively back-crossed into *G. hirsutum* producing 277 BC_1 new genotypes. Growth chamber experiments revealed that the 'G371', a hexaploid bridging line, poses resistance to the reniform nematode. Therefore, resistance to the reniform nematode was controlled by dominant genes.

Trispecies hybrids with *G. thurberi* have been utilized in transferring resistant traits into *G. hirsutum* [67]. This hybrid [(*G. hirsutum* × *G. thurberi*) a hexaploid [2n = 6× = 78, $(AADD)_1 \times D_1$] × *G. longicalyx* (F)] was used in cytogenetic analysis. Fifteen simple sequence repeat (SSR) markers were also utilized in accessing the introgressions in the various hybrid plants through specific bands, which confirmed successful introgressions. Cytogenetic analysis revealed a chromosome configuration 2n = 52 = 14.13 I + 15.10 II + 1.03III + 0.9 IV + 0.03 V + 0.13 VI (I, II, III, IV, V, and VI refer to univalents, bivalents, trivalents, tetravalents, pentavalents, and hexavalents, respectively). Mitotic chromosome analysis provided evidence on the number of chromosome within the genomes of the species and hybrids. The chromosomes varied in number for *G. hirsutum* (52), *G. thurberi* (26), *G. longicalyx* (26), and (*G. hirsutum* × *G. thurberi*) (78), and three-species hybrid [(*G. hirsutum* × *G. herbaceum*) × *G. longicalyx*] (HTL) (52).

Large germplasm lines ('1866' and '907') of *G. hirsutum* and *G. barbadense,* respectively, have been effectively screened in efforts to identify resistance to the reniform nematode [68]. Introgressions from *G. barbadense* into *G. hirsutum* against the reniform nematode, and markers linked to resistance in this pest have been a success [58–60, 68, 69].

Greenhouse assays also complement field screening of germplasm lines for nematode resistance in these lines [70]. In one of these assays, a single test plant was screened against six susceptible and resistant plants of *G. hirsutum*, 'Deltaple-16' and moderately resistant *G. barbadense* 'TX-1348', respectively [51]. Screening assays revealed about 5 and 12% of *G. hirsutum* and *G. barbadense* accessions having lower numbers of reniform nematodes compared to as susceptible check 'TX-1348', respectively. Moderate resistance was observed in the *G. barbadense* cultivar 'TX-110' (PI 163608) and *G. barbadense* accession 'GB 713' (PI 608139). Among the various *G. barbadense* accessions screened with moderate resistance to *M. incognita,* none of these was resistant to the reniform nematode.

Texas AgriLife Research released two breeding lines 'TAM RKRNR-9' (Reg. No. GP-941; PI 662039) and 'TAM RKRNR-12' (Reg. No. CP-942; PI 662040) of Upland cotton in 2010 [58]. Both of these lines poses resistance to *M. incognita* and the reniform nematode. These germplasm lines were developed through the crosses between 'M-315 RNR', an *M. incognita* resistant *G. hirsutum* line, and a reniform nematode-resistant *G. barbadense* line 'TX-110'. Both germplasm lines are commercially available and can be utilized in cotton breeding research. In other collaborative efforts, Research Scientists at the USDA and Mississippi Agricultural and Forestry Experiment Station released three germplasm lines, 'M713 Ren1' (Reg. No. GP-958, PI 665928), 'M713 Ren2' (Reg. No. GP-959, PI 665929), and 'M713 Ren5' (Reg. No. GP-960, PI 665930) in 2012 [59]. The reniform nematode resistance within these lines was from the *G. barbadense accession* 'GB 713'.

SSR markers associated with reniform nematode quantitative trait loci (QTLs) involved in resistance are known [69]. This was achieved through genotyping of 300 F_2 populations of 'GB713' × 'AcalaNem-X' crosses. QTLs were localized to chromosomes 21 and 18, respectively. The QTLs on chromosome 21 were on map positions 168 (LOD 28.0) and 182.7 (LOD 24.6), with the specific SSR markers BNL 1551_162 and GH 132_199 on position 154.2 and 177.3 and BNL 4011_155 and BNL 3279_106 on positions 180.6 and 184.5 associated with these loci, respectively. However, the only single QTL on chromosome 18 was on the map position 39.6 (LOD 4.0) with the specific SSR markers BNL 1721_178 and BNL 569_131 on positions 27.6 and 42.9, respectively. The authors, therefore, suggested the following designations Ren^{barb1} and Ren^{barb2} for QTLs located on chromosome 21 and Ren^{barb3} for those on chromosome 18. Further experiments in controlled environments on 'GB-713' showed a reduction in reniform and *M. incognita* numbers by 90% [60].

5. Functional analysis of reniform nematode infection in cotton

5.1. Parasitism genes

Sequencing of the nematode parasitome usually involves gene products that the nematode secretes during its cycle; critical study of genes will enhance the understanding of the nature of damage caused by nematodes to host plants [22]. Majority of these genes encode cell wall-modifying proteins such as galactosidases, xylanases, pectinases, and expansins [71]. Isolation of the parasitome from plant–parasitic nematodes, for example, β-1-4-endoglucanases (cellulases) was from the subventral glands of *Heterodera glycines* and *Globodera rostochiensis* [72, 73]. These proteins were the first isolated molecules in plant–parasitic nematodes. Cellulases are needed by nematodes to degrade cell walls for easy penetration to the roots [74].

Cellulase genes have been identified within reniform nematode [75–77], *H. glycines* [78], *G. tabacum* [79], *Pratylenchus penetrans* [80], *M. incognita* [81], and *H. schachtii* [82]. Within the cyst nematode, cellulase activity has been observed in J2 juveniles, but rarely in J3 juveniles [78]. These cellulases are associated with the glycosyl hydrolase family 5, with two domain structures (i.e., a catalytic domain with and without a cellulose-binding domain). The cellulase gene (*RR-ENG-1*) of 1341-bp length has also been molecularly characterized in the reniform nematode. This gene had a 19-bp 5′-untranslated region (UTR), a 1245-bp open-reading frame (ORF), and an 80-bp 3′-UTR region [75]. Multiple sequence alignment of the cDNA and genomic sequences revealed seven introns and eight exons for *RR-ENG-1* gene.

Further BLAST analysis gave hits to *HG-ENG-6* mRNA in *H. glycines*. Semiquantitative RT-PCR used in studying gene expression revealed *RR-ENG-1* highly expressed in the second-stage juvenile (J2) and adult vermiform life stages. However, expression levels in the adult female were much lower. Recent characterization of the reniform nematode genome revealed hits to *HG-ENG-6* and *ENG-1* genes in *H. glycines* (Accession # AA025506) and *Radophilus similis* (Accession# ACB38289), respectively [77]. Similarly, transcriptome sequencing of the reniform nematode revealed hits to *ENG-2* (Accession # AAK21881.1 and AAK21883.2), *ENG-1* (Accession # AAD45868.1), and *ENG-7* (Accession # AAK21887.1) genes in *Meloidogyne* spp. [76].

Two cellulase cDNAs (*HG-ENG-1* and *GR-ENG-1*), that code for a secretion of signal peptide, cellulase catalytic domain, cellulose binding domain (CBD), and a small peptide linker, are within the cyst nematode genome. Secretion of these cellulases was within the subventral esophageal gland cells, and their presence was confirmed through mRNA in situ hybridization and immunolocalization. The cellulase activity is usually enhanced by the presence of the CBD. In *G. rostochiensis,* characterization of its cellulase cDNA (*GR-ENG-2*) showed absence of a CBD, which inhibits synthesis of crystalline cellulose [72, 83]. Horizontal gene transfer from prokaryotic microbes such as bacteria to nematodes is known [84]. Cyst nematode cellulases are similar to those found in bacteria, and theories of horizontal gene transfer to ancestor cyst nematodes have been proposed [26, 85]. This phenomenon has also been observed in *Meloidogyne* species EST data and the existence of associations to parasitism [86]. Two *Meloidogyne* genes of rhizobial origin encode L-threonine aldolase (mi01644) and a protein of unknown function (mi00109). Sympatric organisms share the same soil ecological niche and both *Meloidogyne* and rhizobia fall into this class [87]. Another group of parasitism genes characterized in the reniform nematode genome are the C-type lectins (CTLs) [76, 77, 88]. The C-type lectins (CTLs) are a family of Ca^{2+}-dependent carbohydrate-binding proteins with roles in innate immune response. A 5′- and 3′-RACE analysis was used in the identification of 11 reniform nematode CTL transcripts (*RR-CTL-1–RR-CTL-11*), and these ranged from 1083 to 1194 bp with 93–99% sequence identity with the other [88]. Multiple sequence alignment of cDNA and genomic sequences showed three intronic regions. Specific BLAST hits were to *Heligmosomoides polygyrus* and *H. glycines*. The genes *RR-CTL-1, RR-CTL-*2, and *RR-CTL-*3 expressions were constant in the life cycle of the reniform nematode. The Rr-ctl transcripts were not constant in the various juvenile stages and were 839-fold higher in sedentary female nematodes compared to any other juvenile stage. A previous expresses sequence tag (EST) study [89] revealed C-type lectin domain peptides. These groups of peptides are carbohydrate-binding proteins, and therefore, calcium is a requirement for their effective functioning [90] and it is found in metazoans [91]. The *CTL* genes have been characterized in some animal–parasitic nematodes, *Heligmosomoides polygyrus, Toxocara canis,* and *Nippostrongylus brasiliensis* [92, 93]. These CTLs have also been identified in the subventral glands of *M. graminicola* [94]. Characterization of the reniform nematode genome and transcriptome through 454 sequencing showed hits to *BM1_02750* (Accession # XP_001892052) and *CLEC-180* (Accession #NP_501229.2) in *Brugia malayi* and *Caenorhabditis elegans,* respectively [77].

5.2. Parasitism proteins

Parasitism proteins released from the cell of nematodes induce changes in host cell physiology through specific signals in the nucleus within the host cells [95]. The regulation of the host's cells by nematodes occurs during transcription and direct interaction between nematode-secreted protein and plant-protein target has been observed. In the root knot nematode (RKN), a 13-aa secretory peptide 16D10 has interactions with two SCARECROW-like transcription factors [96].

The root knot and cyst nematodes both secrete chorismate mutase (CM) which affects the cellular shikimic acid pathway [71]. An overexpression of this protein in *M. javanica* in plant roots influences indole acetic acid (IAA) secretion which may result in improper tissue development [97]. Other proteins (14-3-3, sxp-ral-2, and ranbpm-like family proteins) influence cell-cycle, calcium binding, and defense regulation mechanisms in plants [71]. The 14-3-3 proteins have also been identified in reniform ESTs and these had homologies to 14-3-3 sequences of *C. briggsae* (Accession # XP_002643936.1) and *C. elegans* (Accession# NP_509939.1) [76]. Within the reniform, nematode genomic sequence hits to 14-3-3 sequences were observed in *Bursaphelenchus xylophilus* (Accession# ACZ13351), *Ancylostoma caninum* (Accession # ACO59962), and *M. incognita* (Accession# AAR85527) [77].

Expansin-like proteins in the potato cyst nematode (*G. rostochiensis*) can imitate some of their host genes in their function. An example is the hg-syv46 parasitism gene with a C-terminus having a similar function to CLAVATA3/ESR (CLE), a conserved domain in *Arabidopsis thaliana* [98, 99]. Three reniform nematode genes that code for putative CLE motifs (rr-cle-1, rr-cle-2, and rr-cle-3) have been isolated [100]. These peptides have an amino-terminal signal peptide with specific roles in secretion and pose a C-terminal CLE motif which can be associated with that of *Heterodera* spp. The parasitism gene (16D10) is a conserved gene found in root knot nematode species controlling signaling events in RKN and its host associations. A double-stranded RNA (dsRNA) within the genomes of nematodes produces RNA interference (RNAi) of the targeted transcript. The technique of RNAi was first studied in *C. elegans* [101] and has been applied in gene silencing of variety organisms [102]. There are *in vitro* assays that facilitate stimulation of parasitic J2 nematodes to intake dsRNA from solutions through the nematodes stylet for RNAi induction [96, 103]. Specific nematode parasitism genes that are targeted could be easily knocked out and their functions effectively studied at the molecular level through RNAi approach [103].

5.3. Host-pathogen interactions

Plant host-pathogen interactions have fascinated plant pathologists over hundreds of years [104]. Contemporary studies on interactions began with seminal work on the gene-for-gene concept in plant host-pathogen interactions [105]. The gene-for-gene concept states that for every host R (resistance) gene, a corresponding Avr (avirulence) gene exists; thus, a successful host-defensive response requires a successful interaction [105]. The ranbpm-like family proteins and chorismate mutase (CM) interact with plant R genes, indicating nematode parasitism proteins act as avirulence genes [106, 107].

Proteins made by animal parasitic nematodes have been found in some plant parasitic nematode genomes and they are conserved [108]. These proteins function to challenge the host's immune system invoking specific responses [109]. The last two decades have advanced the global approach to studying gene expression. We now have advanced recombinant DNA technologies to study gene expression at the mRNA or total RNA (transcriptome) and protein (proteome) levels. Approaches employed in the study of plant response to nematode parasitism include differential display [110, 111], promoter-reporter gene fusions [112–114], RNA blotting, protein immunolocalization, *in situ* hybridization [79, 115], and differential library screening [116]. Identification of genes playing useful roles in parasitism have been achieved through development of cDNA libraries from esophageal gland cells of the soybean cyst nematode [117, 118]. Other techniques used in the study of gene expression in plants at a single time point during early stages of infection of nematodes include oligonucleotide and cDNA microarrays [119, 120]; for example, in soybean cyst nematode, 1358 cDNAs from the esophageal glands were identified in expression analysis [121].

Recently, RNA-Seq analysis has been used in transcriptome sequencing of cotton (*G. hirsutum* L.) genotypes to measure comparative transcript abundance in reniform nematode susceptible ('DP90' & 'SG747'), resistant ('BARBREN-713'), and hypersensitive ('LONREN-1') genotypes of cotton (*G. hirsutum* L.) with and without reniform nematode infestation [122]. Several resistance genes that encode proteins known to be tightly linked to pathogen perception and resistance, for example, LRR-like and NBS-LRR domain-containing proteins were identified.

Most gene expression is a regulated process with genes being active in some situations and inactive in others. Gene expression relates to the physical signals from the environment and developmental cues of the organism in question. The rate of protein synthesis was once thought to be proportional to the concentration of mRNA; therefore, gene expression regulation depends on the regulation of the steady-state concentration of mRNAs [123]. However, mRNA levels and protein concentrations only partially correlate, a finding based on thoroughly composed reference datasets accounting for factors where ribosome occupancy and density and open-reading frame (ORF)-specific translation elongation rates were considered [124]. Therefore, many regulatory mechanisms involved with gene expression operate at many levels. The mechanisms influence on alterations in DNA structure, modification of transcription, stability, or translation of mRNA, or alterations in protein activity through post-translational modification.

Plants display varying levels of resistance to most pathogens in their environment, often being able to recognize pathogens through specifically distinct methods of detection [125]. A series of mechanisms of defense have been developed by plants, some of which can be constitutive or inducible. Resistance in plants is defined as the inability of a pathogen to propagate and spread on a host plant, usually involving a response referred to as the hypersensitive response (HR) [125]. The lines between a plant and its pathogens are truly battlegrounds where there are deployments of defense. The most current description of the action that takes place applies also to cotton-reniform interactions. Inducible defense responses in this type of interaction follow the 'zigzag' model [126].

According to the model suppression of immune-associated macroscopic programmed cell death (PCD) triggered by MAPK cascades or by the ETI cognate elicitors R3a/Avr3a occurs in susceptible hosts [126, 127]. The study showed that nematodes injected into the plant, thereby suppress PAMP-triggered immunity (PTI) or effector-triggered immunity (ETI) that are associated with the activation of PCD. Therefore, resistance is the ability of the host plant to evade the suppression of PCD. In other words, the host is resistant when its cells are able to undergo PCD and susceptible when the cells cannot undergo PCD.

6. Conclusion

There has been much progress and success made by researchers in introgression of reniform nematode resistance into Upland cotton from distant and close relatives. However, introgressed genotypes, solely developed to withstand reniform nematode parasitism, may have low crop yields in fields where mixed-populations of nematodes occur. The challenge now is to develop germplasm lines that may be able to withstand more than two nematode types in the same field. The rapid advances in genomics, transcriptomics, and proteomic analysis provide huge datasets, from which several resistance genes to the reniform nematode and other nematodes have been identified. These genes could be further explored and transferred into Upland cotton with various trials initiated in specific cotton-producing localities, for this overarching goal to be achieved.

Author details

Seloame T. Nyaku[1*], Yonathan Tilahun[2], Kathy Lawrence[3], Venkateswara R. Sripathi[4], Abreeotta J. Williams[4] and Govind C. Sharma[4]

*Address all correspondence to: stnyaku@ug.edu.gh; seloame.nyaku@gmail.com

1 Crop Science Department, College of Basic and Applied Sciences, University of Ghana, Legon-Accra, Ghana

2 Extension, School of Agriculture & Applied Sciences, Langston University, Langston, OK, USA

3 Department of Entomology and Plant Pathology, Auburn University, Auburn, AL, USA

4 Center for Molecular Biology, Alabama A&M University, Normal, AL, USA

References

[1] Smith AL. Distribution and relation of meadow nematode, *Pratylenchus praunsis*, to *Fusarium* wilt of cotton in Georgia. Phytopathology. 1940; 30:710. doi: 10.12691/wjar-1-4-1.

[2] Lawrence GW. Managing the reniform nematodes with nematicides. In: Proceedings of the Beltwide Cotton Conference, 6–10 January 1999; Orlando, FL. p. 100–101.

[3] Lawrence GW, McLean KS. The reniform nematode. In: Kirkpatrick TL, Rothrock CS, editors. Compendium of Cotton Diseases. APS Press, St. Paul, MN; 2001. p. 42–44.

[4] Blasingame D. Cotton disease loss estimate committee report. In: Proceedings of the Beltwide Cotton Conference, 3–6 January 2006; San Antonio, TX. p. 155–157.

[5] Robinson AF, Percival, AE. Resistance to *Meloidogyne incognita* race 3 and *Rotylenchulus reniformis* in wild accessions of *Gossypium hirsutum and G. barbadense* from Mexico. Journal of Nematology. 1997; 29:746–755.

[6] Linford MB, Oliveira JM. *Rotylenchulus reniformis* nov. gen., n. sp., a nematode parasite of roots. In: Proceedings of the Helminthological Society of Washington; 1940. p. 35–42.

[7] Riddle DL, Bird AF. Responses of the plant parasitic nematodes *Rotylenchulus reniformis, Anguina agrostis,* and *Meloidogyne javanica* to chemical attractants. Parasitology. 1985; 91:185–195. DOI: 10.1017/S0031182000056626.

[8] Yik CP, Birchfield W. *Gossypium* germplasm resistant to the reniform nematode. Journal of Nematology. 1981; 13:465. (Abstr.).

[9] Khan RM, Khan MW. Histopathology of cauliflower roots infected with reniform nematode. Pakistan Journal of Nematology. 1985; 3:83–85. (Abstr.).

[10] Rebois RV, Madden PA, Eldridge BJ. Some ultrastructural changes induced in resistant and susceptible soybean roots following infection by *Rotylenchulus reniformis*. Journal of Nematology. 1975; 7:122–139.

[11] Vovlas N, Ekanayake HMRK. Histological alterations induced by *Rotylenchulus reniformis* alone or simultaneously with *Meloidogyne incognita* on banana roots. Nematropica. 1985; 15:9–17.

[12] Gaur HS, Perry RN. The biology of the plant parasitic nematode *Rotylenchulus reniformis*. Agricultural Zoology Reviews.1991; 4:177–212.

[13] Sivakumar CV, Seshadri AR. Life history of the reniform nematode *Rotylenchulus reniformis* Linford and Oliveira, 1940. Indian journal of Nematology. 1971; 1:7–20.

[14] Radewald JD, Takeshita G. Desiccation studies on five species of plant-parasitic nematodes of Hawaii. Phytopathology. 1964; 54: 903–904.

[15] Birchfield W. Host-parasite relations of *Rotylenchulus reniformisonreniformis* on *Gossypium hirsutum,* Phytopathology. 1962; 52:862–865.

[16] Mai WF. Plant-parasitic nematodes: their threat to agriculture. In: Sasser J, Carter CC, editors. An Advanced Treatise on *Meloidogyne*. North Carolina State University Graphics, Raleigh, USA;1985. 1:11–17.

[17] Sasser JN. Root-knot nematode: a global menace to crop production. Plant Disease. 1980; 64:36–41.

[18] Hussey RS. Host-parasite relationships and associated physiological changes. In: Sasser J, Carter CC, editors. An Advanced Treatise on *Meloidogyne*. 1985; 1:143–153.

[19] Jones MGK. Early stages of nematode-induced giant-cell formation in roots of *Impatiens balsamina*. Journal of Nematology. 1978; 10:70–84.

[20] Sijmons PC, Atkinson HJ, Wyss U. Parasitic strategies of root nematodes and associated host cell responses. Annual Review of Phytopathology. 1994; 32:235–259. doi: 10.1146/annurev.py.32.090194.001315.

[21] Hussey RS, Davis EL, Baum TJ. Secrets in secretions: genes that control nematode parasitism in plants. Brazilian Journal of Plant Physiology. 2002; 14:183–194. doi: 10.1590/S1677-04202002000300002.

[22] Gheysen G, Fenoll C. Gene expression in nematode feeding sites. Annual Review of Phytopathology. 2002; 40: 191–219. doi: 10.1146/annurev.phyto.40.121201.093719.

[23] Williamson VM, Gleason, CA. Plant-nematode interactions. Current Opinion Plant Biology. 2003; 6:327–333. doi: 10.1016/S1369-5266(03)00059-1.

[24] Bird DM. Manipulation of host gene expression by root-knot nematodes. Journal of Parasitology. 1996; 82:881–888. doi: 10.2307/3284193.

[25] Davis EL, Mitchum MG. Nematodes: sophisticated parasites of legumes. Plant Physiology. 2005; 137:1182–1188. doi: 10.1104/pp.104.054973.

[26] Davis EL, Hussey RS, Baum TJ. Getting to the roots of parasitism by nematodes. Trends in Parasitology. 2004; 20:134–141. doi: 10.1016/j.pt.2004.01.005.

[27] Cnavar. Cotton varieties planted in 2015 [{internet]. 2016. Available from: https://www.ams.usda.gov/mnreports/cnavar [Accessed: 2016-05-20].

[28] Agudelo PR, Robbins T, Kim KS, Stewart J McD. Histological changes in *Gossypium hirsutum* associated with reduced reproduction of *Rotylenchulus reniformis*. Journal of Nematology. 2005; 37:185–189.

[29] Agudelo P, Robbins RT, Stewart JM, Szalanski AL. Intra-specific variability of *Rotylenchulus reniformis* from cotton-growing regions in the United States. Journal of Nematology. 2005; 37(1):105–114.

[30] Tilahun Y, Soliman K, Lawerence KS, Cseke LJ, Ochieng JW. Nuclear ribosomal DNA diversity of a cotton pest (*Rotylenchulus reniformis*) in the United States. African Journal of Biotechnology. 2008; 7(18):3217–3224.

[31] Nyaku ST, Sripathi VR, Kantety RV, Gu YQ, Lawrence KS, Sharma GC. Characterization of the two intra-individual sequence variants in the 18S rRNA gene in the plant parasitic nematode, *Rotylenchulus reniformis*. PLoS ONE. 2013; 8(4): e60891. doi: 10.1371/journal.pone.0060891.

[32] Nyaku ST, Kantety RV, Tilahun Y, Lawrence KS, Soliman KM, Cebert E, Sharma GC. 18S and ITS1 genomic sequence variations in *Rotylenchulus reniformis* isolates in Alabama. Journal of Cotton Science. 2013; 17:184–194.

[33] Deng D, Zipf A, Tilahun Y, Sharma GC, Jenkins J, Lawrence K. An improved method for the extraction of nematodes using iodixanol (OptiPrep™). African Journal of Microbiology Research. 2008; 2:167–170.

[34] van Den Berg E, Palomares-Rius JE, Vovlas N, Tiedt LR, Castillo P, Subbotin SA. Morphological and molecular characterization of one new and several known species of the reniform nematode, *Rotylenchulus* Linford & Oliveira, 1940 (Hoplolaimidae: Rotylenchulinae), and a phylogeny of the genus. Nematology. 2016; 18:67–107. doi: 10.1163/15685411-00002945.

[35] Sikkens, RB, Weaver DB, Lawrence KS, Moore SR, van Santen E. LONREN upland cotton germplasm response to *Rotylenchulus reniformis* inoculum level. Nematropica. 2011; 41:68–74.

[36] Bhandari B, Myers GO, Indest MO, Overstreet C. Response of five resistant cotton genotypes to isolates of *Rotylenchulus reniformis* collected from reniform nematode infested fields of Louisiana. Nematropica. 2015; 45:252–262.

[37] Koenning SR, Walters SA, Barker KR. Impact of soil texture on the reproductive and damage potentials of *Rotylenchulus reniformis* and *Meloidogyne incognita* on cotton. Journal of Nematology. 1996; 28:527–536.

[38] Sturhan D. Biological races. In: Zuckerman BM, Mai WF, Rohde RA, editors. Plant parasitic nematodes volume II. Academic Press, New York, NY; 1971. p. 51–71.

[39] Leach M, Agudelo P. Genetic variability of *Rotylenchulus reniformis*. Plant Disease. 2012; 96:30–36. doi: 10.1094/PDIS-02-11-0132.

[40] Arias RS, Stetina SR, Tonos JL, Scheffler JA, Scheffler BE. Microsatellites reveal genetic diversity in *Rotylenchulus reniformis* populations. Journal of Nematology. 2009; 41:146–156.

[41] Barker KR. Resistance/tolerance and related concepts/terminology in plant nematology. Plant Disease. 1993; 77:111–113.

[42] Das S, De Mason DA, Ehlers JD, Close TJ, Roberts PA. Histological characterization of root-knot nematode resistance in cowpea and its relation to reactive oxygen species modulation. Journal of Experimental Botany. 2008; 59:1305–1313.doi: 10.1093/jxb/ern036.

[43] Schrimsher DW, Lawrence KS, Sikkens RB, Weaver DB. Nematicides enhance growth and yield of *Rotylenchulus reniformis* resistant cotton genotypes. Journal of Nematology. 2014; 46(4):365–75.

[44] Kohel RJ, Lewis CF, editors. Cotton. Agronomy 24. American Society of Agronomy, Madison, WI; 1984. 605 p.

[45] Percival AE, Wendel JF, Stewart JM. Taxonomy and germplasm resources. In: Smith CW, Cothren JT, editors. Cotton: Origin, History, Technology, and Production. John Wiley & Sons, Inc., New York, NY; 1999. p. 33–63.

[46] Jones JE, Beasley JP, Dickson JL, Caldwell WD. Registration of four cotton germplasm lines with resistance to reniform and root-knot nematodes. Crop Science. 1988; 28:199–200.doi: 10.2135/cropsci1988.199b.rgp.

[47] Cook, CG, Robinson AF, Namken, LN. Tolerance to *Rotylenchulus reniformis* and resistance to *Meloidogyne incognita* race 3 in high yielding breeding lines of upland cotton. Journal of Nematology. 1997; 29:322–328.

[48] Usery SR, Lawrence KS, Lawrence GW, Burmester CH. Evaluation of cotton cultivars and tolerance to *Rotylenchulusreniformis*. Nematropica. 2005; 35: 121–133.

[49] Weaver DB, Lawrence K, van Santen E. Reniform nematode resistance in upland cotton germplasm. Crop Science. 2007; 47:19–24.doi:10.2135/cropsci2006.02.0130.

[50] Yik CP, Birchfield W. Resistant germplasm in *Gossypium* species and related plants to *Rotylenchulus reniformis*. Journal of Nematology. 1984; 16:146–153.

[51] Robinson AF, Percival AE. Resistance to *Meloidogyne incognita* race 3 and *Rotylenchulus reniformis* in wild accessions of *Gossypium hirsutum*and *G. barbadense* from Mexico. Journal of Nematology. 1997; 29:746-755.

[52] McCarty JC, Jenkins JN, Wubben MJ, Hayes RW, LaFoe II. Registration of three germplasm lines of cotton derived from L. accession T2468 with moderate resistance to the reniform nematode. Journal of Plant Registrations. 2012; 6:85–87. doi: 10.3198/jpr2011.07.0381crg.

[53] Robinson AF. Reniform in U.S. cotton: when, where, why, and some remedies. Annual Review of Phytopathology. 2007; 45:263–288. doi: 10.1146/annurev.phyto.45.011107.143949.

[54] Starr JL, Koenning SR, Kirkpatrick TL, Robinson AF, Roberts PA, Nichols RL. The future of nematode management in cotton. Journal of Nematology. 2007; 39:283–294.

[55] Ehou MK. Attempt at utilization of the wild diploid species *G. longicalyx* for the improvement of the cultivated tetraploid species *G. hirsutum* by the method of addition and substitution lines. [thesis] (In French.) Univ. Pierre et Mari Curie, Paris; 1983.

[56] Sacks EJ, Robinson AF. Introgression of resistance to reniform nematode (*Rotylenchulus reniformis*) into upland cotton (*Gossypium hirsutum*) from *G. Arboreum* and a *G. hirsutum*/*G. aridum* bridging line. Field Crops Res. 2009; 112:1–6. doi: 10.1016/j.fcr.2009.01.006.

[57] Romano GB, Sacks EJ, Stetina SR, Robinson FA, Fang DD, Gutiérrez OA, Scheffler JA. Identification and genomic location of a reniform nematode (*Rotylenchulus reniformis*) resistance locus (Renari) introgressed from *Gossypium aridum* into upland cotton (*G.*

hirsutum). Theoretical Applied Genetics. 2009; 120:139–150. doi: 10.1007/s00122-009-1165-4.

[58] Starr JL, Smith CW, Ripple K, Zhou E, Nichols RL, Faske TR. Registration of TAM RKRNR-9 and TAM RKRNR-12 germplasm lines of upland cotton resistant to reniform and root-knot nematodes. Journal of Plant Registrations. 2011; 5:393–396.doi: 10.3198/jpr2011.01.0048crg.

[59] McCarty JC, Jenkins JN, Wubben MJ, Gutiérrez OA, Hayes RW, Callahan FE, Deng D. Registration of three germplasm lines of cotton derived from *Gossypium barbadense* L. accession GB713 with resistance to the reniform nematode. Journal of Plant Registrations. 2013; 7:220–223. doi: 10.3198/jpr2012.08.0024crg.

[60] Bell AA, Robinson FA, Quintana J, Duke SE, Starr JL, Stelly DM, Zheng X, Prom S, Saladino V, Gutiérrez OA, Stetina RS, Nichols RL. Registration of BARBREN-713 germplasm line of upland cotton resistant to reniform and root-knot nematodes. Journal of Plant Registrations. 2015; 9:89–93. doi: 10.3198/jpr2014.04.0021crg.

[61] Robinson AF, Bell AA, Dighe ND, Menz MA, Nichols RL, Stelly DM. Introgression of resistance to nematode *Rotylenchulus reniformis* into upland cotton (*Gossypium hirsutum*) from *Gossypium longicalyx*. Crop Science. 2007; 47:1865–1877. doi: 10.2135/cropsci2006.12.0776.

[62] Bell AA, Robinson AF, Quintana J, Dighe ND, Menz MA, Stelly DM, Zheng X, Jones JE, Overstreet C, Burris E, Cantrell R, Nichols RL. Registration of LONREN-1 and LONREN-2 germplasm lines of upland cotton resistant to reniform nematode. Journal of Plant Registrations. 2014; 8:187–190. doi: 10.3198/jpr2013.11.0069crg.

[63] Sikkens RB, Weaver DB, Lawrence KS, Moore SR, van Santen E. LONREN upland cotton germplasm response to *Rotylenchulus reniformis* inoculum level. Nematropica. 2011;41:68–74.

[64] Weaver DB, Sikkens RB, Lawrence KS, Sürmelioğlu Ç, van Santen E, Nichols RL. REN^{lon} and its effects on agronomic and fiber quality traits in upland cotton. Crop Science. 2013; 53:913–920. doi: 10.2135/cropsci2012.08.0504.

[65] Dighe N, Robinson AF, Bell A, Menz M, Cantrell R, Stelly D. Linkage mapping of resistance to reniform nematode in cotton (*Gossypium hirsutum* L.) following introgression from *G. longicalyx* (Hutch. & Lee). Crop Science. 2009; 49:1151–1164. doi: 10.2135/cropsci2008.03.0129.

[66] Avila CA, Stewart J McD, Robbins RT. Introgression of reniform nematode resistance into upland cotton. In: Proceedings of the Beltwide Cotton Conference; January 3–6, 2006; San Antonio, TX; p. 154.

[67] Konan NO, Baudoin JP, D–Hont A, Mergeai G. Creating a tri-species hybrid cotton resistant to reniform nematode. Cashiers Agriculture. 2007; 16(1), 37–39.

[68] Robinson AF, Bridges AC, Percival AE. New sources of resistance to the reniform (*Rotylenchulus reniformis*) and root-knot (*Meloidogyne incognita*) nematode in upland

(*Gossypium hirsutum* L.) and sea island (*G. barbadense* L.) cotton. Journal of Cotton Science. 2004; 8:191–197.

[69] Gutiérrez OA, Robinson AF, Jenkins JN, McCarty JC, Wubben MJ, Callahan FE, Nichols RL. Identification of QTL regions and SSR markers associated with resistance to reniform nematode in *Gossypium barbadense* L. accession GB713. Theoretical and Applied Genetics. 2011; 122:271–280. doi: 10.1007/s00122-010-1442-2.

[70] Luzzi BM, Boerma HR, Hussy RS. Resistance to three species of root-knot nematode in soybean. Crop Science. 1987; 27:258–262. doi: 10.2135/cropsci1987.0011183X002700020027x.

[71] Mitchum MG, Hussey RS, Davis EL, Baum TJ. Application of biotechnology to understand pathogenesis of nematode plant pathogens. In: Punja ZK, De Boer S, Sanfacon H, editors. Biotechnology & Plant Disease Management. CABI International; Nosworthy Way, Walliford, Oxfordshire, UK; 2007. p. 58–86. doi: 10.1079/9781845932886.0058.

[72] Smant G, Yan Y,Stokkermans JWPG, de Boer JM, Davis EL, Pomp H, Zilverentant JF, Overmars HA, Helder J, Hussey RS, Schots A, Bakker J. Endogenous cellulases in animals: isolation of β-1,4-endoglucanase genes from two species of plant-parasitic cyst nematodes. Proceedings of the National Academy of Sciences. 1998; 95:4906–4911. doi: 10.1073/pnas.1118560109.

[73] Yan Y, Smant G, Stokkermans J, Qin L, Helder J, Baum TJ, Schots A, Davis EL. Genomic organization of four β-1,4-endoglucanase genes in plant-parasitic cyst nematodes and its evolutionary implications. Gene. 1998; 220:61–70. doi: 10.1016/S0378-1119(98)00413-2.

[74] Wang X, Meyers D, Yan Y, Baum TJ, Smant G, Hussey RS, Davis EL. In planta localization of a β-1,4-endoglucanase secreted by *Heterodera glycines*. Molecular Plant-Microbe Interactions. 1999; 12:64–67.doi: 10.1094/MPMI.1999.12.1.64.

[75] Wubben MJ, Ganji S, Callahan FE. Identification and molecular characterization of a β-1,4-endoglucanase gene (*Rr-eng-1*) from *Rotylenchulus reniformis*. Journal of Nematology. 2010; 42:342–351.

[76] Nyaku ST, Sripathi VR, Wiley G, Najar FZ, Cseke LJ, Sharma GC, Roe BA, Cseke SB, Moss E, Kantety RV. The expressed parasitism genes in the reniform nematode (*Rotylenchulus reniformis*). American Journal of Plant Science. 2013; 4:780–791. doi: 10.4236/ajps.2013.44097.

[77] Nyaku ST, Sripathi VR, Kantety RV, Cseke SB, Buyarappu R, Gu YQ, Lawrence K, Senwo Z, Sripathi P, McEwan R, George P, Sharma GC. Characterization of the reniform nematode genome through shotgun Sequencing. Genome. 2014; 57(4):209–21. doi: 10.1139/gen-2014-0019.

[78] Gao B, Allen R, Maier T, Davis EL, Baum TJ, Hussey RS. Identification of a new β-1,4-endoglucanase gene expressed in the subventral gland cells of *Heterodera glycines*. Journal of Nematology. 2002; 33:12–15.

[79] Goellner M, Wang XH, Davis EL. Endo-beta-1,4-glucanase expression in compatible plant-nematode interactions. Plant Cell. 2001; 13:2241–2255. doi: 10.1105/tpc.010219.

[80] Uehara T, Kushida A, Momota Y. PCR-based cloning of two β-1,4-endoglucanases from the root-lesion nematode *Pratylenchus penetrans*. Nematology. 2001; 3:335–341.

[81] Rosso MN, Favery B, Piotte C, Arthaud L, De Boer JM, Hussey RS, Bakker J, Baum TJ, Abad P. Isolation of a cDNA encoding a beta-1,4- endoglucanase in the root-knot nematode *Meloidogyne incognita* and expression analysis during plant parasitism. Molecular Plant-Microbe Interactions. 1999; 12:585–591. doi: 10.1094/MPMI.1999.12.7.585.

[82] de Meutter J, Vanhomle B, Bauw G, Tytgat T, Gheysen G. Preparation and sequencing of secreted proteins from the pharyngeal glands of the plant parasitic nematode *Heterodera schachtii*. Molecular Plant Pathology. 2001; 2:297–301. doi: 10.1046/j.1464-6722.2001.00078.x.

[83] de Boer JM, Yan Y, Bakker J, Davis EL, Baum TJ. In situ hybridization to messenger RNA of *Heterodera glycines*. Journal of Nematology. 1998; 30:309–312.

[84] Hotopp JCD, Clark ME, Oliveira DCSG, Foster JM, Fischer P, Torres MCM, Giebel JD, Kumar N, Ishmael N, Wang S, Ingram J, Nene RV, Shepard J, Tomkins J, Richards S, Spiro DJ, Ghedin E, Slatko BE, Tettelin H, Werren JH. Widespread lateral gene transfer from intracellular bacteria to multicellular eukaryotes. Science. 2007; 317:1753–1756. doi: 10.1126/science.1142490.

[85] Keen NT, Roberts PA. Plant parasitic nematodes: digesting a page from the microbe book. Proceedings of the National Academy of Sciences. 1998; 95:4789–4790. doi: 10.1073/pnas.95.9.4789.

[86] Scholl EH, Thorne JL, McCarter JP, Mck Bird D. Horizontally transferred genes in plant-parasitic nematodes: a high-throughput genomic approach. Genome Biology. 2003; 4:R39.1–R39.11. doi: 10.1186/gb-2003-4-6-r39).

[87] Bird DM, Koltai H. Plant parasitic nematodes: habitats, hormones, and horizontally-acquired genes. Journal of Plant Growth Regulation. 2000; 19:183–194. doi: 10.1007/s003440000022.

[88] Ganji S, Jenkins JN, Wubben MJ. Molecular characterization of the reniform nematode C-type lectin gene family reveals a likely role in mitigating environmental stresses during plant parasitism. Gene. 2014; 537:269–278. doi: 10.1016/j.gene.

[89] Wubben MJ, Callahan FE, Scheffler BS. Transcript analysis of parasitic females of the sedentary semi-endoparasitic nematode *Rotylenchulus reniformis*. Molecular and Biochemical Parasitology. 2010; 172:31–40. doi: 10.1016/j.molbiopara. 2010.03.011.

[90] Zelensky AN, Gready JE. The C-type lectin-like domain superfamily. FEBS Journal. 2005; 272(24):6179–217. doi: 10.1111/j.1742-4658.2005.05031.x.

[91] Drickamer K. C-type lectin domains. Current Opinion in Structural Biology. 1999; 9:585–590. doi: 10.1016/S0959-440X(99)00009-3.

[92] Harcus Y, Nicoll G, Murray J, Filbey K, Gomez-Escobar N, Maizels RM. C-type lectins from the nematode parasites *Heligmosomoides polygyrus* and *Nippostrongylus brasiliensis*. Parasitology International. 2009; 58:461–470. doi: 10.1016/j.parint. 2009.08.011.

[93] Loukas AC, Mullin NP, Tetteh KKA, Moens L, Maizels RM. A novel C-type lectin secreted by a tissue-dwelling parasitic nematode. Current Biology. 1999; 9: 825–828. doi: 10.1016/S0960-9822(99)80366-2.

[94] Haegeman A, Bauters L, Kyndt T, Rahman MM, Gheysen G. Identification of candidate effector genes in the transcriptome of the rice root knot nematode *Meloidogyne graminicola*. Molecular Plant Pathology. 2013; 14(4):379–390. doi: 10.1111/mpp.12014.

[95] Elling AA, Davis EL, Hussey RS, Baum TJ. Active uptake of cyst nematode parasitism proteins into the plant cell nucleus. International Journal of Parasitology. 2007; 37:1269–1279. doi:10.1016/j.ijpara.2007.03.012.

[96] Huang G, Dong R, Allen R, Davis EL, Baum TJ, Hussey RS. A root-knot nematode secretory peptide functions as a ligand for a plant transcription factor. Molecular Plant–Microbe Interactions. 2006; 19:463–470. doi: 10.1094/MPMI-19-0463.

[97] Doyle EA, Lambert KN. 3. *Meloidogyne javanica* chorismate mutase 1 alters plant cell development. Molecular Plant Microbe–Interactions. 2003; 6:123–131. doi: 10.1094/MPMI.2003.16.2.123.

[98] Olsen AN, Skriver K. Ligand mimicry? A plant-parasitic nematode polypeptide with similarity to CLAVATA3. Trends Plant Science. 2003; 8:55–57. doi: 10.1016/S1360-1385(03)00003-7.

[99] Wang X, Mitchum MG, Gao BL, Li C, Diab H, Baum TJ, Hussey RS, Davis EL. A parasitism gene from a plant-parasitic nematode with function similar to CLAVATA3/ESR (CLE) of *Arabidopsis thaliana*. Molecular Plant Pathology, 2005; 6:187–191. doi: 10.1111/J.1364-3703.2005.00270.x.

[100] Wubben MJ, Gavilano L, Baum TJ, Davis EL. Sequence and spatiotemporal expression analysis of CLE-Motif containing genes from the reniform nematode (*Rotylenchulus reniformis* Linford& Oliveira). Journal of Nematology. 2015; 47(2):159–165.

[101] Fire A, Xu S, Montgomery MK, Kostas SA, Driver SE, Mello CC. Potent and specific genetic interference by double-stranded RNA in *Caenorhabditis elegans*. Nature. 1998; 391:806–811. doi: 10.1038/35888.

[102] Hannon GJ. RNA interference. Nature. 2002; 418:244-251. doi: 10.1038/418244a.

[103] Lilley CJ, Bakhetia M, Charlton WL, Urwin PE. Recent progress in the development of RNA interference for plant parasitic nematodes. Molecular Plant Pathology. 2007; 8:701–711. doi: 10.1111/j.1364-3703.2007.00422.x.

[104] Ward HM. On the relations between host and parasite in the bromes and their brown rust, *Puccinia dispersa* (Erikss). Annals of Botany. 1902; 16:233–316.

[105] Flor HH. Current status of the gene-for-gene concept. Annual Review of Phytopathology. 1971; 9:275–296. doi: 10.1146/annurev.py.09.090171.001423.

[106] Moffett P, Sacco M. A nematode avirulence determinant and a co-factor for a disease resistance protein converge on the Ran signaling pathway. Phytopathology. 2006; 96:S80. doi: 10.1094/PHYTO.2006.96.6.S1.

[107] Lambert KN, Bekal S, Domier LL, Niblack TL, Noel GR, Smyth CA. Selection of *Heterodera glycines* chorismate mutase-1 alleles on nematode-resistant soybean. Molecular Plant-Microbe Interactions. 2005; 18:593–601. doi: 10.1094/MPMI-18-0593.

[108] Baum TJ, Hussey RS, Davis EL. 2006. In: Setlow JK, editor. Root-knot and cyst nematode parasitism genes: the molecular basis of plant parasitism. Genetic Engineering, volume 28. p. 17–43. doi: 10.1007/978-0-387-34504-8_2.

[109] Jasmer DP, Goverse A, Smant G. Parasitic nematode interactions with mammals and plants. Annual Review of Phytopathology. 2003; 41:245–270. doi: 10.1146/annurev.phyto.41.052102.104023.

[110] Hermsmeier D, Hart JK, Byzova M, Rodermel SR, Baum TJ. Changes in mRNA abundance within *Heterodera schachtii*-infected roots of *Arabidopsis thaliana*. Molecular Plant-Microbe Interactions. 2000; 13:309–315. doi: 10.1094/MPMI.2000.13.3.309.

[111] Vercauteren I, Van Der Schueren E, Van Montagu M, Gheysen G. Arabidopsis thaliana genes expressed in the early compatible interaction with root-knot nematodes. Molecular Plant-Microbe Interactions. 2001; 14:288–299. doi: 10.1094/MPMI.2001.14.3.288.

[112] Goverse A, Biesheuvel J, Wijers GJ, Gommers FJ, Bakker J, Schots A, Helder J. *In planta* monitoring of the activity of two constitutive promoters, CaMV 35S and in developing feeding cells induced by *Globodera rostochiensis* using green fluorescent protein in combination with confocal laser scanning microscopy. Physiological and Molecular Plant Pathology. 1998; 52:275–284. doi: 10.1006/pmpp.1998.0154.

[113] Mazarei M, Lennon KA, Puthoff DP, Rodermel SR, Baum TJ. Expression of an *Arabidopsis* phosphoglycerate mutase homologue is localized to apical meristems, regulated by hormones, and induced by sedentary plant-parasitic nematodes. Plant Molecular Biology. 2003; 53:513–530. doi: 10.1023/B:PLAN.0000019062.80459.80.

[114] Mazarei M, Lennon KA, Puthoff DP, Rodermel SR, Baum TJ. Homologous soybean and Arabidopsis genes share responsiveness to cyst nematode infection. Molecular Plant Pathology. 2004; 5:409–423. doi: 10.1111/j.1364-3703.2004.00241.x.

[115] Niebel A, Engler JD, Tire C, Engler G, Van Montagu M, Gheysen G. Induction patterns of an extension gene in tobacco upon nematode infection. Plant Cell. 1993; 5:1697–1710. doi: 10.1105/tpc.5.12.1697.

[116] Gurr SJ, McPherson MJ, Scollan C, Atkinson HJ, Bowles DJ. Gene expression in nematode-infected plant roots. Molecular and General Genetics. 1991; 226:361–366.

[117] Gao B, Allen R, Maier T, Davis EL, Baum TJ, Hussey RS. The parasitome of the phytonematode *Heterodera glycines*. Molecular Plant Microbe Interactions. 2003; 16:720–726. doi: 10.1094/MPMI.2003.16.8.720.

[118] Wang X, Allen R, Ding X, Goellner M, Maier T, de Boer JM, Baum TJ, Hussey RS, Davis EL. Signal peptide-selection of cDNA cloned directly from the esophageal gland cells of the soybean cyst nematode *Heterodera glycines*. Molecular Plant Microbe Interaction. 2001; 14:536–544. doi: 10.1094/MPMI.2001.14.4.536.

[119] Puthoff DP, Nettleton D, Rodermel SR, Baum TJ. Arabidopsis gene expression changes during cyst nematode parasitism revealed by statistical analyses of microarray expression profiles. The Plant Journal. 2003; 33:911–921. doi: 10.1046/j.1365-313X.2003.01677.x.

[120] Khan R, Alkharouf N, Beard H, MacDonald M, Chouikha I, Meyer S, Grefenstette J, Knap H, Matthews B. Microarray analysis of gene expression in soybean roots susceptible to the soybean cyst nematode two days post invasion. Journal of Nematology. 2004; 36:241–248.

[121] De Boer JM, McDermott JP, Wang X, Maier T, Qui F, Hussey RS, Davis EL, Baum TJ. The use of DNA microarrays for the developmental expression analysis of cDNAs from the esophageal gland cell region of *Heterodera glycines*. Molecular Plant Pathology. 2002; 3:261–270. doi: 10.1046/j.1364-3703.2002.00122.x.

[122] Li R, Rashotte AM, Singh NK, Lawrence KS, Weaver DB, Locy RD. Transcriptome analysis of cotton (*Gossypium hirsutum* L.) genotypes that are susceptible, resistant, and hypersensitive to reniform nematode (*Rotylenchulus reniformis*). PLoS One. 2015; 10:1–27. doi: 10.1371/journal.pone.0143261.

[123] D'haeseleer P, Liang S, Somogyi R. Genetic network inference: from co-expression clustering to reverse engineering. Bioinformatics. 2000; 16:707–726.

[124] Brockmann R, Beyer A, Heinisch JJ, Wilhelm T. Posttranscriptional expression regulation: what determines translation rates? PLoS Computational Biology. 2007; 3:0531–0539. doi: 10.1371/journal.pcbi.0030057.

[125] Odjakova M, Hadjiivanova C. The complexity of pathogen defense in plants. Bulgarian Journal of Plant Physiology. 2001; 27:101–109.

[126] Jones JDG, Dangl JL. The plant immune system. Nature. 2006; 444:323–329. doi: 10.1038/nature05286.

[127] Niu J, Liu P, Liu Q, Chen C, Guo Q, Yin J, Yang G, Jian H. Msp40 effector of root-knot nematode manipulates plant immunity to facilitate parasitism. Scientific Reports. 2016; 6:1–13. doi: 10.1038/srep19443.

Chapter 10

Science Behind Cotton Transformation

Abdul Qayyum Rao, Muhammad Azam Ali,
Muhammad Azmat Ullah Khan,
Kamran Shahzad Bajwa, Adnan Iqbal, Tahir Iqbal,
Ahmad Ali Shahid, Idrees Ahmad Nasir and
Tayyab Husnain

Additional information is available at the end of the chapter

http://dx.doi.org/10.5772/64888

Abstract

The introduction of foreign genes into plant has made possible to bring out desired traits into crop of our own interest. With the advancement in cell biology, regeneration of plants from single cell and advent of different procedures for gene transformation to the plants have opened new avenues for the efficient and applicable implementation of biotechnology for the modifications of desired crop characteristics. Identifications and isolation of different genes for various traits from different organisms have made possible to get the crop plants with modified characters. Over time improvement has been made in transformation technology depending upon the crop of interest. The efficiency of plant transformation has been increased with advances in plant transformation vectors and methodologies, which resulted in the improvement of crops. A detailed discussion on advanced techniques for genetic modification of plants with their handy use and limitation has been focused in this chapter.

Keywords: *Agrobacterium*, biolistic gun, infiltration, microinjection, transformation

1. Introduction

Cell theory of Schleiden established the framework of modern plant biotechnology [1], and Schwann's cell theory [2] was based upon phenomenon that cell is the basic unit of living organisms.

The idea of totipotency has been originated from the concept of cell theory, which later on laid the foundation of plant biotechnology. Hernalsteens [3] further provided the evidence and forecasted the production of somatic embryos from vegetative cells.

Among the key discoveries of plant biotechnology, gene transformation in crop plants and regeneration of plants from callus are the most significant achievements. In 1980s, chimeric genes were produced, which resulted in further expansion of genetic modification technology of the plants [1]. It led to the development of new transformation vectors [2], which ultimately changed the ways of DNA delivery systems [3]. Genetic transformation of crop plant can be achieved by a number of ways like *Agrobacterium* Ti plasmid vectors, microinjection, microprojectile bombardment, electroporation of protoplasts, and/or chemical (PEG) treatment of protoplasts. All of these methods have certain merits over each other with some demerits, but transformation using *Agrobacterium* and microprojectile bombardment is currently the most extensively used methods [4]. Due to regeneration ability of tobacco, as done by Skoog and Miller [5] in 1957, tobacco is the first and model plant to be used for genetic transformation. It provided the basis for tissue culture [6]. The ongoing technological expansions in rice, barley, wheat, and cotton may prove to be a hindrance in commercial release of novel GM cereals. Below, a concise narration of all methodologies used in transformation has been presented.

2. Plant regeneration

A number of attempts were made during 1950 to provide clear understanding of the phenomenon of totipotency but it was 1954 when Muir et al. [7] demonstrated the possible aspects of culturing of single plant cell. The cell divisions obtained by him from callus of tobacco placed on a small piece of filter paper provided the basis for totipotency. Davidonis and Hamilton further confirmed the results by obtaining similar results from single cell and group of cells suspended in the agar medium. It was the extension of these experiments when Jones et al. compared with many other crops, reported that it is more difficult to obtain somatic embryogenesis and plant regeneration from cotton except Coker 312. Davidonis and Hamilton [8] first described that plant regeneration from 2-year-old callus of *Gossypium hirsutum* L. [9] was able to grow single isolated cell in microculture chamber providing devised nutrient medium. For the survival and growth of isolated cells, the role of nurse or nutrition medium becomes evident from these studies.

Rao et al. [12] in 2009 were the first who provide the clear evidence of totipotency and its use during regeneration from callus of plants when they were able to regenerate isolated single cells into flowering plants of tobacco, cultured in microchambers, without the aid of nurse cells or conditioned media. Verdiel et al. [9] in 2007 demonstrated that stem cells in meristematic regions are pluripotent and are dependent, whereas those that are present in embryogenic regions are totipotent and hence are independent.

3. Embryo formation

Improvements of many plants, such as cereals, soybean, cotton, canola, cassava, and woody tree species, are dependent on the development of somatic embryos; therefore, the formation of competent embryogenic cultures is imperative for the success of plant biotechnology. Somatic embryogenesis in cotton species has been reported to be the most difficult to regenerate [10, 11]. Regeneration in cotton has not been achieved rapidly, with the report of regeneration of *G. hirsutum* [12]. Plants obtained from embryogenic cultures are free from any variations phenotypically or genotypically because they are formed from single cells and during the process of embryogenesis normal cells are selected rigorously [13]. Nowadays, embryogenic cultures of extensive range of plant species can be grown on synthetic media due to ever-increasing information about the physiological aspects and genetic regulation of zygotic as well as somatic embryogenesis [14]. In most cases, embryogenic cultures are initiated by using 2,4-dichlorophenoxyacetic acid (2,4-D), and when such plant cell cultures are relocated to media that contains no or very low quantity of 2,4-D they develop into somatic embryos.

4. Binary vectors

In 1984, Braybrook [14] constructed the first binary vector pBIN19, since then efforts are being made to modify binary vectors in order to amplify their efficacy and transformation effectiveness. Japonica rice was successfully transformed using *Agrobacterium* bearing the super binary vector pTOK233 constructed by taking *virB, virG,* and *virC* genes from pTiBo542 and cloning them into pGA472 [15]. Afterwards, maize, javanica rice, indica rice [16], Sorghum, and *Allium cepa* [17] transformation was also performed by the same method. The misconception that monocots cannot be transformed by *Agrobacterium*-mediated transformation has been cleared now. Lately, mung bean has been transformed using *Agrobacterium* bearing pTOK233 binary vector [18].

Complete sequencing of pBIN19 has been performed [19]. A modified version pBIN20 has more single restriction sites within the multiple cloning site (MCS) [20]. A newly developed types of pPZP vectors are small and are steady in *Agrobacterium* cells [21]. pCAMBIA series of vectors are extensively used for the transformation of rice. These have kanamycin resistance (neomycin phosphotransferase II; *NPTII)* or bialaphos herbicide resistance (*BAR*) genes as selection markers and beta-glucuronidase *(GUS)* or green florescence protein (*GFP*) as reporter genes and were constructed by using the backbone of pPZP vector.

Plant expression vectors of pRT100 series with a polyA signal under CaMV 35S promoter were developed by Töpfer et al. [22]. Making single-restriction sites available in the expression cassette holding the target gene is usually a very difficult task. Hou and Guo [23] constructed a set of pART7 and pART27 plasmids to deal with this problem. A MCS is present between CaMV35S promoter and OCS polyA signal of the shuttle plasmid pART7. NofI sites (an infrequent 8 bp recognition site) are present on both sides of the expression cassette. In pART27, the coding sequence of a target gene has been cloned in its MCS. NotI is used to cut the expression cassette, which is then cloned in the Not I site of pART27, a binary vector. In pART27 vector, *NPTII* gene is positioned next to the left border to make sure that the selection marker is transferred in the last in the plants. Zapata et al. [24] reported the use of gramineous expression vectors pGU4AGBar and pGBIU4AGBar [23]. Twenty transformants of winter wheat showed protein expression after transforming the snowdrop lectin (*Galanthus nivalis agglutinin; GNA)* gene in them through the pollen tube pathway. This method confirms that whole T-DNA containing the target gene would be present in the transformed plants having kanamycin selection.

5. Methods involved in transformation

Transformation methods can be divided in two main categories: (1) direct and (2) indirect transformations, which are detailed in below sections.

5.1. Indirect transformation

In these methods, plants are transformed using *Agrobacterium tumefaciens* or *Agrobacterium rhizogenes* to introduce the plasmid construct carrying the target gene into the target cell.

5.2. Direct transformation

In direct methods of transformation, bacterial cells are not used. The most frequently used direct methods include microprojectile bombardment or protoplast transformation. Problems with plant regeneration low transient expression of transgenes arise as a result of protoplast transformation (mostly in monocots).

The chemical substances used to disintegrate the cell walls and electrical field protoplasts lose their viability and ability to divide. In cotton, some attempts have been made to transform cells directly in the shoot apex either through the gene gun or *Agrobacterium* [24], but these methods suffer from extremely low transformation efficiencies. Others have used particle bombardment of suspension cultures of cotton. This method suffers from the fact that additional time is required for establishment of suspension cultures [25]. The most distinguishing limiting factor of using the gene gun is that it causes the presence of multiple copies of the target genes, which may lead to alteration or concealing of the expression. In addition, gene gun is a very expensive method. The usage of in vitro cultures for plant transformation may give rise to few somaclonal changes. Due to this, they cannot be used in further studies, and analysis of the transformants becomes quite complex. As a result of the limitations mentioned, many new transformation methods are being introduced as substitutes. Most commonly mentioned methods out of them are (a) silicon carbide fiber-mediated transformation; (b) microinjection; (c) infiltration; (d) electrophoresis of embryos; (e) transformation through the pollen tube pathway; (f) electroporation of cells and tissues; and (g) liposome-mediated transformation.

6. Overview of transformation techniques

6.1. Protoplasts and somatic hybridization

In 1970 and 1971, two major advances were made, which proved the beneficial role of protoplasts in the enhancement of plants: (i) somatic hybrid cells and novel hybrid plants are developed by inducing fusion of protoplasts of different species having no taxonomic relationships between them [26], and (ii) use of cultured protoplasts in regeneration of plants [27].

Geerts et al. [28] initiated the micropod culture and Schryer et al. [29] improved it [29]. In grain legumes, protoplast fusion is not well studied [30], but today, a variety of plants can be regenerated from protoplasts. Likewise, vast ranges of somatic hybrids are developed among related as well as unrelated plant species. However, functional hybrids have been developed in case of small number of plants such as Citrus, Solanum, and Brassica. A significant role has been played by protoplasts in the successful genetic transformation of variety of plants [31] including cereal crops [32]. Limitation of protoplast transformation method is given below; Protoplast transformation method consists of variable frequencies of gene transfer in both cases within or between experiments. Therefore, the results of this transformation method are not accurately assessed. This transformation method is recommended only to those plants species which have quality of callus regeneration [33].

6.2. Direct gene transformation through imbibitions

Desiccated plant tissues can uptake foreign DNA through the process of imbibition [34]. Numerous asserts and disproof can be found in literature regarding this method. During the process of desiccation, various physiological and substantial alterations take place such as bursting of the cell wall, leakiness and changes in structure of the cell membrane, quick expansion of the cell, and development of a huge water flow among the peripheral solution and the dehydrated tissue. Uptake and transitory expression, by the cereal and legume seed embryos, of the DNA plasmid bearing the *NPTII* gene through the process of imbibition were confirmed by Töpfer et al. [22].

Permeability of the membrane is a key factor in this process. This was proved by an increase in uptake and expression of the DNA as a result of using 20% DMSO during the process. Successive studies have led to 70% transitory *GUS* expression in dehydrated somatic embryos of alfalfa [35]. Yoo and Jung have also stated a stability of transformation in rice through the process of imbibition. From 30% to 50% incidence of transient expression of *GUSA* and *NPT* genes was observed using vectors, where insertions were driven by CaMV35S promoter. Meristematic regions of the roots and leaf vascular bundles are the major locations for the expression of *GUSA* gene. Different PCR techniques and southern blot analysis of genome showed the uptake, incorporation, and expression of the *HPT* gene in rice. *Hygromycin phosphotransferase* (*HPT*) DNA was not found as a plasmid but rather it was present in an incorporated form in the genome of rice [36]. This method is the easiest of all the direct gene transformation techniques because the formation of target plant tissues is quite uncomplicated and no professional equipment is needed to perform it. Few drawbacks of this transformation method are given below; this method cannot be applied to very specific organs or tissues such as new pollinated flowers or hydrating embryos.

6.3. *Agrobacterium*-mediated transformation

A. tumefaciens causes the crown gal disease in plants. Pett et al. [37] in 1958 performed an experiment and proposed that tumor-inducing property of this soil bacterium is responsible for transformation in plants. Bacteria-free tumor cells contain large number of opines, which is a new class of metabolites.

Chilton et al. [39] introduced the idea of virulent strain of *Agrobacterium*, which leads to the discovery of mega plasmid. The plasmid were called tumor-inducing plasmid and only a small portion of that plasmid known as T-border is considered responsible for tumor induction [38] and was found to be present in the nuclear DNA of the tumor-inducing cells [39].

Ti plasmid is an integrated part of the plant genome during tumor formation (transformation), suggesting that the plasmid could be used as a vector to transfer other genes. It was reported that various methods were tested to insert genes into the Ti plasmid. Transformed crown-gall tumor tissues, which were grown on hormone-free media, only formed highly aberrant shoots in culture [40]. This was related to the presence of genes controlling the expression of auxin and cytokinin synthesis. Deletion of these genes resulted in the production of transformed tissues that required media supplemented with auxin and cytokinin for continued growth and regeneration of normal shoots and plants. Nadolska-Orczyk et al. [43] showed that efficient *Agrobacterium*-mediated transformation of *Metrosideros polymorpha* provide molecular techniques to facilitate comparative genomics. It was reported that above-discussed facts led to the use of Ti plasmid of *Agrobacterium* as a vector for plant transformation and kanamycin resistance genes as selection marker for transformed cells, and then transformed plants are regenerated [41] (**Figures 1** and **2**). *Agrobacterium*-mediated transformation followed by somatic embryogenesis remains the method of choice for most cotton transformation. However, regeneration aspect of the transformation process remains more difficult and choices are limited in case of cotton, one of the most difficult crop for transformation [42].

As *Agrobacterium* is highly attracted to phenolics, this method of transformation is not preferable for monocots due to production of phenolics, whereas it can be used for dicots. However, recently, *Agrobacterium*-mediated transformation has been optimized and becomes the best method for transformation of monocots [43].

6.4. Biolistic transformation

In early 1980s, direct DNA delivery methods for protoplast were developed [44], especially for the economically important cereal crops, which were not subjected to the umbrella *Agrobacterium*-mediated transformation [45]. In this procedure, osmotic or electric shocks are applied to the protoplasts suspended in solutions containing DNA. After that planting on selection media is performed. Transformation based on embryogenic cell suspension cultures produced the first transgenic cereals [13]. The use of protoplasts for genetic transformation became less striking once it was shown that monocots could be transformed by co-cultivation of embryonic tissues and supervirulent strains of *Agrobacterium* in the presence of acetosyringone [15]. In case of Ricinus (castor oil plant), transformation through gene gun is dependent on many factors such as helium pressure, target distance, osmoticum, microcarrier type and size, DNA quantity, explant type, and number of bombardments had significant influence on transformation efficiency (**Figure 2**). Recommended distance is 6.0 cm, helium pressure of 1100 psi, 0.6-μm gold microcarriers, furthermore single bombardment has shown

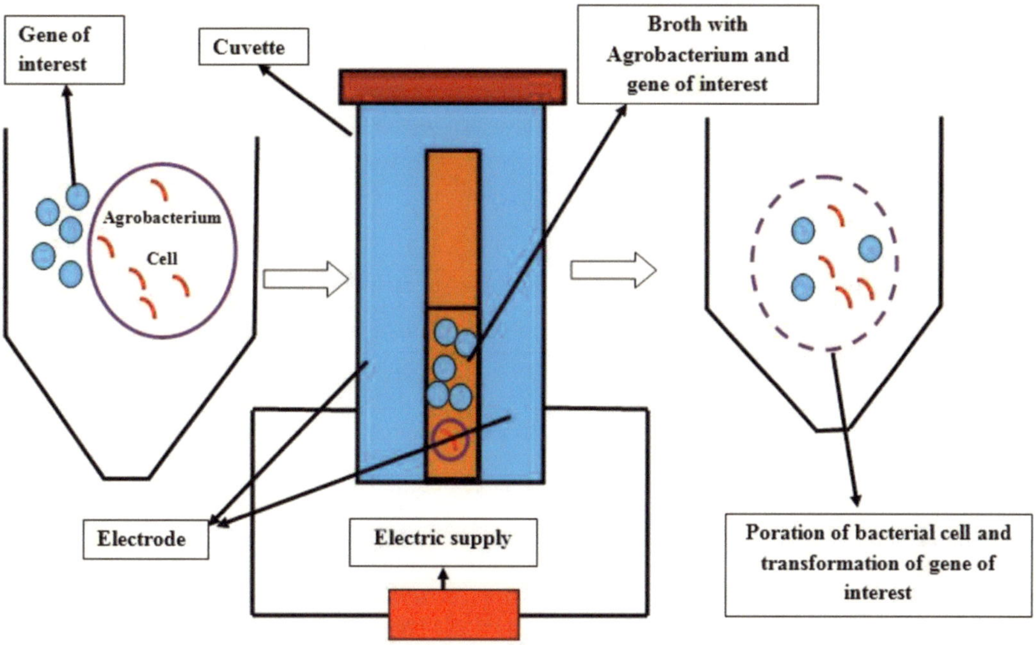

Figure 1. Basic concept of gene transformation through *Agrobacterium*.

positive results [46]. Finer and McMullen [47] demonstrated the successful recovery of transgenic cotton plants by biolistic bombardment of embryogenic suspension cultures and reported a transient to stable conversion frequency of about 0.7%. Biolistic method is not recommended for the crops, which cannot be tissue cultured.

6.5. Biolistic with *Agrobacterium*

Limitations of *Agrobacterium*-mediated transformation and difficulties involved in isolation and maintaining of embryogenic cultures have led to the discovery of universal transformation method redundant [48]. However, not a single transformation technique had proved satisfactory to be universal; therefore, a novel transformation technique for transformation was developed by Sanford et al. [49]. DNA-coated gold or tungsten particles are bombarded with high velocity to the intact cells or tissues. Combination of *Agrobacterium* and biolistics methods of transformation is most widely used method. However, choice depends on the individual researcher or plant tissue/ sample [50]. **Figure 2** explains the schematic overview of biolistic gene transformation in plants.

6.6. Chemical method

To enhance the uptake of DNA, a combination of polybrene-spermidine treatment is used to obtain non-chimeric transgenic cotton plants. Polybrene-spermidine combination treatment for plant genetic transformation has the advantage because it is less toxic than the other chemicals; furthermore, it also protects condensation effect, DNA shearing, and integration of the plasmid with host genome [35]. To deliver plasmid DNA into cotton suspension culture obtained from

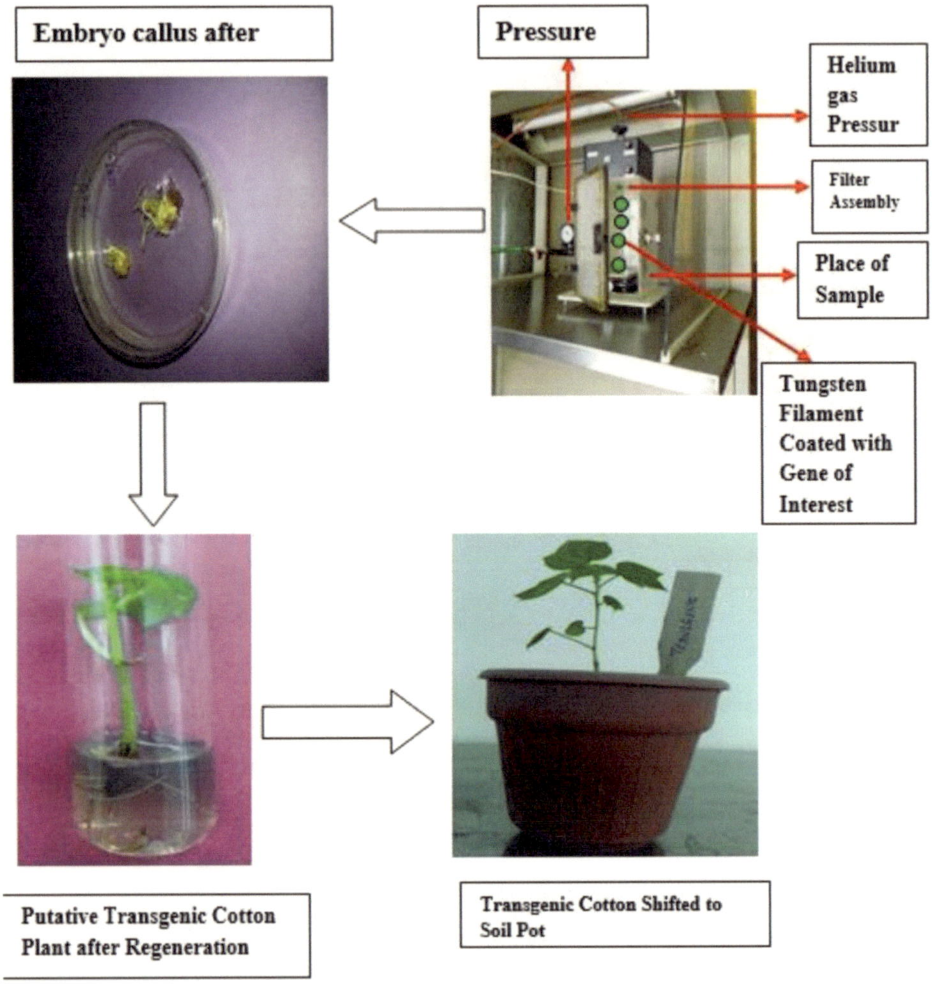

Figure 2. Schematic overview of gene transformation through gene gun.

cotyledon-induced callus, polybrene and/or spermidine treatments were used. Researchers have also regenerated and analyzed the cotton plants containing *HPT* genes as a selectable marker [51]. Major limitation in chemical transformation technique is its low efficiency when compared to other transformation techniques.

6.7. Microinjection

Microinjection technique is based on introducing DNA in the cells using injection pipette of microcapillary glass [51]. This operation requires a micromanipulator. In this case, cells are immobilized by holding glass and gentle suction. Both pipettes are filled with mineral oil.

Microinjection is mostly used for animal cells, while with plants, a cell wall causes hindrance for transformation by microinjection as it works as barrier for microglass tools. Using

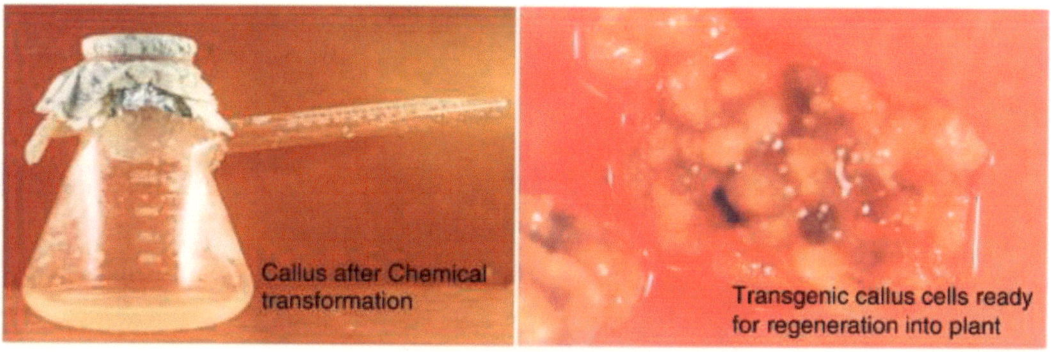

Figure 3. Schematic overview of gene transformation through chemical [12].

microinjection technique for protoplast, there is a risk of toxic compounds to be released, which may cause sudden death of the protoplast. It is also possible to remove vacuoles before microinjection but regeneration and division may be decreased [52].

Protoplast microinjection involves different methods for immobilization, in which instead of using sucking poly-L-lysine is coated to the protoplasts. One of the major advantages of the microinjection is that it not only allows the transformation of the DNA plasmid but also the whole chromosome [53]. This technique is being used for the cellular mechanism and functions of the plant cells and to study the physiology of the plastids especially for tobacco [54] (**Figure 3**). Major limitation of microinjection method involves the use of expensive micromanipulator and it is a time-consuming procedure. Furthermore, frequency of transformation is very low and dependent on the species, i.e., proved to be successful in tobacco [55], Petunia [53], Rape [56], and Barley [57].

6.8. The pollen tube pathway method

Transformation by pollen tube pathway has got great intention in molecular breeding [58]. After pollination, a foreign DNA/plasmid is applied to the styles. To reach ovule, DNA uses the pollen tube pathway. This method of transformation was first used by Luo et al. [60] in rice [59]. In case of rice, a high frequency of transgenic plants was obtained, and this method was then applied to the other commercially important crops, such as wheat [60], soybean [61], *Petunia hybrid* [62], and watermelon [63]. At the premeiotic stage, bacterial inoculum can be applied to the inflorescence without removing the stigma. Pena et al. [65] used this protocol for transformation in rye. Limitation of pollen tube pathway method reported by Shou et al. [66] collected pollens from the genetically engineered plants and reported 10-fold less efficiency in soybean. It was concluded that pollen tube pathway is not reproducible in case of cotton and soybean (**Figure 4**).

6.9. Liposomes

Direct transformation of the foreign DNA into the plant cells using liposomes was Employed in the 1980s. Liposomes are phospholipids with spherical shape, carry nucleic acid, and

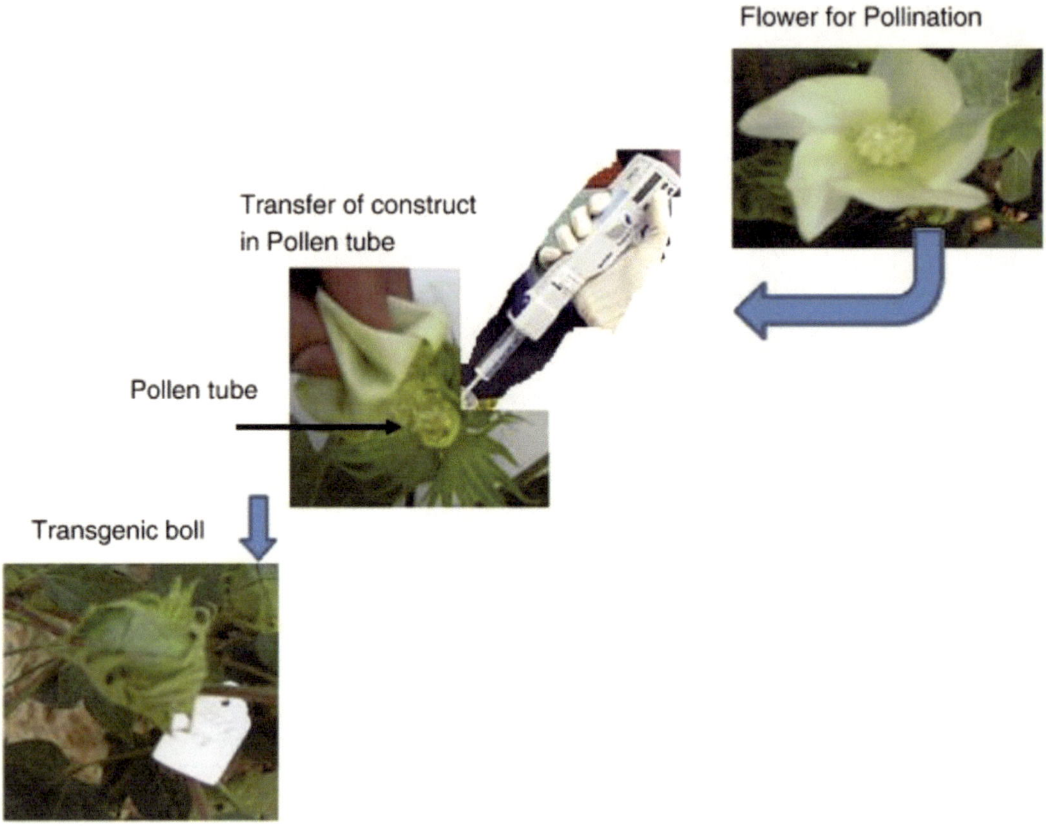

Figure 4. Schematic overview of gene transformation through pollen tube [12].

internally aqueous. Liposomes were put in a nutshell with the DNA fragments to get attached to the cell membranes. Thus, in this way DNA enters the cell and then to the nucleus. For the transfer of the bacterial, plant, and animal genes, lipofection has been a very competent technique. Lipofection takes place by fusion through membrane, and it has improved transformation efficiency because the genetic material used for lipofection is not naked as used in conventional techniques [64, 65]. In spite of cheap and less equipment demanding technique, liposome transformation is not so common. Major limitations in this technique are its low efficiency and being so hectic. Therefore, success story for liposome-mediated transformation have been published so far only for tobacco [66] and wheat [67].

6.10. Shoot apex method of transformation

Transformation by shoot apex method is a rapid method of transformation in cotton, and it is a genotype independent method. In this method, shoots are isolated from the plant and subjected to a virulent strain of *A. tumefaciens*, an antibiotic selection is also applied, and shoots are regenerated *in vitro*. In shoots, dedifferentiation does not take place and is less prone to mutations. Rooting occurs in 6–10 days depending on the cotton cultivar [68]. The shoot apex gives hairy transformed roots because it is most reactive to develop tumor. Shoot apex method is a substitute method for *Agrobacterium*-mediated transformation of dicotyledonous cultivars in which regeneration by protoplasts, leaf disks, or epidermal strips does not take place. This technique offers a rapid method for transformation with less risk of mutations [27]. Katageri et al. [59,71] transformed an Indian variety with shoot apex method and showed a great potential for transformation. Shoot apex transformation method is a time consuming and laborious method for transformation, and there are higher rates of somaclonal variations.

6.11. Sonication-assisted *Agrobacterium*-mediated transformation (SAAT)

SAAT method is based on principle of causing thousands of wounds by ultrasound. These wounds allow the *Agrobacterium* to infect and cause gall formation. The chance of transformation of gene of interest is increased in sonication-assisted method due to infecting deeper plant cells. For the *GUSA*, transient expression protocol was optimized. This method has shown competitive advantage for being used as a routine method [10]. A sonication-assisted method of transformation was used to improve the transformation efficiency of the flax. These wounds created by the ultrasounds allow the uptake of the plasmid DNA into the flax hypocotyls and cotyledons, and its efficiency is dependent on duration and frequency of the sonication applied. SAAT could be a potential tool for increasing transformation efficiency in flax [11]. Due to low efficiency of *Agrobacterium*-mediated method in cotton, an alternative method was required to overcome the barrier of efficiency. SAAT should be a valuable and alternative method for demonstrating the stable cotton transformation [69].

6.12. Infiltration

In vitro culture is required for some transformation procedures. Some transformation procedures do not require *in vitro* culture. In the case of infiltration, plant parts at meiotic or mitotic stages are applied with bacterial inoculums. This method is mainly applied for *Arabidopsis* species for the past many years.

This simple procedure in which plant at the early stages is placed upside down in the beaker containing 5% sucrose solution with *A. tumefaciens* in such a way that only the inflorescences are submerged in the inoculum. Beakers are placed in vacuum chamber with usually 0.05 bar pressure. Seeds are collected and sown on selected media under sterile condition in order to protect from microbial contamination. Up to 95% plants with transgenic seeds can be obtained by keeping optimal conditions.

Vacuum infiltration was applied for the first time in 1993 for transformation of *Arabidopsis* [11]. Over the next 5 years, the optimal conditions were improved and efficiency increased about 2%. Another version of this protocol is to use optimum concentration of sucrose and bacterial inoculum by the surfactant, Silwet L-19 [70]. This modified protocol, which was optimized by Clough and Bent, gives the best result in transformation of *Arabidopsis* [71]. Modified infiltration method was replaced the vacuum infiltration, and the protocol was modified a bit by immersing flowering plant in bacterial culture or spraying bacterial culture on plant. In another study, which was performed by Chung et al. [72], there is a comparison of the classical vacuum infiltration and new version which include modification. The results indicated that plants with bacterial suspension produced much better results, i.e., 2.41% vs. 1.76% for vacuum infiltration and 2.09% for immersion.

Infiltration method is most suitable to plants which have smaller genome. Vacuum infiltration is excluded for plants having genome greater than *Arabidopsis*. Attempts were failed with Chinese cabbage so far. Hence this technique is species specific [12].

6.13. Silicon carbide-mediated transformation (SCMT)

SCMT is less complicated method of plant transformation. Silicon carbide fibers are added to a suspension containing plant tissue (cell clusters, immature embryos, and/or callus) and plasmid DNA; it is mixed and then vortexed. Kaeppler et al. [73] demonstrated that DNA-coated fibers penetrate the cell wall in the presence of small holes created by collisions between the plant cells and fibers. The fibers mostly used in this procedure are single crystals of silica organic minerals like silicon carbide, elongated in shape having a length of 10–80 mm, and a diameter of 0.6 mm and show a high resistance to expandability.

The factors controlling the efficiency of SCMT are fiber size, vortexing parameters, shape of the vessels used, the plant material, and the characteristics of the plant cells, especially the thickness of the cell wall. The main advantages of this procedure are the low expenses and its usefulness for various plant materials. Disadvantages of this method are low transformation efficiency, damage to cells negatively influencing their further regeneration capability, and the necessity of obeying extraordinarily rigorous precaution protocols during laboratory work, as breathing the fibers in, especially asbestos ones, can lead to serious sicknesses [74].

Transgenic forms, cell colonies, or plants were derived from maize [75], and rice [76], from wheat [77], from tobacco [78], and from *Lolium multiflorum, Lolium perenne, Festuca arundinacea,* and *Agrostis stolonifera* [79]. Maize variety Black Mexican Sweet (BMS) cell suspension was transformed with the plasmid carrying the *BAR* gene [73]. They found that 3.4% transgenic cell lines were expressing both transgenes from a 300 ml of packed cell volume, which shows that the integration of transgenes occurred in one per one million cells. The efficiency was significantly lower as described earlier by the same team or other authors employing micro bombardment for transformation. Vortexing with silicon carbide fibers caused the damage to cells decreasing their viability about 29% and causing the decrease in the efficiency of transformation. However, SCMT is speedy and cost-effective with easy to perform. Therefore, this method may prove an alternative method for plant transformation where gene gun method is restricted (i.e., most of monocots). It was suggested that SCMT system of using commercial shakers, which has been reported for maize, seemed to be very good for commercial large-scale transformation [80]. Frame et al. [81] obtained first fertile transgenics for maize in 1994. Out of 22 independent transgenic cell lines, 311 transgenic plants were derived, and 8 of those turned out to be stable transformants. The efficiency of SCMT was 5- to 10-fold lower than gene gun-mediated transformation. Petolino et al. [79] reported that efficiency is much lower in comparison with micro bombardment. The authors concluded that silicon carbide fibers cause damage to transformed cells that is why the results obtained were unsatisfactory [75].

6.14. Electroporation of intact plant cells and tissues

The principles of electroporation are the same for plant cells and protoplasts. However, difference may exist in other plant tissues such as pollen, microspores, leaf fragments, embryos, callus, seeds, or buds. During electroporation, the material used can be in the form of plasmid DNA and *Agrobacterium* inoculums. To check the transient expression of transgenes, different efforts were performed in early 1990s by applying electroporation technology.

Protocols were established for successful electroporation in cell suspensions, e.g., in tobacco [82], rice [24], and in wheat [83]. In early 1990s, experiments were performed to obtain transgenic plants. It was reported that the best results were obtained for maize. Researchers transformed immature embryos and embryogenic callus type I, which were treated by a solution of pectolytic enzymes, and then transferred into electroporating cuvettes [66]. The electroporation efficiency was relatively high when compared with micro bombardment conducted for same species, and about 90 transgenic plants were regenerated from 1440 embryos (6.25%) and 31 plants from 55 callus clusters (54.6%).

Laursen et al. [86] obtained similar results for this species. The authors estimated that the integration of transgenes took place approximately in one per 10,000 cells. Sorokin et al. [87] reported that much lower efficiency, i.e., about three transgenic plants from 1080 immature embryos (0.28%), was observed in the case of wheat electroporation. The transformation efficiency could be increased by the post-pulse addition of ascorbic acid or another ascorbate without any negative influence on cell viability [69]. Tissues were electroporated in liquid media containing 8 mg/L benzyl adenine that showed maximal regeneration through secondary somatic embryogenesis. DaSilva et al. [88] reported that the secondary somatic embryos regenerated from electroporation were positive for *GUS* expression. PCR analysis was positive for the *GUS* and *BAR* genes at torpedo shape somatic embryos. For some species, electroporation is an effective method but it is not widely used for plant transformation.

6.15. Electrophoresis

At the end of the 1980s, Songstad et al. [78] developed a method employing electrophoresis for the transformation of immature embryos, especially in monocotyledonous plants. This method was adopted as an alternative for transformation, but it is very expensive and yield poor results when compared with micro-projectile bombardment [53]. Transfected embryos were placed between the tip of two pipettes and connected to electrodes. The pipette connected to the anode was filled with agar / agarose followed by an EDTA containing electrophoresis buffer.

The pipette connected to the cathode contained agar that was mixed with DNA and an electrophoresis buffer. This pipette was in contact with the apical meristem of the embryo, whereas the second one was located near basal apical part of embryo. Electrophoresis-mediated transformation efficiency depends on various factors, such as electrical field parameters, duration of electrophoresis, contents of electrophoresis buffer, and physicochemical properties of the embryonic tissues. Voltage of 25 mV and an amperage of 0.5 mA for 15 minutes are mostly used for electrophoresis program [74]. In spite of its simplicity, electrophoresis is not considerable method in plant transformation, and the reason behind is less viability of treated embryos. Ahokas et al. [84] showed that none of the plants showed expression of transgene inserted. Griesbach et al. [85] obtained successfully transformed plants of *Calnthe orchid* L.

7. Conclusion

Plant transformation is an essential tool for incorporating new characteristics in crop plant like cotton. Cotton is recalcitrant crop hence a reproducible regeneration is not available in local cotton varieties. Among all strategies developed by different researchers, a little success in cotton (*G. hirsutum*) genetic modification has been reported using *Agrobacterium*-mediated shoot apex cut method of cotton or embryo and sonication-assisted *Agrobacterium*-mediated transformation, except Coker genotypes, where regeneration potential leads to the use of particle bombardment or even *Agrobacterium*-mediated gene transformation as the best procedure. Limitations of gene transformation in cotton are observed in almost all of other procedures. One the most listed limitations of their application is the decreased viability of cells. Infiltration is the main transformation method for *Arabidopsis*, whereas SCMT is for maize, which does not have much success in cotton. With optimizing conditions, these transformation procedures might soon be available for a broad spectrum of plant transformation. The investigations like RNAseq of cotton regeneration in comparison with Coker genotypes or 2D-gel electrophoresis of embryogenic callus of cotton in comparison with control can give better insight to further improve the regeneration potential of cotton cultivars for improvement of cotton regeneration and for better cotton genetic modification in future.

Author details

Abdul Qayyum Rao[1]*, Muhammad Azam Ali[1], Muhammad Azmat Ullah Khan[2], Kamran Shahzad Bajwa[1], Adnan Iqbal[1], Tahir Iqbal[1], Ahmad Ali Shahid[1], Idrees Ahmad Nasir and Tayyab Husnain[1]

*Address all correspondence to: qayyumabdul77@yahoo.com

1 National Center of Excellence in Molecular Biology, University of the Punjab, Lahore Pakistan

2 Faculty of Life Sciences, University of Central Punjab, Lahore, Pakistan

References

[1] Fraley RT, Rogers SG, Horsch RB, Sanders PR, Flick JS, Adams SP Bittner ML, Brand LA, Fink CL, Fry JS. Expression of bacterial genes in plant cells. Proceedings of the National Academy of Sciences. 1983;**80**:4803-4807. DOI: 6308651

[2] Hoekema A, Hirsch P, Hooykaas P, Schilperoort R. A binary plant vector strategy based on separation of vir-and T-region of the *Agrobacterium tumefaciens* Ti-plasmid. Nature. 1983;**303**:179-180. DOI: 10.1038/303179a0

[3] Hernalsteens J, Van Vliet F, De Beuckeleer M, Depicker A, Engler G, Lemmers M, et al. The *Agrobacterium tumefaciens* Ti plasmid as a host vector system for introducing foreign DNA in plant cells. 1980. Biotechnology (Reading, Mass). 1992;**24**:374. DOI: 10.1038/287654a0

[4] Dai S, Zheng P, Marmey P, Zhang S, Tian W, Chen S, et al. Comparative analysis of transgenic rice plants obtained by *Agrobacterium*-mediated transformation and particle bombardment. Molecular Breeding. 2001;**7**:25-33. DOI: 10.1023/A:1009687511633

[5] Skoog F, Miller C, editors. Chemical regulation of growth and organ formation in plant tissue cultured in vitro. Symposia of the Society for Experimental Biology. 1957;**11**:118-131.

[6] Azam S, Samiullah TR, Yasmeen A, ud Din S, Iqbal A, Rao AQ, et al. Dissemination of Bt cotton in cotton growing belt of Pakistan. Advancements in Life Sciences. 2013;**1**:18-26.

[7] Muir W, Hildebrandt A, Riker A. Plant tissue cultures produced from single isolated cells. Science. 1954;**119**:877-878. DOI: 10.1126/science.119.3103.877-a

[8] Davidonis GH, Hamilton RH. Plant regeneration from callus tissue of *Gossypium hirsutum* L. Plant Science Letters. 1983;**32**:89-93. DOI: 10.1016/0304-4211(83)90102-5

[9] Verdeil J-L, Alemanno L, Niemenak N, Tranbarger TJ. Pluripotent versus totipotent plant stem cells: dependence versus autonomy? Trends in Plant Science. 2007;**12**:245-252. DOI: 10.1016/j.tplants.2007.04.002

[10] Larkin P, Ryan S, Brettell R, Scowcroft W. Heritable somaclonal variation in wheat. Theoretical and Applied Genetics. 1984;**67**:443-455. DOI: 10.1007/BF00263410

[11] Rao AQ, Hussain SS, Shahzad MS, Bokhari SYA, Raza MH, Rakha A, et al. Somatic embryogenesis in wild relatives of cotton (*Gossypium* Spp.). Journal of Zhejiang University Science B. 2006;**7**:291-298. DOI: 10.1631/jzus.2006.B0291

[12] Rao AQ, Bakhsh A, Kiani S, Shahzad K, Shahid AA, Husnain T, et al. The myth of plant transformation. Biotechnology Advances. 2009;**27**:753-763. DOI: 10.1016/j.biotechadv.2009.04.028

[13] Vasil IK. A history of plant biotechnology: from the cell theory of Schleiden and Schwann to biotech crops. Plant Cell Reports. 2008;**27**:1423-1440. DOI: 10.1007/s00299-008-0571-4

[14] Braybrook SA, Stone SL, Park S, Bui AQ, Le BH, Fischer RL, et al. Genes directly regulated by LEAFY COTYLEDON2 provide insight into the control of embryo maturation and somatic embryogenesis. Proceedings of the National Academy of Sciences of the United States of America. 2006;**103**:3468-3473. DOI: 10.1073/pnas.0511331103

[15] Hiei Y, Ohta S, Komari T, Kumashiro T. Efficient transformation of rice (*Oryza sativa* L.) mediated by *Agrobacterium* and sequence analysis of the boundaries of the T-DNA. The Plant Journal. 1994;**6**:271-282. DOI: 10.1046/j.1365-313X.1994.6020271.x

[16] Kumria R, Waie B, Rajam M. Plant regeneration from transformed embryogenic callus of an elite indica rice via *Agrobacterium*. Plant Cell, Tissue and Organ Culture. 2001;**67**:63-71. DOI: 10.1023/A:1011645315304

[17] Zheng S-J, Khrustaleva L, Henken B, Sofiari E, Jacobsen E, Kik C, et al. *Agrobacterium tumefaciens*-mediated transformation of *Allium cepa* L.: the production of transgenic onions and shallots. Molecular Breeding. 2001;7:101-115. DOI: 10.1023/A:1011348229189

[18] Jaiwal PK, Kumari R, Ignacimuthu S, Potrykus I, Sautter C. *Agrobacterium tumefaciens*-mediated genetic transformation of mungbean (Vigna radiata L. Wilczek)—a recalcitrant grain legume. Plant Science. 2001;**161**:239-247. DOI: 10.1016/S0168-9452(01)00352-1

[19] Frisch DA, Harris-Haller LW, Yokubaitis NT, Thomas TL, Hardin SH, Hall TC. Complete sequence of the binary vector Bin 19. Plant Molecular Biology. 1995;**27**:405-409. DOI: 10.1007/BF00020193

[20] Hennegan KP, Danna KJ. pBIN20: an improved binary vector for shape *Agrobacterium*-mediated transformation. Plant Molecular Biology Reporter. 1998;**16**:129-131. DOI: 10.1023/A:1007444100898

[21] Hajdukiewicz P, Svab Z, Maliga P. The small, versatile pPZP family of *Agrobacterium* binary vectors for plant transformation. Plant Molecular Biology. 1994;**25**:989-994.

[22] Töpfer R, Gronenborn B, Schell J, Steinbiss H-H. Uptake and transient expression of chimeric genes in seed-derived embryos. The Plant Cell. 1989;**1**:133-139. DOI: 10.1105/tpc.1.1.133

[23] Hou W-S, Guo S-D, Lu M. Development of transgenic wheat with a synthetical insecticidal crystal protein gene via pollen-tube pathway. Acta Agronomica Sinica. 2003;**29**:806-809.

[24] Zapata C, Park S, El-Zik K, Smith R. Transformation of a Texas cotton cultivar by using *Agrobacterium* and the shoot apex. Theoretical and Applied Genetics. 1999;**98**:252-256. DOI: 10.1007/s001220051065

[25] Wilkins TA, Rajasekaran K, Anderson DM. Cotton biotechnology. Critical Reviews in Plant Sciences. 2000;**19**:511-550.

[26] Power J, Cummins S, Cocking E. Fusion of isolated plant protoplasts. Nature (London). 1970;**225**:1016-1018. DOI: 19701607260

[27] Takebe I, Labib G, Melchers G. Regeneration of whole plants from isolated mesophyll protoplasts of tobacco. Naturwissenschaften. 1971;**58**:318-320. DOI: 10.1007/BF00624737

[28] Geerts P, Sassi K, Mergeai G, Baudoin J-P. Development of an in vitro pod culture technique for young pods of *Phaseolus vulgaris* L. In Vitro Cellular & Developmental Biology-Plant. 2000;**36**:481-487. DOI: 10.1007/s11627-000-0086-3

[29] Schryer P, Lu Q, Vandenberg A, Bett K. Rapid regeneration of *Phaseolus angustissimus* and *P. vulgaris* from very young zygotic embryos. Plant Cell, Tissue and Organ Culture. 2005;**83**:67-74. DOI: 10.1007/s11240-005-2586-7

[30] Ochatt S, Abirached-Darmency M, Marget P, Aubert G. The Lathyrus paradox:"poor men's diet" or a remarkable genetic resource for protein legume breeding. Breeding of Neglected and Under-Utilised Crops, Spices and Herbs. 2007. INRA, C.R, de Dijon, URLEG, B.P.86510, 21065 Dijon cedex, France pp. 41-60.

[31] Davey M, Cocking E, Freeman J, Pearce N, Tudor I. Transformation of Petunia protoplasts by isolated *Agrobacterium* plasmids. Plant Sciencc Letters. 1980;**18**:307-313. DOI: 10.1016/0304-4211(80)90121-2

[32] Vasil IK. Molecular improvement of cereals. Plant Molecular Biology. 1994;**25**:925-937.

[33] Waldron C, Malcolm S, Murphy E, Roberts J. A method for high-frequency DNA-mediated transformation of plant protoplasts. Plant Molecular Biology Reporter. 1985;**3**:169-173. DOI: 10.1007/BF02886753

[34] Hess D. Transformation experiments in higher plants-reproducibility of anthocyanin induction in petunia and preliminary characterization of transforming principle. Zeitschrift Fur Pflanzenphysiologie. 1969;**61**:286-298.

[35] Muzaffar A, Kiani S, Khan MAU, Rao AQ, Ali A, Awan MF, et al. Chloroplast localization of Cry1Ac and Cry2A protein-an alternative way of insect control in cotton. Biological Research. 2015;**48**:1. DOI: 10.1186/s40659-015-0005-z

[36] Yoo J, Jung G. DNA uptake by imbibition and expression of a foreign gene in rice. Physiologia Plantarum. 1995;**94**:453-459. DOI: 10.1111/j.1399-3054.1995.tb00953.x

[37] Pett A, Delhaye S, Tempe J, Morel G. Recherches sur les guanidines des tissus de crown gall. mise en evidence d'une relation biochimique specifique entre le souches d'*Agrobacterium tumefaciens* et les tumeurs qu'elles induisent. Physiologie Végétale. 1970.

[38] Chilton M-D, Drummond MH, Merlo DJ, Sciaky D, Montoya AL, Gordon MP, et al. Stable incorporation of plasmid DNA into higher plant cells: the molecular basis of crown gall tumorigenesis. Cell. 1977;**11**:263-271. DOI: 10.1016/0092-8674(77)90043-5

[39] Chilton M-D, Saiki RK, Yadav N, Gordon MP, Quetier F. T-DNA from *Agrobacterium* Ti plasmid is in the nuclear DNA fraction of crown gall tumor cells. Proceedings of the National Academy of Sciences. 1980;**77**:4060-4064.

[40] Van Haute E, Joos H, Maes M, Warren G, Van Montagu M, Schell J. Intergeneric transfer and exchange recombination of restriction fragments cloned in pBR322: a novel strategy for the reversed genetics of the Ti plasmids of *Agrobacterium tumefaciens*. The EMBO Journal. 1983;**2**:411.

[41] Bevan M, Flavell R, Chilton M. A chimaeric antibiotic resistance gene as a selectable marker for plant cell transformation. 1983. Biotechnology (Reading, Mass). 1992;**24**:367. DOI: 10.1038/304184a0

[42] Thomas JC, Adams DG, Keppenne VD, Wasmann CC, Brown JK, Kanost MR, et al. Protease inhibitors of Manduca sexta expressed in transgenic cotton. Plant Cell Reports. 1995;**14**:758-762. DOI: 10.1007/BF00232917

[43] Nadolska-Orczyk A, Orczyk W, Przetakiewicz A. *Agrobacterium*-mediated transformation of cereals—from technique development to its application. Acta Physiologiae Plantarum. 2000;**22**:77-88. DOI: 10.1007/s11738-000-0011-8

[44] Shillito R. Methods of genetic transformation: electroporation and polyethylene glycol treatment. Molecular Improvement of Cereal Crops. Springer Netherlands; 1999. p. 9-20. DOI: 10.1007/978-94-011-4802-3_2

[45] Vasil IK. The story of transgenic cereals: the challenge, the debate, and the solution—a historical perspective. In Vitro Cellular & Developmental Biology-Plant. 2005;**41**:577-583. DOI: 10.1079/IVP2005654

[46] Sailaja M, Tarakeswari M, Sujatha M. Stable genetic transformation of castor (*Ricinus communis* L.) via particle gun-mediated gene transfer using embryo axes from mature seeds. Plant Cell Reports. 2008;**27**:1509-1519. DOI: 10.1007/s00299-008-0580-3.

[47] Finer JJ, McMullen MD. Transformation of cotton (Gossypium hirsutum L.) via particle bombardment. Plant Cell Reports. 1990;**8**:586-589. DOI: 10.1007/BF00270059

[48] Zhao T-J, Zhao S-Y, Chen H-M, Zhao Q-Z, Hu Z-M, Hou B-K, et al. Transgenic wheat progeny resistant to powdery mildew generated by *Agrobacterium* inoculum to the basal portion of wheat seedling. Plant Cell Reports. 2006;**25**:1199-1204. DOI: 10.1007/s00299-006-0184-8

[49] Sanford JC, Klein TM, Wolf ED, Allen N. Delivery of substances into cells and tissues using a particle bombardment process. Particulate Science and Technology. 1987;**5**:27-37. DOI: 10.1080/02726358708904533

[50] Altpeter F, Baisakh N, Beachy R, Bock R, Capell T, Christou P, et al. Particle bombardment and the genetic enhancement of crops: myths and realities. Molecular Breeding. 2005;**15**:305-327. DOI: 10.1007/s11032-004-8001-y

[51] Crossway A, Oakes JV, Irvine JM, Ward B, Knauf VC, Shewmaker C. Integration of foreign DNA following microinjection of tobacco mesophyll protoplasts. Molecular and General Genetics MGG. 1986;**202**:179-185. DOI: 10.1007/BF00331634

[52] Lörz H, Paszkowski J, Dierks-Ventling C, Potrykus I. Isolation and characterization of cytoplasts and miniprotoplasts derived from protoplasts of cultured cells. Physiologia Plantarum. 1981;**53**:385-391. DOI: 10.1111/j.1399-3054.1981.tb04517.x

[53] Griesbach R. Chromosome-mediated transformation via microinjection. Plant Science. 1987;**50**:69-77. DOI: 10.1016/0168-9452(87)90032-X

[54] Knoblauch M, Hibberd JM, Gray JC, van Bel AJ. A galinstan expansion femtosyringe for microinjection of eukaryotic organelles and prokaryotes. Nature Biotechnology. 1999;**17**:906-909. DOI: 10.1038/12902

[55] Schnorf M, Neuhaus-Url G, Galli A, Iida S, Potrykus I, Neuhaus G. An improved approach for transformation of plant cells by microinjection: molecular and genetic analysis. Transgenic Research. 1991;**1**:23-30. DOI: 10.1007/BF02512993

[56] Neuhaus G, Spangenberg G, Scheid OM, Schweiger H-G. Transgenic rapeseed plants obtained by the microinjection of DNA into microspore-derived embryoids. Theoretical and Applied Genetics. 1987;**75**:30-36. DOI: 10.1007/BF00249138

[57] Holm PB, Olsen O, Schnorf M, Brinch-Pedersen H, Knudsen S. Transformation of barley by microinjection into isolated zygote protoplasts. Transgenic Research. 2000;**9**:21-32. DOI: 10.1023/A:1008974729597

[58] Song X, Gu Y, Qin G. Application of a transformation method via the pollen-tube pathway in agriculture molecular breeding. Life Science Journal. 2007;**4**:77-79.

[59] Luo Z, Wu R. A simple method for the transformation of rice via the pollen-tube pathway. Plant Molecular Biology Reporter. 1989;**7**:69-77. DOI: 10.1007/BF02669590

[60] Mu H-M, Liu S-J, Zhou W-J, Wen Y-X, Zhang W-J, Wei R-X: [Transformation of wheat with insecticide gene of arrowhead proteinase inhibitor by pollen tube pathway and analysis of transgenic plants] [In Process Citation]. Yi chuan xue bao= Acta Genetica Sinica. 1998;**26**:634-642.

[61] Hu C-Y, Wang L. In planta soybean transformation technologies developed in China: procedure, confirmation and field performance. In Vitro Cellular & Developmental Biology-Plant. 1999;**35**:417-420. DOI: 10.1007/s11627-999-0058-1

[62] Tjokrokusumo D, Heinrich T, Wylie S, Potter R, McComb J. Vacuum infiltration of Petunia hybrida pollen with *Agrobacterium tumefaciens* to achieve plant transformation. Plant Cell Reports. 2000;**19**:792-797. DOI: 10.1007/s002990050009

[63] Chen WS, Chiu CC, Liu HY, Lee TL, Cheng JT, Lin CC, et al. Gene transfer via pollen-tube pathway for anti-fusarium wilt in watermelon. IUBMB Life. 1998;**46**:1201-1209. DOI: 10.1080/15216549800204762

[64] Shou H, Palmer RG, Wang K. Irreproducibility of the soybean pollen-tube pathway transformation procedure. Plant Molecular Biology Reporter. 2002;**20**:325-334. DOI: 10.1007/BF02772120

[65] Murakawa T, Kajiyama S, Ikeuchi T, Kawakami S, Fukui K. Improvement of transformation efficiency by bioactive-beads-mediated gene transfer using DNA-lipofectin complex as entrapped genetic material. Journal of Bioscience and Bioengineering. 2008;**105**:77-80. DOI: 10.1263/jbb.105.77

[66] Dekeyser RA, Claes B, De Rycke RM, Habets ME, Van Montagu MC, Caplan AB. Transient gene expression in intact and organized rice tissues. The Plant Cell. 1990;**2**:591-602. DOI: 10.1105/tpc.2.7.591

[67] Zhu Z, Sun B, Liu C, Xiao G, Li X. Transformation of wheat protoplasts mediated by cationic liposome and regeneration of transgenic plantlets. Chinese Journal of Biotechnology. 1992;**9**:257-261.

[68] Yaqoob A, Shahid AA, Samiullah TR, Rao AQ, Khan MAU, Tahir S, et al. Risk assessment of Bt crops on the non-target plant-associated insects and soil organisms.

Journal of the Science of Food and Agriculture. 2016;**96**:2613-2619. DOI: 10.1002/jsfa.7661

[69] Hussain SS, Husnain T, Riazuddin S. Sonication assisted *Agrobacterium* mediated transformation (SAAT): An alternative method for cotton transformation. Pakistan Journal of Botany. 2007;**39**:223.

[70] Clough SJ, Bent AF. Floral dip: a simplified method *forAgrobacterium*-mediated transformation of *Arabidopsis thaliana*. The Plant Journal. 1998;**16**:735-743. DOI: 10.1046/j.1365-313x.1998.00343.x

[71] Ye GN, Stone D, Pang SZ, Creely W, Gonzalez K, Hinchee M. Arabidopsis ovule is the target for *Agrobacterium* in planta vacuum infiltration transformation. The Plant Journal. 1999;**19**:249-257. DOI: 10.1046/j.1365-313X.1999.00520.x

[72] Chung M-H, Chen M-K, Pan S-M. Floral spray transformation can efficiently generate *Arabidopsis*. Transgenic Research. 2000;**9**:471-486. DOI: 10.1023/A:1026522104478

[73] Kaeppler H, Somers D, Rines H, Cockburn A. Silicon carbide fiber-mediated stable transformation of plant cells. Theoretical and Applied Genetics. 1992;**84**:560-566. DOI: 10.1007/BF00232262

[74] Songstad D, Somers D, Griesbach R. Advances in alternative DNA delivery techniques. Plant Cell, Tissue and Organ Culture. 1995;**40**:1-15. DOI: 10.1007/BF00041112

[75] Petolino J, Hopkins N, Kosegi B, Skokut M. Whisker-mediated transformation of embryogenic callus of maize. Plant Cell Reports. 2000;**19**:781-786. DOI: 10.1007/s002999900180

[76] Nagatani N, Honda H, Shimada T, Kobayashi T. DNA delivery into rice cells and transformation using silicon carbide whiskers. Biotechnology Techniques. 1997;**11**:471-473. DOI: 10.1023/A:1018497529493

[77] Brisibe EA, Gajdosova A, Olesen A, Andersen SB. Cytodifferentiation and transformation of embryogenic callus lines derived from another culture of wheat. Journal of Experimental Botany. 2000;**51**:187-196. DOI: 10.1093/jexbot/51.343.187

[78] Kaeppler HF, Gu W, Somers DA, Rines HW, Cockburn AF. Silicon carbide fiber-mediated DNA delivery into plant cells. Plant Cell Reports. 1990;**9**:415-418. DOI: 10.1007/BF00224152

[79] Dalton S, Bettany A, Timms E, Morris P. Transgenic plants of *Lolium multiflorum, Lolium perenne, Festuca arundinacea* and *Agrostis stolonifera* by silicon carbide fibre-mediated transformation of cell suspension cultures. Plant Science. 1998;**132**:31-43. DOI: 10.1016/S0168-9452(97)00259-8

[80] Bullock W, Dias D, Bagnal S, Cook K, Teronde S, Ritland J, et al., editors. A high efficiency maize "whisker" transformation system. Plant and Animal Genomes IX Conference, San Diego, CA; 2001.

[81] Frame BR, Drayton PR, Bagnall SV, Lewnau CJ, Bullock WP, Wilson HM, et al. Production of fertile transgenic maize plants by silicon carbide whisker-mediated transformation. The Plant Journal. 1994;**6**:941-948. DOI: 10.1046/j.1365-313X.1994.6060941.x

[82] Abdul-Baki AA, Saunders JA, Matthews BF, Pittarelli GW. DNA uptake during electroporation of germinating pollen grains. Plant Science. 1990;**70**:181-190. DOI: 10.1016/0168-9452(90)90132-8

[83] Zaghmout O, Trolinder NL. Simple and efficient method for directly electroporating *Agrobacterium* plasmid DNA into wheat callus cells. Nucleic Acids Research. 1993;**21**:1048. DOI: PMC309253

[84] Ahokas H. Transfection of germinating barley seed electrophoretically with exogenous DNA. Theoretical and Applied Genetics. 1989;**77**:469-472. DOI: 10.1007/BF00274265

[85] Griesbach R. An improved method for transforming plants through electrophoresis. Plant Science. 1994;**102**:81-89. DOI: 10.1016/0168-9452(94)03936-4

[86] Laursen, C. M., Krzyzek, R. A., Flick, C. E., Anderson, P. C., & Spencer, T. M. Production of fertile transgenic maize by electroporation of suspension culture cells. *Plant Molecular Biology*, (1994). **24**(1), 51-61. DOI: 10.1007/BF00040573

[87] Sorokin AP, Ke XY, Chen DF, Elliott MC. Production of fertile transgenic wheat plants via tissue electroporation. Plant Science. 2000 28;**156**(2):227-33. dx.doi.org/10.1016/S0168-9452(00)00260-0

[88] Da Silva RF, Menéndez-Yuffá A. Transient gene expression in secondary somatic embryos from coffee tissues electroporated with the genes gus and bar. Electronic Journal of Biotechnology. 2003 **6**(1):11-2. dx.doi.org/10.4067/S0717-34582003000100006

Section 4

Cotton Based Products and Textile Research

Chapter 11

UV Treatments on Cotton Fibers

Franco Ferrero, Gianluca Migliavacca and

Monica Periolatto

Additional information is available at the end of the chapter

http://dx.doi.org/10.5772/63796

Abstract

Ultraviolet (UV) radiations can act in different ways on the functionalization of textiles, through pre- or posttreatments, in order to modify their behavior in dyeing and finishing processes. In cotton fiber, unlike the wool, the UV absorption is not due to any of the structural groups of the normal cellulosic chains and can only be attributed to "impurities" or "faults" bearing carbonyl and/or carboxyl groups. In fact, UV irradiation coupled with mild oxidation can improve some properties of the cotton fibers such as pilling resistance, water swelling, and dyeability. Therefore, the process of differential dyeing with direct and reactive dyes assisted by UV irradiation was studied and interesting differential chromatic effects were obtained by a UV posttreatment capable to fade dyeing. On the other hand, the surface modification of cotton fabrics by UV curing and UV grafting with suitable chemicals was pursued to obtain finishing treatments able to confer oil and/or water repellency. Finally, antimicrobial finishing by chitosan UV grafting was proposed as valid environmental friendly method to confer a satisfactory washing-resistant antimicrobial activity to cotton fabrics even with low polymer add-on.

Keywords: cotton, dyeing, finishing, UV curing, UV grafting, UV radiation

1. Introduction

Cotton fiber differs markedly from other cellulose fibers in morphological traits. Due to its many features, cotton, even though it was discovered later than other fibers, gained a high position and strongly stimulated the development of textile industry. Cotton today is the most used textile fiber in the world. Its current market share is 56% for all fibers used for apparel and home furnishings; another contribution is attributed to nonwoven textiles and personal care items. It is generally recognized that most consumers prefer cotton fiber for personal care items to those containing synthetic fibers.

Soft hand, good absorbency, and color retaining are among the advantages of cotton fabric; it is easy to print, handle, and sew; it is machine-washable and dry-cleanable; and it has good strength and hangs well. These are all the desirable properties for a textile but, for some applications, they can show drawbacks, which suggested modifications of the fibers achievable with chemical or physical treatments. Among the latter, ultraviolet (UV) irradiation was experimented.

UV radiations can act in different ways on the functionalization of textiles, through pre- or post-treatments, in order to modify their behavior in dyeing and finishing processes.

The UV treatments applied in textile field, in addition to required specific effects, should also have the following advantages: (1) easy application, not needing expensive and sophisticated equipment; (2) durability and fastness of the degree of treatment looking at the future uses; (3) limited treatment costs, without precluding any market segment; and (4) environmentally friendly requirements, for sustainable textile processes. Many research works were developed with the aim to utilize the effects of UV radiations on various natural as well as synthetic fibers [1–6]. Most of these studies were devoted to the surface modification of wool, but even cotton fiber was considered.

In cotton, unlike the wool, the true origin of the UV absorption, which is not due to any of the structural groups that make up the normal cellulosic chains, is uncertain and can only be attributed to "impurities" or "faults" bearing carbonyl and/or carboxyl groups.

Naturally pigmented green cotton fiber derives its color from caffeic acid that is deposited in alternating layers with cellulose around the outside of the fiber. The isolated compound is fluorescent (287 and 310 nm absorption wavelengths), and it has been theorized that its purpose is to absorb UV radiation in order to protect the seed. Brown and tan cottons derive their color from tannin vacuoles in the lumen of the fiber cells rather than in the wax layer as in green cotton. The brown color appears after the fibers are exposed to oxygen and sunlight, which happens when the seed pod opens.

The gray cotton fiber contains the above-cited impurities, so one or more pretreatment processes before dyeing are applied to attain its full textile exploitation. The pretreatment processes of cotton fabrics include scouring to get off noncellulosic impurities, pigments, and waxes. An oxidative bleaching is carried out to wipe out natural coloring matter for white or dyeing, while singing is applied to eliminate the protruding loose fibers [7].

Mansuri et al. [8] claimed that cotton-knitted fabric padded in a solution of hydrogen peroxide and then irradiated with UV lamp showed a significant pilling reduction, comparable to that obtained with industrial system of biopolishing. Moreover, Millington said that Siroflash® treatment (UV irradiation coupled with mild wet oxidation with hydrogen peroxide) is highly effective against pilling formation of wool as well as of cotton fiber [9]. In the latter case, the application of Siroflash® process would require the presence of a sensitizer or a photoinitiator to absorb UV radiation in the primary photochemical step. Such a photoinitiator must be odor-free, nontoxic, low expensive, and easily removable by aqueous washing. This rules out many of the commercial UV photoinitiators, but hydrogen peroxide is able to absorb UV radiations below 300 nm to produce highly reactive hydroxyl radicals. One would expect these radicals to reduce the strength of knitted cotton fabric by breaking the cellulose chains. In fact, significant dry-burst strength losses were observed in dependence on hydrogen peroxide concentration, but some fabric strength loss would be acceptable if the limiting factor is an unacceptable level of pills.

Mercerization is the treatment of cotton yarns, fabrics, and knit goods with cold, strong caustic soda bath under tension to give increased luster, smoothness, dye and finishing chemical uptake, dimensional constancy, and better mechanical properties. Zuber et al. [10] demonstrated that UV rays have a similar effect, on cellulosic fibers, as the alkaline treatment; irradiated cellulosic fibers showed higher swelling in comparison with any concentration of soda treatment, but tear and tensile strength were worse compared to the untreated and to the alkali-treated ones. They emphasized that UV rays do not produce loss in weight after exposure of cotton fabrics, and affinity for direct dyes is slightly enhanced in comparison with that found with mercerization. However, with a reactive dye it is found that UV irradiation not only enhanced the strength of dye on irradiated fabric but also improved the dyeing properties [11]. The reason for this might be that the exposure of cotton fiber to UV radiation in the presence of oxygen causes cellulose oxidation to carboxylic acids and opens spaces between the fibers causing imbibition of more dye, hence the interaction for dyeing becomes more significant [12].

Iqbal et al. [13] and more recently Adeel et al. [14] observed that UV radiation not only enhances the uptake and fastness of natural dyes on pre-irradiated cotton fabric using low concentrations of dye but also with a low concentration of mordant.

Cotton fiber immersed in water develops a negative surface potential, which consequently gives rise to electrostatic repulsion of anionic dyes. Therefore, a large amount of electrolyte, such as sodium sulfate or chloride, is required in order to reduce the repulsion between the negatively charged fibers and the anionic dyes. Moreover, the complete dye exhaustion is not normally reached, causing environmental problems due to the discharge of colored effluent having a high salt concentration. To overcome these problems, the cationization of cotton fiber was applied to increase the substantivity of anionic dyes by introducing positively charged sites on the fibers. Pretreatments with glycidyltrimethylammonium chloride and other cationization reagents were reported. However, cationic polymerizable monomers, such as methacryloyl quaternary ammonium compounds, have also been fixed onto cotton fabric using UV radiation with a view to producing print-patterned dyeings [15].

Instead, Jang et al. [16] have examined the potential of photografting cationic monomers onto crease-resistant cross-linked cotton fabric by incorporation of a water-soluble photoinitiator to improve grafting. In fact, whereas untreated cotton is readily dyeable with anionic dyes in the presence of salt, the cross-linked fiber is undyeable to a comparable deep shade, since the diffusion of relatively large dye molecules into the cross-linked substrate is hindered by a low swelling under aqueous conditions. The dyeability of cationized cotton fiber by three classes of dyes (direct, reactive, and sulfur dyes) has been significantly improved owing to the increased ionic attraction between dyes and cationized cellulose, even in the absence of salts [17].

On the other hand, Dong and Jang [18] proposed the direct photografting of wool-reactive dyes themselves onto cotton fabric. This coloration utilizes the photoreactivity of certain dyes under UV irradiation, through photopolymerization, photografting, and photocross-linking processes, to form a polymerized and cross-linked dye network. Thus, a single class of dye can color almost any textile substrate since no specific affinity of particular dyes to individual fibers is required. Reactive dyes containing an α-bromoacrylamido reactive group are among the most successful metal-free dyes for protein fibers because of their brilliant color and high wet-fastness properties. However, these reactive dyes hardly react with cotton fiber under similar conditions owing to the rather low nucleophilicity of the hydroxyl groups in cellulose compared with the thiol and amino groups in proteins. Therefore, dyes containing α-bromoacrylamido groups were employed as grafting monomers to be photografted onto cellulose under continuous UV irradiation. This novel approach may realize the photoactive coloration of cotton fiber even with dyes of low affinity for conventional reactive dyeing. Furthermore, the coloration does not require large amounts of salt, time, and energy, which makes it an alternative process of excellent environmental friendliness.

2. Differential dyeing on cotton fabric by UV irradiation

2.1. Differential dyeing

Textile world is always looking for new color effects, both for artistic questions and in order to meet the current fashion demands; for these reasons, differential dyeing effects mainly on wool fibers were studied. These can be achieved by surface modification on selected areas of fabric by a physical surface treatment such as plasma [19] or UV irradiation on one side followed by a conventional dyeing [20]. Moreover, patterning effects can be obtained if a suitable mask is interposed between energy source and fabric for selective surface modification. This represents an alternative and less expensive method than the usual production of patterned fabrics by printing or color weaving.

In the Sun-Wash method patented by Nearchimica with Stamperia Emiliana (Italy) [21], the continuous UV pretreatment of wool fabric on one face before dyeing has been proposed to obtain different shades on the two faces or patterning effects. A careful selection of dyes is needed to obtain satisfactory tone-on-tone effects and even more to produce double-face effects with different colors. These suggestions inspired the experiments on differential dyeing of wool by UV irradiation carried out by Migliavacca et al. [22]. A good final shade uniformity was obtained, with an acceptable color difference ($\Delta E \geq 5.0$) between UV-treated and untreated fabric area (double-face effect), due to an increased dye-fiber affinity of the side previously treated with UV radiation.

The same type of chromatic effect was also wanted for cellulosic fibers, in particular for cotton [23]. An unscoured 100% cotton yarn was chosen (N_m = 2/34), and from this material many knitted fabrics were prepared in order to do dyeing tests with direct dyes. At first, these fabrics were subjected to a dynamic UV irradiation under a Hg-medium pressure vapor lamp, with the following parameters:

UVA irradiance:	430 mW/cm^2
source working length:	0.6 m
radiant exposure:	8.6 J/cm^2
fabric speed:	11 m/min
no. of irradiation steps:	6
total irradiation time:	30 s

Colorimetric measurements were made comparing the UV-treated fabric with the untreated one, using a reflectance spectrophotometer Datacolor Check II Plus, with the results reported in **Table 1**.

Sample	ΔL	Δa	Δb	ΔE
UV treated	−0.65	−0.18	2.86	2.94

Table 1. CIE L a b difference parameters for unscoured cotton fabric after UV treatment.

In these conditions of treatment, a global fiber-yellowing effect is observed, mainly due to a process that involves both photodegradation and photochromic reactions; chemical species probably involved in this phenomenon are quinol and phenylcoumaran residues (belonging to lignin impurity).

2.2. Dyeings performed with direct dyes

Dyeing tests were carried out on cotton fabrics (UV irradiated and not) using Solophenyl® (Huntsman) direct dyes for cellulosic fibers applied on 0.1% o.w.f. (on the weight of fabric), 1:40 material to liquor ratio, with 2.0 g/L Albatex UNI as leveling agent, and 1.0 g/L NaCl. The dyeing was performed at 100°C for 30 min, then the samples were cooled at 80°C, and maintained at 80°C for 15 min. The irradiation conditions were the same as reported in Section 2.1.

The final bath exhaustion was about 70% for all the dyes, and the resulted dyeings showed good color level and chromatic homogeneity. However, the color differences between UV-treated and untreated fabrics were minimal, as shown in **Table 2**, where a color difference greater than 5.0 ΔE units was evidenced only with Navy Solophenyl BLE, evidenced in bold.

Increasing the dyeing depth over 0.1%, the chromatic differences between UV-treated and untreated fabrics would increase; however, the wet fastness of dyed cotton fabric would be less, then not acceptable. Therefore, this dye selection seems not to be suitable for the differential dyeing.

Dye	ΔL	Δa	Δb	ΔE
Orange Solophenyl TGL 182%	0.58	−1.0	−1.20	1.68
Bordeaux Solophenyl 3BLE	1.20	−0.75	0.52	1.51
Blue Solophenyl FGLE 220%	1.30	0.75	2.30	2.75
Navy Solophenyl BLE 250%	4.94	0.06	3.58	**6.10**

Table 2. Color difference parameters for 0.1% dyeings with Solophenyl dyes.

On the other hand, differential dyeing effects can be pursued applying UV irradiation on dyed samples, just using the discoloration induced by radiation. In this case, the fading ability of the dyes on cotton yarn was exploited and in many cases significant color differences (Δ*E* higher than 5.0) were found between UV-irradiated and untreated samples.

2.3. Differential dyeing performed with UV fading of reactive dyes

Fading of dyed cotton yarns was carried out on dyed yarn samples wrapped on cardboard where one side was exposed for half area to UV rays. The irradiation condition and color evaluation were the same as reported in Section 2.1.

Two series of reactive dyes for cellulosic fibers were investigated, at first reactive dyes namely Kayacelon React® (Nippon Kayaku) and Kemacelon® (Kem Color) having reactive groups belonging to triazinyl betaine (**Figure 1**).

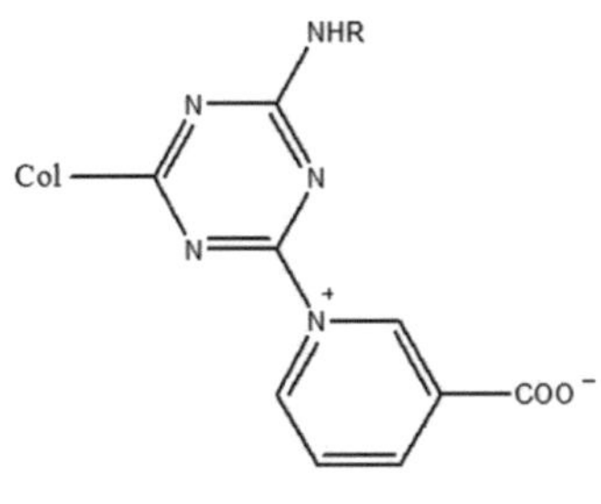

Figure 1. Triazinyl reactive group.

These dyes were applied at 1.0% o.w.f. with liquor ratio of 1:20, in the presence of an alkali donor (1.0 g/L of Buslid 509, which slowly releases hexamethylenetetramine increasing pH) and 40 g/L Na_2SO_4 working at 90°C for 60 min. The results are reported in **Table 3**.

Even this series of reactive dyes presents only a term (Kayacelon React Red CN-3B, evidenced in bold) with acceptable color difference for a differential dyeing between UV-treated and untreated samples.

The chromatic investigation was continued with the reactive dyes Avitera SE® (Huntsman), constituted by a chromogen with three reactive groups (chemical structure still under patent), applied at 0.5% o.w.f., 1:20 liquor ratio, and 50 g/L NaCl working at 60°C for 30 min adding 9 g/L of Na_2CO_3 divided into three aliquots (1/6, 2/6, 3/6), always working at 60°C for another 30 min. The results are reported in **Table 4**.

Dye	Δ*L*	Δ*a*	Δ*b*	Δ*E*
Kayacelon React Yellow CN-RL	−0.18	0.79	−0.48	0.94
Kayacelon React Yellow CN-ML	1.11	−0.49	−0.33	1.26
Kayacelon React G. Yellow CN-GL	−0.02	0.45	−2.43	2.47
Kayacelon React Red CN-3B	2.28	−6.84	2.27	**7.56**
Kayacelon React Blue CN-MG	1.19	0.55	3.68	3.91
Kayacelon React Dark Blue CN-R	3.36	1.78	3.1	4.92

Table 3. Color difference parameters for 1.0% dyeings with Kayacelon React dyes.

Dye	Δ*L*	Δ*a*	Δ*b*	Δ*E*
Avitera Yellow SE	0.86	−0.77	−2.48	2.74
Avitera Red SE	4.92	−10.0	4.02	**11.8**
Avitera deep Blue SE	5.39	4.14	5.06	**8.47**

Table 4. Color difference parameters for 0.5% dyeings with Avitera dyes.

This series of reactive dyes presents only two terms, evidenced in bold, with acceptable values for differential dyeing effects. It was then decided to consider other series of DyStar reactive dyes, based on the monochloro-difluoro-pyrimidine reactive group, Levafix type (**Figure 2a**), and β-sulfatoethylsulfonic reactive group, Remazol type (**Figure 2b**).

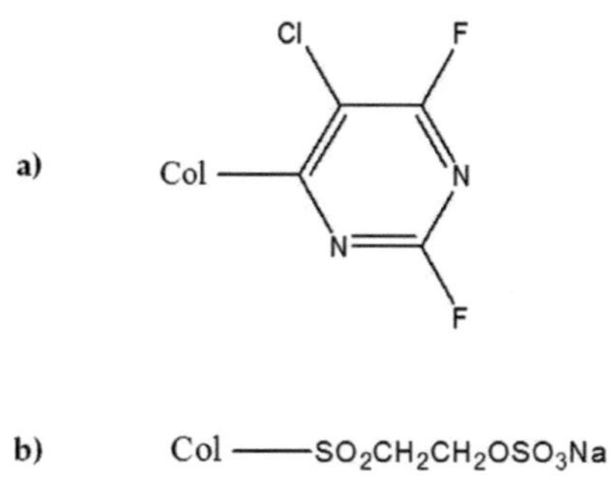

Figure 2. Molecular structure of dyes with monochloro-difluoro-pyrimidine reactive group (a) and β-sulfatoethylsulfonic reactive group (b).

In accordance with the works carried out by Batchelor et al. [24] about photofading, it was observed that light fastness (and therefore also the fading ability toward UV radiations) is instead related to the chemical structure of the chromogen; they showed that fading is caused by both visible and UV light, with visible light responsible for azo dyes and UV light responsible for phthalocyanines.

Generally speaking, the photofading is mainly due to singlet oxygen development, $^1O_2$, which can be formed by the quenching of excited states of dyes by the triplet ground state of oxygen, $^3O_2$:

$$\text{dye} \xrightarrow{\text{light}} \text{dye}^* + {}^3O_2 \xrightarrow{\text{quench}} \text{dye} + {}^1O_2$$

Color index	Commercial name	Light fastness (1/6 SD)	Structure	Reactive group
R.Y. 160	Yellow br. Remazol 4GL	5	Azo	Vinylsulfone
R.Y. 176	Yellow Remazol 3RS	5	Unknown	Unknown
R.O. 107	G. yellow Remazol RNL 150%	4/5	Azo	Vinylsulfone
R.O.16	Orange br. Remazol 3R spec.	4/5	Azo	Vinylsulfone
Unknown	Scarlet Levafix CA	4	Azo	Triazinyl + vinylsulfone
Unknown	Red Levafix CA	4	Azo	Triazinyl + vinylsulfone
R.R. 180	Red br. Remazol F-3B	3/4	Azo	Vinylsulfone
R.Bl. 21	Turquoise Remazol G 133%	5	Phthal.	Vinylsulfone
Unknown	Navy Levafix CA	3/4	Azo	Triazinyl + vinylsulfone
R.Bk. 5	Black Remazol B 133%	3/4	Disazo	2 vinylsulfone
Unknown	Yellow Remazol RR	4	Unknown	Unknown
Unknown	Orange Remazol RR	4	Unknown	Unknown
Unknown	Red Remazol RR	4	Unknown	Unknown
Unknown	Blue Remazol RR	4	Unknown	Unknown
R.Y. 217	Yellow Avitera SE	5/6	Unknown	3 reactive groups
R.R. 286	Red Avitera SE	4	Unknown	3 reactive groups
R.Bl. 281	Deep blue Avitera SE	4	Unknown	3 reactive groups
Unknown	Blue Farbofix SP-BRF 150%	4/5	Unknown	Unknown
Unknown	Navy Farbofix SP-BRK/N	3/4	Unknown	Unknown
R.Bl. 225	Navy Levafix E-BNA	2/3	Unknown	Unknown
Unknown	Blue br. Neareafix AC-BRF 150%	5	Unknown	Unknown

Table 5. Light fastness, structure, and groups of commercial dyes experimented.

Table 5 shows light fastness and structure types of the investigated reactive dyes (data derived from color charts of the producers).

Table 6 shows the measured color differences between UV-irradiated and untreated cotton yarns of the dyeings carried out with 0.5% Levafix dyes, while **Table 7** reports those obtained with 0.5% Remazol dyes (in both tables $\Delta E > 5$ are evidenced in bold).

Dye	ΔL	Δa	Δb	ΔE
Levafix Yellow CA	−0.65	−0.36	−3.94	4.01
Levafix Amber CA	2.09	−3.27	−4.98	**6.31**
Levafix Scarlet CA	4.02	−3.80	−1.12	**5.64**
Levafix Red CA	4.37	−5.21	3.15	**7.49**
Levafix Rubin CA	3.05	−4.66	0.42	**5.58**
Levafix Blue CA	1.77	−0.42	4.69	**5.03**
Levafix Navy CA	4.47	2.61	4.35	**6.76**

Table 6. Color difference parameters for 0.5% dyeings with Levafix dyes.

Dye	ΔL	Δa	Δb	ΔE
Remazol Yellow br. 4GL	−1.05	0.99	−1.33	1.96
Remazol Yellow RR	−0.17	−0.10	−0.53	0.56
Remazol Orange RR	3.05	−5.94	−5.63	**8.93**
Remazol Red RB 133%	4.65	−11.50	3.69	**12.90**
Remazol Red RR	9.62	−13.17	4.10	**16.80**
Remazol Red 3BS 150%	3.39	−7.62	2.33	**8.66**
Remazol Blue RR	6.50	2.40	5.21	**8.67**
Remazol Navy GG 133%	2.77	3.90	2.83	**5.56**
Remazol Black B 133%	4.58	2.76	4.76	**7.16**

Table 7. Color difference parameters for 0.5% dyeings with Remazol dyes.

Specifically, it was noted that the chromogens more difficult to fade under UV radiations are those providing yellow shades, typically made up of pyrazolone. Only the amber tone (Levafix) is interesting as a yellow, but it is an orange yellow; the fading ability increases going from orange shades (azo) toward red (azo), while in the case of shades provided by diazo dyes the fading ability increases going from navy until the maximum value in the case of Remazol Blue RR, as demonstrated in **Table 7** (Remazol dyeings).

A selection of dyes sensitive toward UV-generated fade was thus performed offering a combination of the six terms reported in **Table 8**.

Dye	ΔE
Levafix Amber CA	**6.31**
Remazol Orange RR	**8.93**
Remazol Red RB 133%	**12.90**
Remazol Navy GG 133%	**5.56**
Remazol Black B 133%	**7.16**
Remazol Blue RR	**8.67**

Table 8. Total color difference (Δ*E*) for 0.5% selected dyeings.

It is possible to observe, as reported in **Tables 6** and **7**, that the total color difference (Δ*E*) is due not only by an achromatic fading (ΔL) but also results from a variation of chromatic parameters (Δ*a* and Δ*b*), because a tone change after UV exposure occurs.

The selection shown in **Figure 3** has characteristics of good mutual combinability and synchronism in dye exhaustion, together with a color difference higher than 5.0 units of Δ*E*.

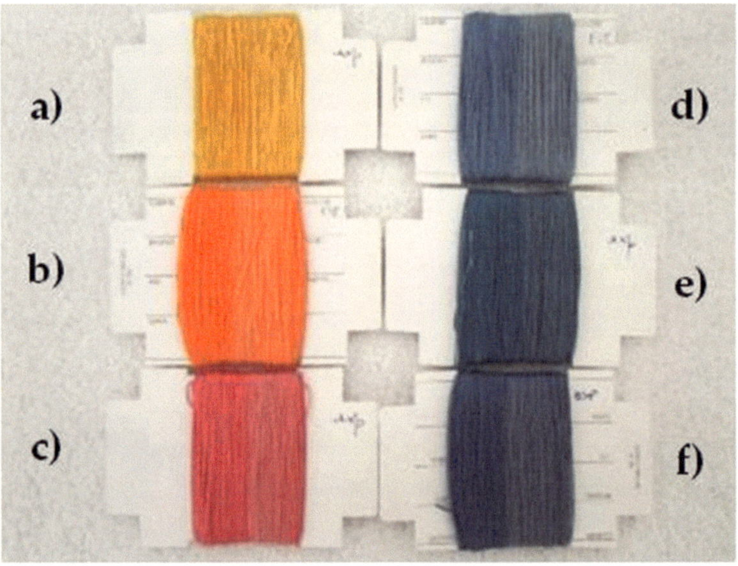

Figure 3. Dyeings with 0.5% selected dyes: (a) Levafix Amber CA, (b) Remazol Orange RR, (c) Remazol Red RB 133%, (d) Remazol Navy GG 133%, (e) Remazol Black B 133%, (f) Remazol Blue RR (for each shade: untreated yarn on the left side, UV faded on the right side).

In conclusion, on cotton fibers, unlike wool, a UV pretreatment does not substantially change the dyeing affinity, but a UV posttreatment is capable to fade dyeing, allowing to obtain interesting differential chromatic effects.

http://dx.doi.org/10.5772/63796

3. Surface modification of cotton fabrics by UV curing and UV grafting

Cotton fabrics often find its application in producing home furnishing, such as table linen, clothing, or work wear with high hygienic requirements. The high concentration of hydroxyl groups on cotton fabric surface makes the fabrics water adsorbent and easily stained by liquids. Moreover, the chemical composition and morphological properties of cellulosic fibers provide an excellent medium for bacterial growth. To overcome these limits, a finishing treatment is required on cotton fabrics to confer oil and/or water repellency and antibacterial activity.

Usually, the desired properties are achieved by thermal polymerization, regardless of energy consumption and costs of the process [25]. Fluorinated or silicone monomers, applied to the fabrics by padding, can confer oil and water repellency, while Triclosan, quaternary ammonium salts, and silver ions [26] are commonly used as antibacterial agents [27].

Ferrero et al. [3] proposed the UV curing as eco-friendly and cheap alternative to thermal curing of functional monomers onto cotton fibers. In UV-curing processes, a suitable photoinitiator is able to interact with UV radiations yielding radical or cationic species, which induce a rapid curing of reactive monomers and oligomers at low temperature, with lower environmental impact and lower cost than thermal process.

For textile applications on cotton fabrics, if a mixture of monomer and initiator is absorbed by the fibers and subsequently UV-irradiated, the polymeric chains can form inside the textile structure, establishing also graft bonds (UV grafting) with the cellulose macromolecules and making the treatment solid and water resistant. Moreover, the interpenetration of components and homogeneous distribution of monomers, even at a low concentration, contribute to obtain textile materials with modified surface properties without high add-on of polymer. In this way, the bulk properties of the fibers, such as mechanical and thermal resistance, are not affected and also the fabric breathability can be kept unvaried.

3.1. Water- and oil-repellent finishing of cotton fabrics by UV radiation

Water and oil repellency are among the most common functional properties that need to be assessed for protective clothing. This property can be conferred by the modification of the surface energy of textile fibers, possibly confined to a thin surface layer, so that the bulk properties of the textile fabric such as mechanical strength, flexibility, breathability, and softness should remain uncompromised.

Hydrophobic or oleophobic surfaces are difficult to wet by water or apolar liquids, respectively, and are called low-energy surfaces. Wetting primarily comes from the non-ideality of solid substrates that are both rough and chemically heterogeneous. The surface modification of textile fibers to confer these properties can be achieved by physical or chemical methods or by the combination of both. Plasma treatments and exposure to radiations, often accomplished in the presence of reactive gases or after impregnation with suitable chemicals, are mainly representative of physical methods, while chemical treatments can generally be carried out with oxidants or other finishing agents, followed by thermal treatment or by sol-gel techniques.

Polysiloxanes are widely used for textile finishing to impart desirable properties such as softness, crease resistance, and water repellency, depending on the nature of organic functional groups incorporated in the polymer structure. The application of a polymeric coating to a cotton fabric in the form of a thin film ensures waterproof properties, but the fabric could lose comfort characteristics, such as handling and breathability. Therefore, hydrorepellency obtained by homogeneous adsorption of monomers onto each fiber and followed by a radiation curing method should be preferred. This was proposed by Ferrero et al. [3], which obtained water-repellent cotton fabrics by radical UV curing of silicone and urethane acrylates. The values of contact angle (**Table 9**), wettability, and moisture adsorption showed that a low resin add-on on the fabric is enough to confer water repellency, while scanning electron microscopy (SEM) analysis confirmed that UV curing yields a coating layer onto each single fiber than a film on the fabric surface (**Figure 4**) without damage of breathability.

Resin	Chemical nature	Weight on cotton (%)	Contact angle (°)
Coatosil 3503	Silicone (medium) acrylate	1.3	143
Coatosil 3509	Silicone (high) acrylate	2.9	114
Tego Rad 2600	Polysiloxane epoxy	2.6	100
Ucecoat 7849	Urethane acrylate (MW = 10,000)	2	100

Table 9. Hydrorepellent finishing of cotton fabrics by radical UV curing of silicone and urethane acrylates.

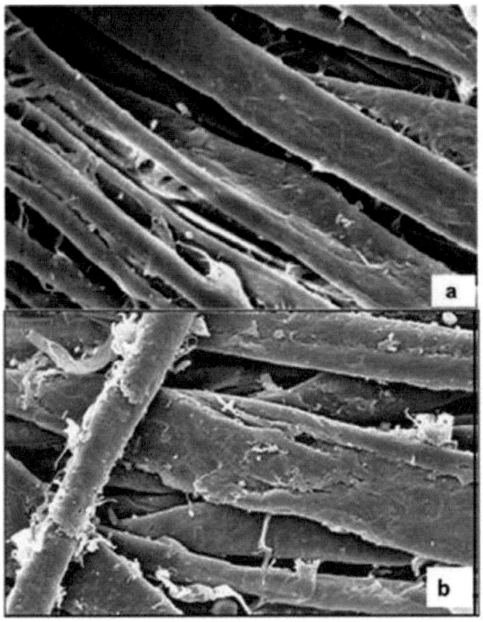

Figure 4. SEM images of cotton fibers untreated (a) and treated by radical UV curing of a silicone acrylate resin 3% add-on (b).

http://dx.doi.org/10.5772/63796

Periolatto et al. [28] recently investigated the application by UV grafting of polyhedral oligomeric silsesquioxanes (POSSs) and a polysilazane (KION 20) to cotton fabrics to confer hydrorepellency.

POSSs are polyhedral clusters yielded by hydrolytic condensation of trifunctional silanes. The generic formula is $(RSiO_{1.5})_n$, where each silicon atom is bound on average to one and a half oxygen atoms and to one hydrocarbon group. The single nanoparticle may be represented as a silica cage core (diameters in the range of 1–3 nm) bearing organic functional groups attached to the corners of the cage (**Figure 5a**).

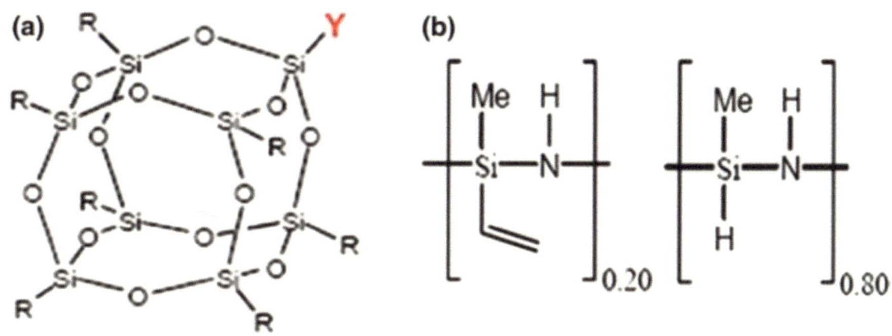

Figure 5. Molecular structures of polyhedral oligomeric silsesquioxanes (POSSs), where R = i-butyl, Y = methacryloisobutyl functional groups (a) and KION 20 structural units (b).

KION polysilazane contains repeating units in which silicon and nitrogen atoms are bonded in an alternating sequence. Both of these units contain cyclic and linear features. In addition, KION 20 contains fewer low-molecular-weight polysilazane components (**Figure 5b**).

For what concerns the hydrorepellency, it was clearly conferred by the treatment, as confirmed by water contact angles measured on the as-prepared samples higher than 90°, for both POSS- and KION-treated samples. Measurements on aged samples revealed that KION-treated samples could maintain better properties during time, with respect to POSS treated. Moreover, for these two oligomers, higher contact angles were measured on samples treated with solutions at higher concentration. In particular, samples treated with 1- and 5-g/L POSS solutions, although showing an initial water contact angle higher than 100°, after aging immediately absorb the water drop, denouncing the total loss of hydrorepellency.

Many research papers have been published on the production and application of different types of fluorochemicals to textile finishing [29]. Fluorochemicals are organic compounds consisting of perfluorinated carbon chains, which impart water and oil repellency to the fiber surface when incorporated into polymer backbone with perfluoro groups as side chains. The old fluorochemicals used were based on C8 carbon chains, which release highly hazardous and toxic substances, such as perfluoro-octanoic acid and perfluoro-octanesulfonates. Nowadays, C6 fluorochemicals are still in use although the rules on this topic became more stringent, banding also C6 fluorochemicals, so studies about the performance conferred by C2–C3 products are of great interest [30].

Fluorochemical finishings are commercially available as water emulsions and are applied to fabrics by the pad-dry-cure method, with a thermal-curing step at 150–175°C in hot flue for some minutes. As alternative, Ferrero et al. [2, 6] proposed the UV curing of perfluoro-alkyl-polyacrylate resins (Repellan EPF and NFC by Pulcra Chemicals and Oleophobol CP-C by Huntsman), in water emulsions, able to impart water as well as oil repellency to cotton fabrics, and the results were compared with those obtained by thermal polymerization. A radical photoinitiator was added in the proper amount, then the solution was diluted with water, mixed, and applied by dipping or spraying onto strips of fabric that were dried in an oven. Final weight add-ons of 3 and 5% o.w.f. were usually applied in order to obtain the desired properties without loss of fabric handling. Then, the samples were UV radiated on both sides by a medium pressure mercury lamp (about 60 mW/cm^2) under inert atmosphere for 30–60 s. Thermally cured fabrics were considered as reference, treated for 2–3 min at 140 or 150°C according to the indications of the producer.

			Contact angle (°)					
			Before washing			After washing		
Resin	Add-on (%)	Curing type	θA	θR	Δθ	θA	θR	Δθ
Repellan EPF	3	Thermal	134	126	8	142	136	6
	3	UV	138	129	9	134	131	3
	5	Thermal	145	133	12	143	140	3
	5	UV	142	134	8	138	134	4
Repellan NFC	3	Thermal	140	130	10	139	122	17
	3	UV	140	132	8	137	123	14
	5	Thermal	136	125	9	134	124	10
	5	UV	133	126	7	131	119	12

Table 10. Dynamic water contact angles (average of repeated measurements, standard deviation about 4°, θA = advancing, θR = receding, Δθ = hysteresis) before and after washing on cotton fabrics cured with Repellan EPF and NFC.

The effectiveness of the UV treatment was evaluated by the determination of weight loss in chloroform. Repellan EPF showed the highest yields after UV curing, quite similar to those reached with the thermal treatment (93–96%), whereas Repellan NFC showed lower, although acceptable, yields in UV curing (80–81%) than in the thermal one (98%), without the influence of irradiation time and polymer add-on. However, with Oleophobol CP-C lower yields were obtained in both finishing treatments, and longer UV irradiation time, at least 60 s, is necessary to achieve a yield of 91% with a 3% add-on. Measurements of dynamic contact angles of water

http://dx.doi.org/10.5772/63796

and oil drops allowed comparing the repellent behavior of the cotton fabrics finished with both curing methods before and after five domestic washing cycles (**Table 10**). A hysteresis $\Delta\theta > 0$ is typical of most real surfaces, as confirmed by all the results obtained. The good wash fastness of water repellency was proved by the slight reduction of the advancing contact angles after washing, regardless of the curing type and polymer add-on. Oleophobol (data not reported) gave slightly lower contact angles but was practically unaffected by repeated washings.

In conclusion, the laboratory-scale application of the hydro- and oil-repellent finishing on textile fabrics by UV curing of silica based or fluorocarbon resins, with the optimization of process parameters, followed by a deep characterization of treated samples, confirmed the effectiveness of the treatment.

The study of Ferrero and Periolatto went on with the semi-industrial scale-up of the process: a great number (about 80) of larger fabric samples were padded by foulard with Oleophobol and then were irradiated in air by Sun-Wash®, an apparatus for continuous treatment of fabrics by UV light providing an irradiance of 913 mW/cm^2 on an exposed area of about 120 × 60 cm^2. Samples were exposed to the radiation with a carpet speed of 5 m/min, by five passes, corresponding to an irradiation time of 35 s, on both sides [31]. Fabric add-on was significantly reduced in order to hold down the finishing cost. White and dyed samples of different textile composition were treated and evaluated in terms of conferred repellency, yellowing, or color changes. Most relevant process parameters were investigated, considering the thermal process normally adopted at industrial level as reference. Results were so statistically evaluated by Six Sigma method with Minitab 16 software, to point out the most influencing parameters and the real possibility to replace the thermal treatment with UV. Water and oil drop sorption times higher than 2 h were found on all treated samples, showing that Oleophobol works very well as oil- and water-repellent agent for textiles.

UV process was revealed to work better than thermal one, in fact higher water and oil contact angles were obtained with a lower amount (1% o.w.f.) of finishing agent. Considering the UV process, best results were related to white fabrics, rather than dyed, and medium values of both radiation dose and product concentration, taking into account both contact angles and color reflectance evaluations. Finally, contact angle measurements carried out on aged samples (2 years) showed no variations with respect to fresh samples, meaning that the finishing is not affected by aging. Obtained results were considered encouraging and can open the way for a real application of the UV process to industrial field.

3.2. Antimicrobial finishing by chitosan UV grafting

The textile manufacturing industry is going through a period of severe crisis due to the globalization of the world market. A highly competitive context and stringent ecological regulations make quality and eco-friendly processes the major demands for a company.

A first objective aims to lower water and energy consumption; another relevant factor is the possibility of replacing high-polluting or toxic chemicals with others characterized by lower or zero environmental impact. From this point of view, the products of green chemistry, of natural origin, are particularly interesting for applications in the field of textile finishing.

Increased attention toward health and hygiene, due to frequent diseases and invasive infections, brought the attention of the research in textile field on antibacterial materials, which can not only prevent degradation and discoloration of the fabrics by microorganisms but also effectively prevent the spread of pathogenic bacteria. An antibacterial finishing, by means of a suitable surface chemical modification of fibers, is mainly required on natural fibers for furnishing, technical textiles, medical devices, hygienic textiles, food industry, and packaging. Chemicals bearing functional biocide groups are usually applied by padding, followed by a thermal treatment. Unfortunately, most of these products are toxic or carcinogenic, so the application to textiles is not advisable, also considering a possible release of the antibacterial agent during the use, in skin contact.

For these reasons, a strong chemical grafting to treated fibers is mandatory for a fast, stable, and resistant treatment. However, the finishing should not compromise the hand, appearance, and color of the fabric, considering that finishing processes are normally carried out after dyeing. In this view, the application of natural biopolymers by an eco-friendly and cheap process can be the winning choice to develop bioactive eco-sustainable textiles from renewable sources [32].

Cellulose and chitin, the main components of cotton fibers and crustacean shells, respectively, are the two most abundant polysaccharides in nature. They are mutually compatible, due to their similar structure (**Figure 6**), and biodegradable; it makes them good candidates as eco-friendly and eco-sustainable substrates for textile applications. Chitosan (2-amino-2-deoxy-(1–4)-β-D-glucopyranan) is a carbohydrate biopolymer derived from the deacetylation of the chitin with unique biological, physiological, and pharmacological properties, such as biodegradability, no toxicity, and high antibacterial activity toward both Gram-positive and Gram-negative microorganisms, due to the combined bacteriostatic and bactericide action.

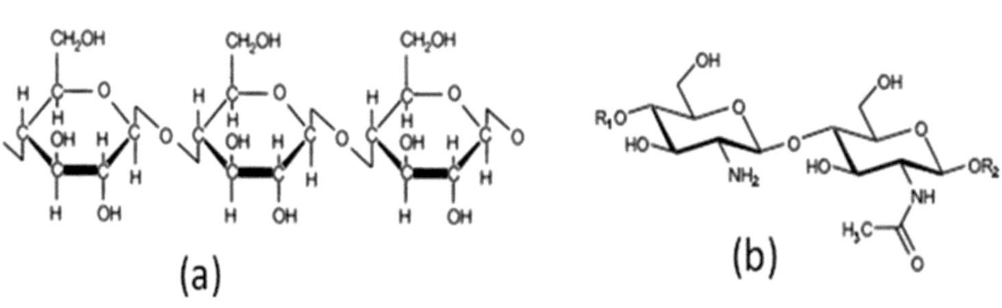

Figure 6. Molecular structures of cellulose (a) and chitosan (b).

In textile field, chitosan is mainly used as a dyeing auxiliary or a finishing agent, but the finishing fastness is limited by the weak interactions between chitosan macromolecules and fibers. To obtain a stable treatment, a thermal wet process is required, with high energy, water consumption, and possible degradation of the treated substrate. Moreover, the addition of cross-linking agents is required. Usually, toxic chemicals bearing aldehyde groups are used in thermal processes; recently, genipin was proposed as natural, nontoxic alternative: encouraging results in terms of fastness improvement were obtained, opening the way for biomedical and pharmaceutical applications [33], but the prohibitive cost of genipin makes it not applicable in textile field.

Ferrero and Periolatto [34] proposed photocuring (UV curing and/or UV grafting) as cheap and eco-friendly process to bind chitosan to textiles by means of radical reactions. Studies about the photodegradation of chitosan macromolecules due to UV exposure confirmed the formation of macroradicals on the polymer. Same radicals can be involved in cross-linking process, promoted by the presence of a suitable radical photoinitiator. Among the substrates considered, there are wool [35], silk [36], polyester, polyamide, and cotton fiber [37], in the form of weft-warp and knitted piquet fabrics [38] but also filter substrates and gauzes with more open structures [39–41].

Focusing on cotton, the research work started with laboratory test on samples of small dimensions, aimed to optimize the process parameters and confirm the treatment efficiency and fastness [36]. A low-viscosity chitosan with deacetylation degree of 75–85% was dissolved in acetic acid solution at pH 4. The solution was added of 2-hydroxy-2-methyl-phenyl-propane-1-one, 4% wt on chitosan, as radical photoinitiator, properly diluted and applied to the fabric surface by dipping, to reach a chitosan add-on ranging from 1 to 3% wt. An impregnation time of 12 h at 25°C or 1 h at 50°C was necessary to obtain 100% process yield.

Chitosan UV curing yielded high antimicrobial properties, against *Escherichia coli* and *Staphylococcus aureus*, on cotton fabrics. The test was carried out according to ASTM E 2149-01 standard test. A microorganism reduction higher than 97% was found on all treated samples, regardless of the application method for chitosan. Moreover, about 2% polymer add-on was enough to confer a strong antibacterial activity to the fabrics without endangerment of hand and breathability. An impregnation time of 12 h at ambient temperature was necessary so that treated fabrics maintained about one half of their own antimicrobial activity after washing with standard ECE detergent, according to UNI-EN ISO 105 C01 standard test, while at lower impregnation time, the antimicrobial activity was more reduced. This was attributed to a not-enough penetration of chitosan inside the fiber structure, due even to the high viscosity of the solution. A prolonged contact time between chitosan solution and fabrics improved this penetration and chitosan could graft to the fibers, showing increased washing fastness. However, this was strongly dependent on the ionic nature of the detergents, and a nonionic surfactant could assure that an antimicrobial activity completely retained after repeated washings.

Semi-industrial scaled tests were carried out on samples of higher dimension, using commercial chitosan powder (Peripret or Chitoclear) dissolved in acetic acid solution [38]. In some cases, a softener (Nearfinish SM/40) or an antioxidant agent (Nearcand) was added to the recipe, while the radical photoinitiator was kept in the same amount. The chitosan add-on was drastically lowered till 0.3% o.w.f, diluting the solution to 0.25% before the impregnation by padding. The as-impregnated samples were dried in a rameuse and finally radiated by Sun-Wash®, as reported in Section 3.1. Results of antibacterial activity tests are reported in **Table 11** and confirmed those previously obtained with samples prepared at laboratory scale.

Sample description	Condition	Microorganism reduction (%)
Untreated		–
Ultrafresh GH-20 2%	Initial	>99.9
	10 washes	>99.9
	30 washes	98.4
Chitosan finishing: 3% Peripret	Initial	>99.9
Wet irradiation	10 washes	>99.9
	30 washes	>99.9
Chitosan finishing 3% Peripret	Initial	>99.9
Dry irradiation	10 washes	>99.9
	30 washes	>99.9
Chitosan finishing: 3% Peripret	Initial	>99.9
With Nearfinish SM/40	10 washes	>99.9
Dry irradiation	30 washes	>99.9
Chitosan finishing: 0.3% Chitoclear	Initial	98.6
Wet irradiation	10 washes	>99.9
	30 washes	>99.9
Chitosan finishing: 0.6% Chitoclear	Initial	99
Wet irradiation	10 washes	>99.9
	30 washes	>99.9
Chitosan finishing: 0.6% Chitoclear	Initial	99.2
With Nearcand	10 washes	>99.9
Wet irradiation	30 washes	>99.9

Table 11. Antibacterial activity of chitosan-treated samples as prepared and after 10 and 30 washing cycles. Quantitative assessment of activity according to ISO 20743: 2007 (E) against *Staphylococcus aureus*.

"Chitosan conferred a strong antibacterial activity, with the total reduction of the microorganism colonies on all the tested samples. Moreover, chitosan treated samples showed optimum washing fastness, maintaining their antibacterial activity unvaried even after 30 washes" [38]. Comparing the results with those related to Ultra-Fresh, a commercial sanitizing agent considered as reference, the performances are similar or even better for chitosan-treated samples after 30 washes. Obtained results are of particular interest considering that the UV exposure was carried out in the presence of oxygen, even on wet samples. *"These are generally considered unfavorable conditions for radical reactions occurring or for photoinitiator effectiveness. Moreover, the strong antibacterial activity and washing fastness were obtained on all treated samples regardless the add-on or the presence of additives* [38]."

"Results obtained with the lowest amount of chitosan on fibers is particularly interesting because makes chitosan competitive with other antibacterial agents commonly used, such as Triclosan, silver ions or quaternary ammonium salts, even from an economical point of view" [38]. The homogeneous distribution of chitosan on fabrics, in particular in correspondence to the sample that presented the best fastness, was confirmed by dyeing tests with an acid dye (**Figure 7**) and by SEM analysis (**Figure 8**) that showed the optimal distribution of the finish on a single fiber surface.

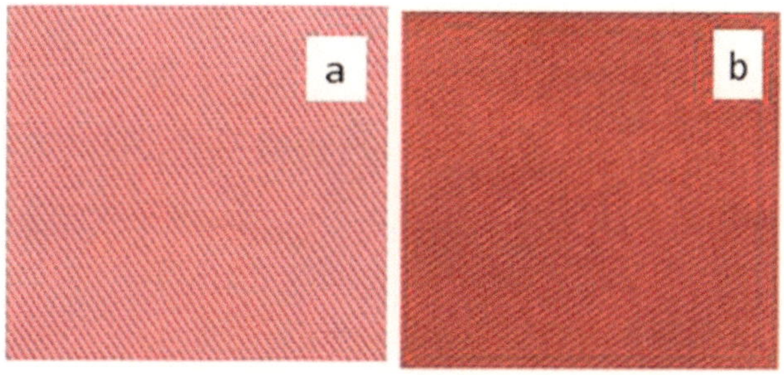

Figure 7. Dyeing test with Direct Red 81: untreated cotton fabric (a), treated with 0.6% wt. chitosan (Peripret CTS) (b).

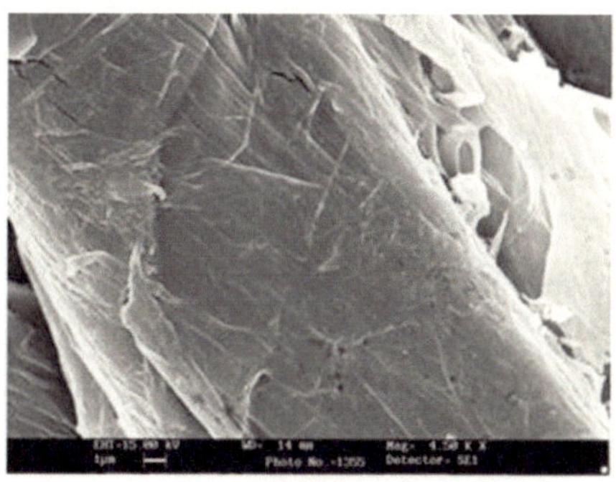

Figure 8. SEM analysis on cotton fabric treated with 3% wt. chitosan (4500×).

4. Conclusion

The UV treatments on cotton fibers can be utilized in dyeing and finishing processes. UV irradiation coupled with mild oxidation can improve some properties of the cotton fibers such as pilling resistance, water swelling, and dyeability. However, significant effects of differential dyeing were obtained by a UV posttreatment capable to fade dyeings with reactive dyes. UV curing and UV grafting with suitable chemical enabled to modify the surface of cotton fibers in order to confer oil and/or water repellency with an eco-friendly and cheap alternative to chemical and thermal finishing treatments. Moreover, the chitosan UV grafting was proposed as valid environmental friendly method to obtain cotton fabrics with a satisfactory washing-resistant antimicrobial activity even with low polymer add-on.

Author details

Franco Ferrero[1*], Gianluca Migliavacca[1] and Monica Periolatto[2]

*Address all correspondence to: franco.ferrero@polito.it

1 Department of Applied Science and Technology, Polytechnic of Turin, Torino, Italy

2 Faculty of Science and Technology, Free University of Bozen, Bolzano, Italy

References

[1] Bhatti IA, Adeel S, Abbas M. Effect of radiation in textile dyeing. In: Hauser P (ed.) Textile Dyeing. Rijeka: InTech; 2011. p. 1–17. Available from: http://www.intechopen.com/books/textile-dyeing/effect-of-radiation-on-textile-dyeing [Accessed: 2016-03-25].

[2] Ferrero F, Periolatto M. Ultraviolet curing for surface modification of textile fabrics. Journal of Nanoscience and Nanotechnology 2011; 11:8663–8669. DOI: 10.1166/jnn.2011.3447

[3] Ferrero F, Periolatto M, Sangermano M, Bianchetto Songia M. Water-repellent finishing of cotton fabrics by ultraviolet curing. Journal of Applied Polymer Science 2008; 107:810–818. DOI: 10.1002/app.27110

[4] Ferrero F, Periolatto M, Bianchetto Songia M. Silk grafting with methacrylic and epoxy monomers: thermal process in comparison with ultraviolet curing. Journal of Applied Polymer Science 2008; 110:1019–1027. DOI: 10.1002/app.28684

[5] Chen W-H, Chen P-C, Wang S-C, Yeh J-T, Huang C-Y, Chen K-N. UV-curable PDMS-containing PU system for hydrophobic textile surface treatment. Journal of Polymer Research 2009; 16:601–610. DOI: 10.1007/s10965-008-9265-4

[6] Ferrero F, Periolatto M, Udrescu C. Water and oil-repellent coatings of perfluoro-polyacrylate resins on cotton fibers: UV curing in comparison with thermal polymerization. Fibers and Polymers 2012; 13:191–198. DOI: 10.1007/s12221-012-0191-z

[7] Bhatti IA, Zia KM, Ali Z, Zuber M, Rehman F-u. Modification of cellulosic fibers to enhance their dyeability using UV-irradiation. Carbohydrate Polymers 2012; 89:783–787. DOI: 10.1016/j.carbpol.2012.04.010

[8] Mansuri AH., Khoddami A, Rezaei Do A. Using ultraviolet radiation for the bleaching and pilling reduction of knitted cotton fabric. Fibres & Textiles in Eastern Europe 2011; 19: 74–77.

[9] Millington K. Using ultraviolet radiation to reduce pilling of knitted wool and cotton. Textile Research Journal 1998; 68:413–421. DOI: 10.1177/004051759806800605

[10] Zuber M, Zia KM., Bhatti IA, Ali Z, Arshad MU, Saif MJ. Modification of cellulosic fibers by UV-irradiation. Part II: After treatments effects. International Journal of Biological Macromolecules 2012; 51:743–748. DOI: 10.1016/j.iibiomac. 2012.07.001

[11] Bhatti IA, Adeel S, Siddique S, Abbas M. Effect of UV radiation on the dyeing of cotton fabric with reactive blue 13. Journal of Saudi Chemical Society 2014; 18:606–609. DOI: 10.1016/j.jscs.2012.11.06

[12] Bhatti IA, Adeel S, Parveen S, Zuber M. Dyeing of UV irradiated cotton and polyester fabrics with multifunctional reactive and disperse dyes. Journal of Saudi Chemical Society 2013, DOI: 10.1016/j.jscs.2012.12.014

[13] Iqbal J, Bhatti IA, Adeel S. Effect of UV radiation on dyeing of cotton fabric with extracts of henna leaves. Indian Journal of Fibre & Textile Research 2008;33:157–162.

[14] Adeel S, Bhatti IA, Kausar A, Osman E. Influence of UV radiations on the extraction and dyeing of cotton fabric with *Curcuma longa* L. Indian Journal of Fibre & Textile Research 2012; 37:87–90.

[15] Shin H, Ueda M, Burkinshaw SM. New methods of obtaining patterned dyeings on cellulosic fibres with anionic dyes: photo-modification using a methacryloyl quaternary ammonium compound. Dyes and Pigments 1999; 41:11–17. DOI: 10.1016/S0143-7208(98)00039-4

[16] Jang, J, Ko, SW., Carr, CM. Investigation of the improved dyeability of cationised cotton via photografting with UV active cationic monomers. Coloration Technology 2001;117:139–146. DOI: 10.1111/j.1478-4408.2001.tb00052.x

[17] Bertoniere NR, King WD. Pore structure and dyeability of cotton crosslinked with DMDHEU and with DHDMI. Textile Research Journal 1989; 59:609–615. DOI: 10.1177/004051759206200607

[18] Dong Y, Jang J. Environmentally friendly coloration of cotton by the UV-induced photografting of α-bromoacrylamido dyes. Coloration Technology 2014;130:296–304. DOI: 10.1111/cote.12094

[19] Ratnapandian S, Wang L, Ferguson SM, Naebe M. Effect of Atmospheric Plasma Treatment on Pad-dyeing of Natural Dyes on Wool. Journal of Fiber Bioengineering and Informatics 2011;4:267–276. DOI: 10.3993/jfbi09201106

[20] Millington KR. Potential applications of UV surface treatments in the textile industry. In: Proceedings of RadTech'98 North America UV/EB Conference; 19–22 April 1998; Chicago, IL, p. 601–609.

[21] Sala EE, Camera Magni E, Camera Magni R. Process for treating yarns, fabrics or textile articles of natural and artificial protein or cellulosic fibers and blends thereof with synthetic fibers. Patent WO 2008061947 A1. Stamperia Emiliana srl/Nearchimica SpA, Italy; 2008.

[22] Migliavacca G, Ferrero F, Periolatto M. Differential dyeing of wool fabric with metal-complex dyes after ultraviolet irradiation. Coloration Technology 2014;130:327–333. DOI: 10.1111/cote.12107

[23] Migliavacca G. Applications of ultraviolet radiations in dyeing processes of yarn and fabrics [PhD thesis]. Torino: Politecnico, Italy; 2014.

[24] Batchelor SN, Carr D, Coleman CE, Fairclough L, Jarvis A. The photofading mechanism of commercial reactive dyes on cotton. Dyes and Pigments 2003;59:269–275. DOI: 10.1016/S0143-7208(03)00118-9

[25] Hasanbeigi A, Price L. A technical review of emerging technologies for energy and water efficiency and pollution reduction in the textile industry. Journal of Cleaner Production 2015;95:30–44. DOI: 10.1016/j.jclepro.2015.02.079

[26] Simončič B, Klemenčič D. Preparation and performance of silver as an antimicrobial agent for textiles: a review. Textile Research Journal 2016;86:210–223. DOI: 10.1177/0040517515586157

[27] Shahid-ul-Islam, Faqeer M. High-energy radiation induced sustainable coloration and functional finishing of textile materials. Industrial Engineering Chemistry Research 2015;54:3727–3745. DOI: 10.1021/acs.iecr.5b00524

[28] Periolatto M, Basit A, Ferri A, Bongiovanni R. Wettability and comfort of cellulosic materials modified by photo grafting of non-fluorinated oligomers. Cellulose 2016;23:1447–1458. DOI: 10.1007/s10570-016-0863-8

[29] Chao-Hua X, Shun-Tian J, Jing Z, Jian-Zhong M. Large-area fabrication of superhydrophobic surfaces for practical applications: an overview. Science and Technology of Advanced Materials 2010;11:3, 033002. DOI: 10.1088/1468-6996/11/3/033002

[30] Yang Y, Shen J, Zhang L, Li X. Preparation of a novel water and oil repellent fabric finishing agent containing a short perfluoroalkyl chain and its application in textiles. Materials Research Innovations 2015;19 (sup 8):S8-401–S8-404. DOI: 10.1179/1432891715Z.0000000001708

[31] Periolatto M, Ferrero F, Tempestini L. Hydro and oil repellent finishing of textiles by UV-curing: influence of scaled-up process parameters. In: Book of Abstracts of 9th International Conference on Surfaces, Coatings and NanoStructured Materials (NANOSMAT 2014); 8–11 September 2014; Dublin, p. 170.

[32] Nabil AI, Basma ME. Potential applications of sustainable polymers in functionalization of cellulosic textile materials. In: Thakhur VK, editor. Handbook of Sustainable Polymers: Processing and Applications. Boca Raton, FL: CRC Press; 2016, p. 215–262.

[33] Muzzarelli RAA., El Mehtedi M , Bottegoni C, Aquili A, Gigante A. Genipin-crosslinked chitosan gels and scaffolds for tissue engineering and regeneration of cartilage and bone. Marine Drugs 2015;13:7314–7338. DOI: 10.3390/md13127068

[34] Ferrero F, Periolatto M. Ultraviolet curing for surface modification of textile fabrics. Journal of Nanoscience and Nanotechnology, 2011;11:8663-8669. DOI: 10.1166/jnn.2011.3447

[35] Periolatto M, Ferrero F, Vineis C, Rombaldoni F. Multifunctional finishing of wool fabrics by chitosan UV-grafting: an approach. Carbohydrate Polymers, 2013; 98:624–629. DOI: 10.1016/j.carbpol.2013.06.054

[36] Periolatto M, Ferrero F, Vineis C. Antimicrobial chitosan finish of cotton and silk fabrics by UV curing with 2-hydroxy-2-methylphenylpropane-1-one. Carbohydrate Polymers 2012;88:201–205. DOI: 10.1016/j.carbpol.2011.11.093

[37] Ferrero F, Periolatto M. Antimicrobial finish of textiles by chitosan UV curing. Journal of Nanoscience and Nanotechnology, 2012;12:4803–4810. DOI: 101166/jnn.2012.4902

[38] Ferrero F, Periolatto M, Ferrario S. Sustainable antimicrobial finishing of cotton fabrics by chitosan UV-grafting: from laboratory experiments to semi industrial scale-up. Journal of Cleaner Production 2015;96:244–252. DOI: 10.1016/j.jclepro.2013.12.044

[39] Ferrero F, Tonetti C, Periolatto M. Adsorption of chromate and cupric ions onto chitosan-coated cotton gauze. Carbohydrate Polymers 2014;110:367–373. DOI: 10.101016/j.carbpol.2014.04.016

[40] Ferrero F, Periolatto M, Vineis C, Varesano A. Chitosan coated cotton gauze for antibacterial water filtration. Carbohydrate Polymers, 2014;103:207–212. DOI: 10.1016/j.carbpol.2013.12.037

[41] Periolatto M, Ferrero F. Cotton filter fabrics functionalization by chitosan UV-grafting for removal of dyes. Chemical Engineering Transactions, 2013;32:85–90. DOI: 10.3303/CET1332015

Chapter 12

Glandless Cottonseed Protein for Environmentally Friendly Bioplastics

Hangbo Yue, Guoqiang Yin and Yingde Cui

Additional information is available at the end of the chapter

http://dx.doi.org/10.5772/64045

Abstract

Environmentally friendly bioplastics have attracted renewed attention over the last few decades due to the ever-growing awareness of the environmental impact of petroleum-based polymers and the rising costs of raw materials. Cottonseed protein (CP) extracted from cottonseed meal has abundant amino acid components and nutrition value, but are not carefully considered in non-feed industries. For the purpose of being explored, glandless cottonseed flour is utilized in this work, as a raw material, to prepare cottonseed protein bioplastics (CPBs) as environmentally friendly products. The optimum synthesis conditions of CPBs were firstly investigated, followed by the analysis of protein modification and cross-linking mechanism, with a close view on changes of their micro- or chemical structures. Detailed morphologies, element composition and biodegradabilities of CPBs were characterized via scanning electron microscopy, energy dispersive spectroscopy (EDS) and soil-burial test, respectively, pointing out its structural heterogeneity as well as nature of biodegradability. Characterizations of the thermal stability and thermomechanical relaxation of thermal-treated CPBs and its interaction with molecule revealed the presence of different thermal relaxation behaviours and different water states. Concluding remarks shortly summarize the importance of the work and point out possible solutions to addressing future potential challenges.

Keywords: biodegradability, bioplastics, cottonseed protein, synthesis, water states

1. Introduction

The soaring consumption of organically synthesized polymers in agriculture and a wide variety of industries around the globe poses a great threat to our living environment, mainly because of the non-biodegradability of such polymers. The increased awareness of environmental impact of using petroleum-derived polymers and the rising costs of chemical raw materials shift people's attention to seeking out environmentally friendly polymers for sustainable development. In the course of this searching over the last few decades across the world, protein-based bioplastics (PBBs) have attracted renewed attention due to the following reasons: they can be completely degraded through regular composting, readily obtained from abundant natural resources (i.e. plant and animal proteins such as soy, corn zein, wheat gluten, sunflower, peanut, cottonseed, milk casein, fish gelatin, feather quill and serum albumin) [1–4], as well as easily modified and manufactured. All these advantages together make PBBs suitable alternatives to petroleum-based plastics, which are being considered or have already fabricated in many environmentally sensitive industries, including agriculture (e.g. mulch films, greenhouse films, flower pots, planting pots, etc.), green packaging (one-time or short-term use before disposal) and possible biomedical industries (e.g. soft-tissue scaffold, superabsorbent) [2, 5–7].

In addition, tons of wasted protein from cottonseed, feather quill, soya residue and animal keratin are being utilized to fabricate bioplastics, which have even emerged as a new family of renewable and sustainable plastics, known as 'Second-generation bioplastics' [1, 8, 9] owing again mostly to their low cost, availability and biodegradability.

Cottonseed proteins (CPs) extracted from cottonseed meal after degreasing and peeling process contain rich amino acid components enjoying nutrition value, thereby they were used mostly as dairy-cattle feeding products. However, this type of protein has not been considered as non-feed industries, especially being used as a raw material for producing biodegradable plastics. The main component of cottonseed protein is globulin, approximately 90%, which contains 60% of globulins with gossypin (11S) and congossypin (7S) and 30% of albumins (2S) [10], resembling soy protein, the most studied material for bioplastic synthesis. In addition, the processability of CP with respect to plasticizer efficiency (PE) calculated from the relative contents of amino acids was similar to that of other proteins that have already been synthesized into various bioplastics [9]. Good amino acid composition together with a relatively high PE value (>5) makes cottonseed protein a good candidate as a renewable raw material for bioplastics production. However, little research to date has been carried out on cottonseed protein bioplastics (CPBs) while most studies focus on soy protein and wheat gluten bioplastics. Casting of CP films has been achieved by Marquié [11], but this process is time consuming and film formation is very limited. On the contrary, hot compression moulding is a more efficient strategy in achieving protein films.

In this chapter, a series of CPBs were synthesized starting from glandless cottonseed flour purified from cottonseed meal that was subjected to the processes of protein denaturation, plasticizing, cross-linking and hot compression; they showed good biodegradability, thermal stability and a low degree of water absorption (WA), but they are structurally heterogeneous even after thorough mixing and dispersion. The results of this study should provide important theoretical guidance on the development of environmentally friendly protein-derived bioplastics with improved properties, and necessary steps to pave the way towards expanding non-feed industry of cottonseed protein after oil extraction.

2. Synthesis of glandless CPBs

2.1. Optimum synthesis conditions

The synthesis route of the bioplastics is demonstrated in **Figure 1**. A typical synthesis experiment includes the following steps in sequences: (i) glandless cottonseed flour was placed into a beaker where deionized water was added at a solid-liquid weight ratio of 1:6, followed by the addition of 1-M urea solution. Denatured cottonseed protein (DCP) was obtained after the mixture was agitated by a magnetic stirrer for 4 h at room temperature; (ii) using 1 N NaOH solution, acidity/alkalinity of the DCP solution was adjusted to pH 11 with stirring for 10 min; (iii) the alkaline solution was kept in a water bath at 70°C, stirred for a further 30 min, and a cross-linking agent (formaldehyde (FA), glyoxal (GX) or glutaraldehyde (GA)) at 10 wt% of cottonseed flour was added; (iv) the resultant mixture was vacuum-dried for 10 h at 80°C prior to further fabrication; (v) glycerol was added to the dried denatured protein and then homogenized in a high-speed mixer (HR1704, PHILIPS Ltd.) for 5 min; (vi) the mixture was then ground and processed for three to five times using a three-roller (at a speed of 9:3:1) mill with the clearance of the outlet roller less than 1 mm; (vii) this mixture was then further conditioned in a desiccator at room temperature for 24 h; (viii) the conditioned mixture was placed on the surface of a stainless steel plate covered with aluminium (Al) foil with a layer of Al foil mounted on the back side; then the mixture was hot pressed at 20 MPa, 130°C for 5 min; and (ix) after cooling, the prepared CPBs were carefully removed from the mould, and then stored in desiccators at room temperature for further uses.

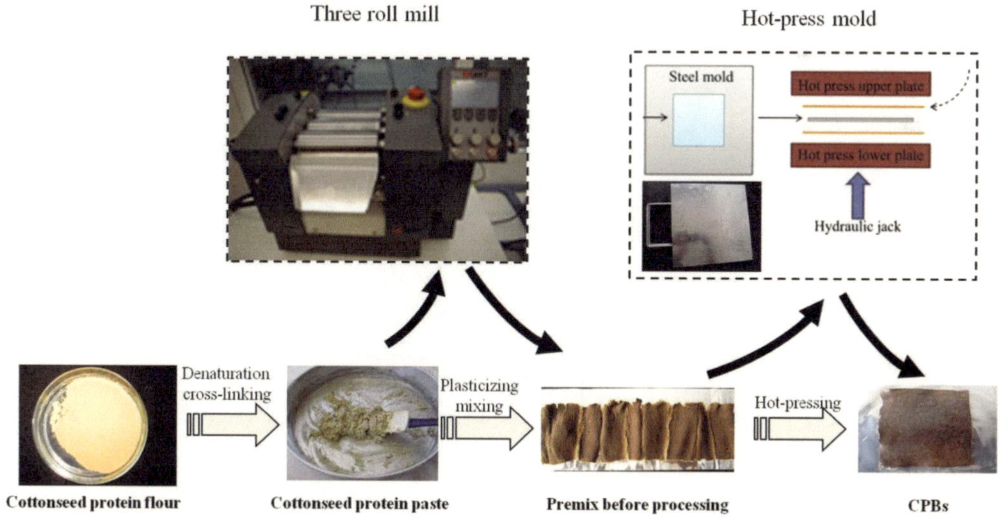

Figure 1. Diagram of cottonseed protein bioplastic preparation, primarily including protein denaturation and cross-linking, plasticizing, homogenization and hot-press moulding.

Regulation and optimization of synthesis and processing conditions are particularly important for improving the comprehensive properties of the bioplastic products. Macroscopic properties and/or microscopic structure of the CPBs are influenced by a series of experimental conditions: the CP flour dosage, solid-liquid ratio of protein solution, concentration of the denaturation agents (urea), cross-linker (aldehyde) content, concentration of the plasticizer (glycerol), reaction temperature and solution pH value. At the same time, a good mixing and homogeneous dispersion of the precursors are necessary while the hot-press processing parameters (temperature, pressure, time) are reasonably controlled. The optimum CPB synthesis conditions were obtained and summarized as follows: initially, cottonseed protein was denatured using a urea solution, which was then adjusted to pH 11 with NaOH solution, the aldehyde cross-linking agent added, and the mixture vacuum-dried for 10 h at 80°C. Glycerol as plasticizer was then added homogeneously to the dried solid using both a high-speed mixer and a three-roller mill. This mixture was conditioned in a desiccator at room temperature for 24 h and then hot pressed at 20 MPa, 130°C for 5 min.

2.2. Mechanism of protein modification and cross-linking

2.2.1. Protein denaturation induced by urea

A schematic illustrating the denaturation of cottonseed protein in the presence of urea is depicted in **Figure 2a**. It is shown that the process of protein denaturation involves both indirect and direct hydrogen bonding between urea molecules and water molecules as well as protein macromolecules, which has been confirmed by Bennion and Daggett [12] using atomic-resolution molecular dynamics simulation. In case of the indirect denaturation, the presence

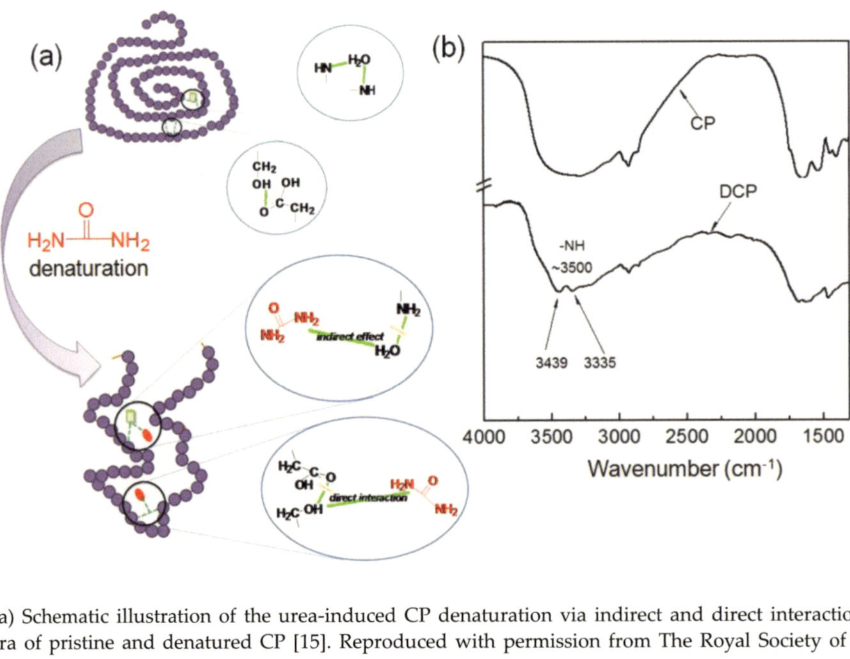

Figure 2. (a) Schematic illustration of the urea-induced CP denaturation via indirect and direct interactions and (b) FTIR spectra of pristine and denatured CP [15]. Reproduced with permission from The Royal Society of Chemistry (2012).

of urea weakens the cohesion of water molecules by reducing the water-water and/or water-protein interactions; as a result, water diffusion is decreased, thus exposing more functional groups in side chains so as to increase water-urea hydrogen bonding. As for the direct denaturation, urea molecules interact with the peptide backbone as well as polar moieties of the protein via direct hydrogen bonding; in particular, the strength of hydrogen bonds between urea and the peptide backbone of CP will largely increase on the condition that the secondary structure of CP is disrupted.

Figure 2b shows Fourier transform infrared (FTIR) spectra of the cottonseed proteins (pristine and denatured CP). Clearly, amide N—H-stretching vibration bands for the CP appear at around 3500 cm^{-1} as a broad absorption, whereas two bands at similar region (3439 and 3335 cm^{-1}) are observed for the denatured cottonseed protein being assigned to the amide N—H-stretching vibration bands in CP and urea, respectively. In addition, the appearance of absorbing band ranging from 1630 to 1680 cm^{-1} can be assigned to the C═O stretch vibrations of the peptide linkages of amide I, the most sensitive spectral area of protein secondary structure [13].

On the contrary, the characteristic amide II band at 1480–1575 cm^{-1} is attributed to in-plane N—H bending and C—N-stretching vibrations. As the position of absorbing amide I and amide II bands is very sensitive to the secondary structure of the protein, the frequency of these bands would be mainly dependent on the hydrogen bonds between C═O and N—H groups. The presence of urea has a noticed impact on the characteristic absorbing band position. For instance, the amide I band shifts from 1648 cm^{-1} (CP) to a lower frequency, 1618 cm^{-1} (DCP), and the amide II band shifts from 1541 cm^{-1} (CP) to 1467 cm^{-1} (DCP), as shown in **Figure 2b**.

2.2.2. Protein cross-linking with aldehyde

Three aldehydes (formaldehyde, glyoxal and glutaraldehyde) react with cottonseed protein molecules in a quite different manner, creating the cross-linked structures. Specifically, methylene bridge formation is responsible for the formaldehyde cross-linked networks (**Figure 3a**) [14]; however, the formaldehyde polymer (in FA solution) cannot generate further methylene bridges. As for the glutaraldehyde cross-linked networks (**Figure 3b**), both GA monomer and GA polymer are able to react with protein molecules via Maillard-driven generation of the imine covalent bond formation [15]. Glyoxal maintains the same mechanism as GA.

This reaction can be accelerated with the increased nucleophilicity as long as the amino groups are deprotonated. In this work, the carbonyl groups in the aldehydes react with the amino groups within CP under an alkaline condition at elevated temperature, leading to the formation of an imine group (—CH═N—), ultimately improving the thermal stability, mechanical strength and moisture resistance of the CPB bioplastics. In addition, Maillard-driven reaction explains the changes in colour and odour [15] before and after the hot press. **Figure 1** shows the colour of the CPBs changing from yellow-brown before preparation to golden-brown after hot compression moulding. Interestingly, the odour was not the same after hot-press moulding. For example, CP-GA smelled like persimmon while the smell of the CP-FA CPBs was a bit malodourous.

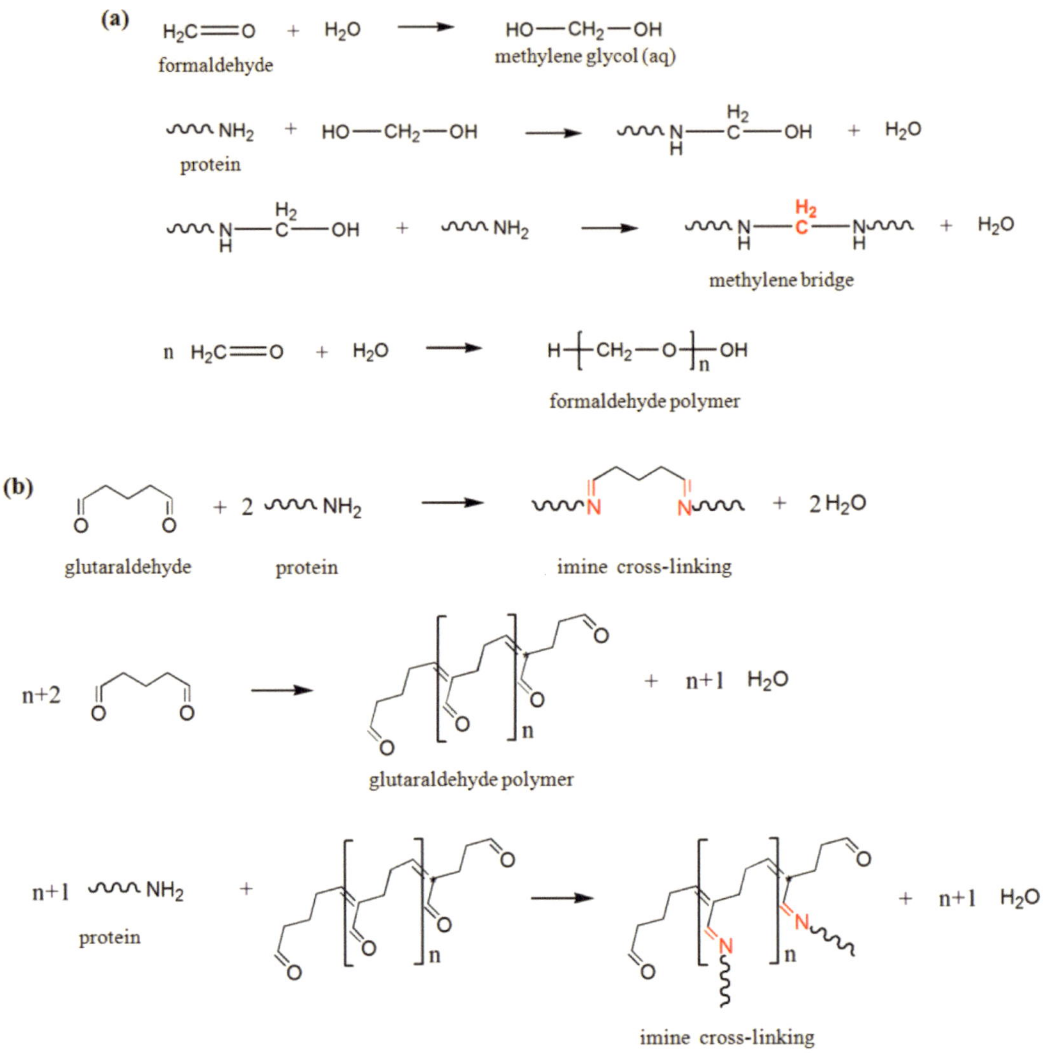

Figure 3. Cross-linking reactions of protein macromolecules with formaldehyde (a) showing the formation of methylene bridge and glutaraldehyde monomer/polymer, and (b) creating imine covalent bonds.

3. Morphology, element composition and biodegradability

Figure 4 shows scanning electron microscopic (SEM) micrographs of the CPBs, including their surface morphology and fracture surface. A fluctuated and continuous structure can be observed from the surface morphology of the cross-linked samples (CP-FA, CP-GX and CP-GA CPBs), compared to the cracks appeared at the smooth surface of CP-0CL indicating its brittle nature. Moreover, the height of the asperities at the fractured surface indicates a ductile failure behaviour for the cross-linked bioplastics, whereas it is discontinuous for the CP-0CL structure.

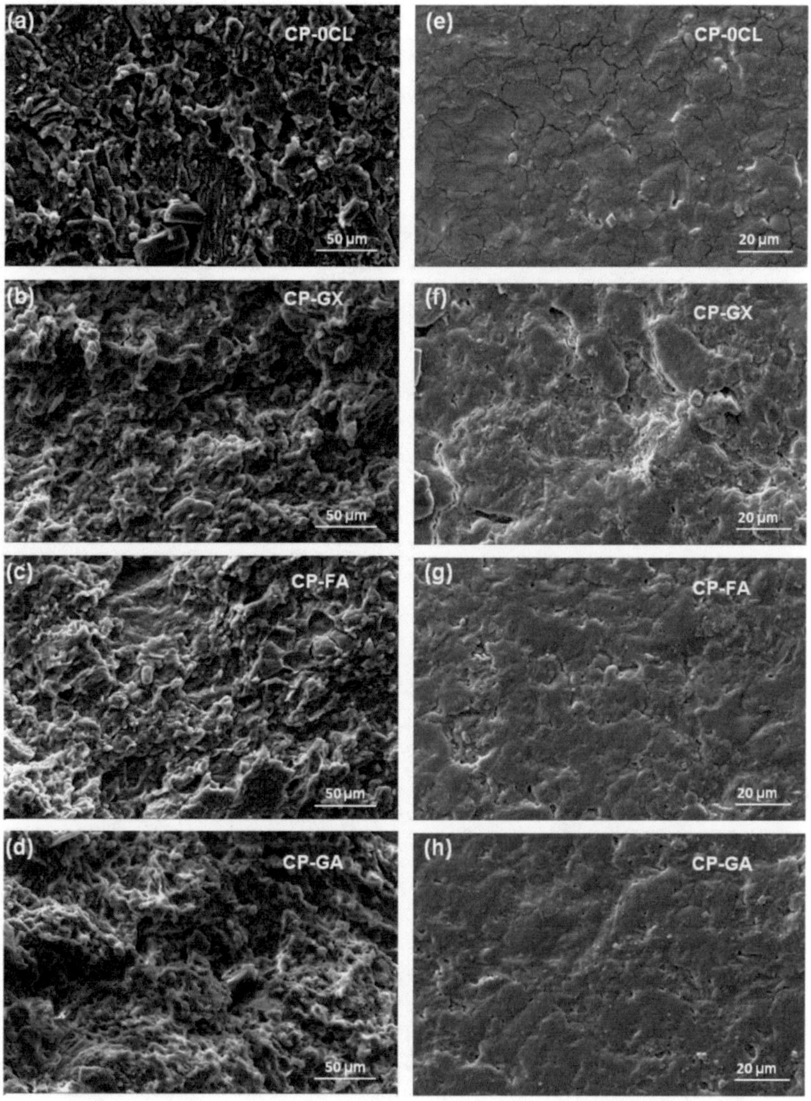

Figure 4. SEM images of the fractured microstructure (a–d) and the surface morphology (e–h) of the CPBs (CP-0CL, CP-FA, CP-GX and CP-GA, respectively) [15]. Reproduced with permission from The Royal Society of Chemistry (2012).

In addition to the ductile characteristics of the cross-linked samples, they exhibit a certain degree of heterogeneity within the whole networks with respect to their element composition distributed as well as the presence of unreacted or partially reacted aldehydes with variable concentration.

3.1. Element composition and heterogeneity feature

The element composition of the CPBs is detected by X-ray energy dispersive spectroscopy (EDS), as shown in **Figure 5**. The dominant presence of three elements, carbon C, nitrogen N and oxygen O, is at an atomic ratio of 4:1:1, or 3:1:1 in weight, while three other elements, magnesium Mg, sulphur S and phosphorus P, are present at a trace amount (weight percentage of <2%, atomic percentage of <1%). All the elements are randomly distributed on the measured surface, especially for Mg, S and P, as can be seen from element mapping (**Figure 6**), suggesting

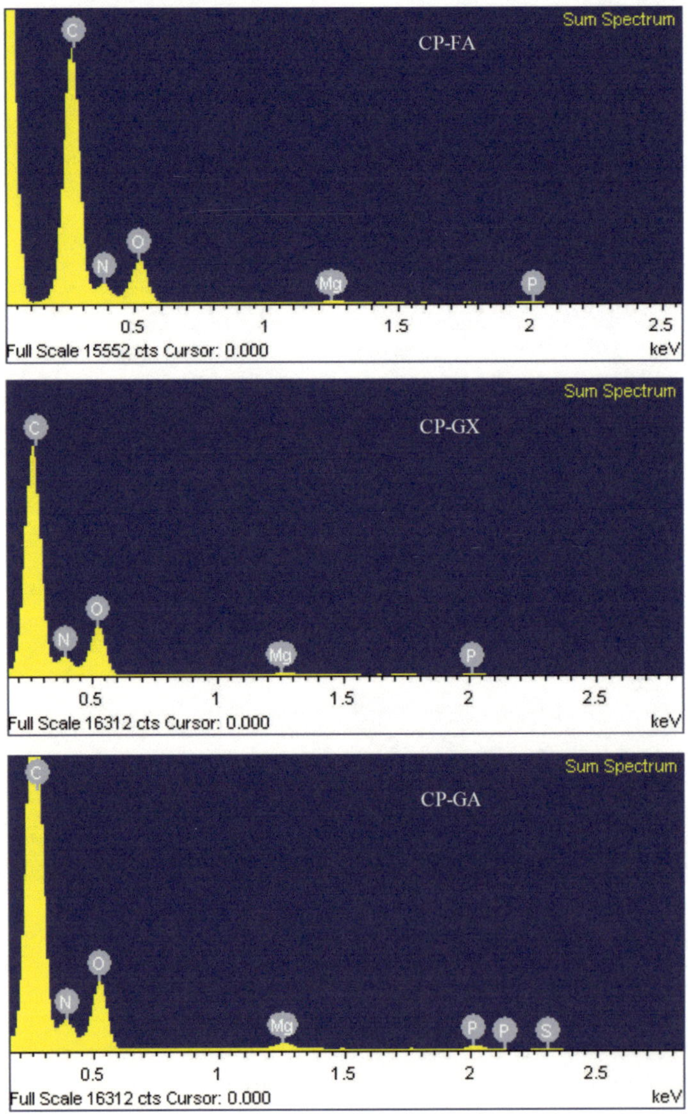

Figure 5. EDS-SEM analysis of the bioplastics, showing all the elements detected.

a characteristic of heterogeneity of the bioplastics. This characteristic is further confirmed by its infrared spectra collected from different locations across the sample surface at micro-scale resolution.

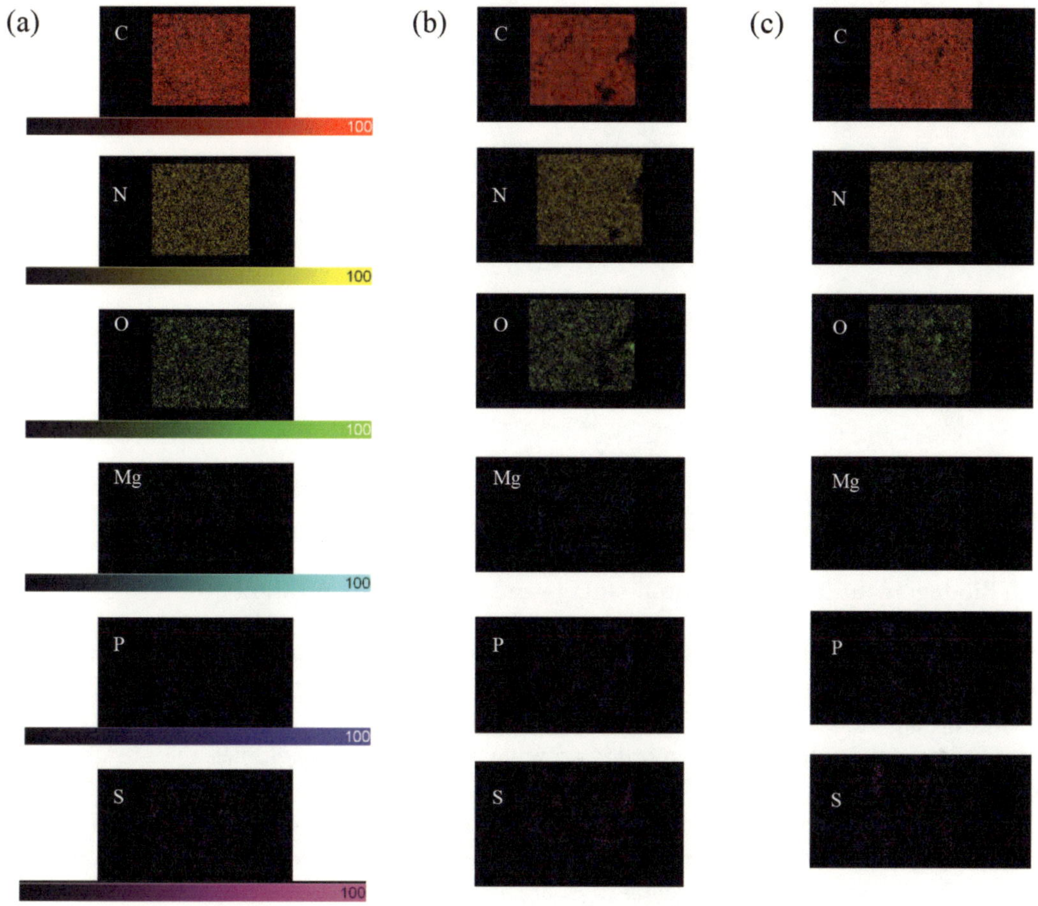

Figure 6. EDS-SEM analysis using element mapping of (a) CP-FA, (b) CP-GX and (c) CP-GA.

Figure 7 shows infrared spectra recorded from various positions on the different samples using an attenuated total reflection (ATR) objective with a Ge crystal with a contact surface of 100-μm diameter. It can be observed that for each cross-linked sample, heterogeneity is observed, notably reflected in the relative intensity of the band appearing around 1697 cm^{-1} associated with carbonyl-stretching vibration (marked) of unreacted or partially reacted aldehyde distributed with variable concentration in the CPB networks.

To develop environmentally friendly protein-derived bioplastics with desired optimized properties, it is expected that a homogeneous distribution of all elements within the sample network and a balanced formula with respect to ideal chemical reaction (in stoichiometry) involved in the synthesis process are initially important. Future studies addressing these two issues are currently under investigation.

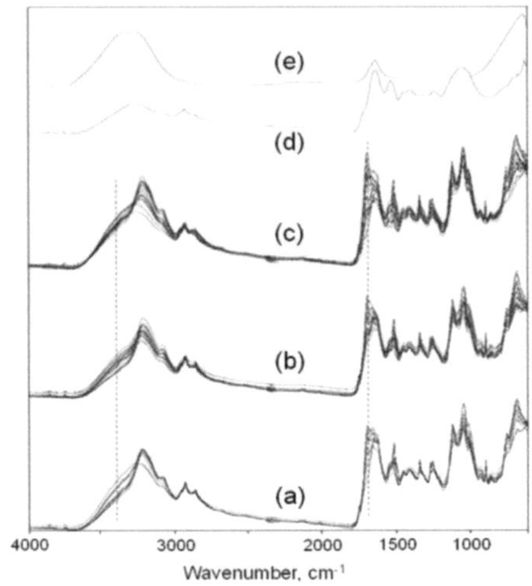

Figure 7. Infrared spectra recorded from different positions of samples (a) CP-FA, (b) CP-GX and (c) CP-GA. Spectrum of (d) water and (e) CPL-0CL is shown for comparison.

3.2. Biodegradability under natural-storage and soil-burial conditions

Biodegradability of the synthesized bioplastics was verified under both natural-storage and soil-burial conditions. Fungi growth on the surface of the CPBs after 6 months under ambient condition is pictured in **Figure 8a** at two different magnifications. It can be seen that filamentous fungi, commonly known as moulds growing as multicellular colonies, lives by absorbing nutrients from the contacting organic matter (the bioplastic). In fact, the natural-storage condition—room temperature and 40% relative humidity—is an unfavourable environment for mould growth for the reason that, on one hand, only a limited number of filamentous fungi such as *Bacillus subtilis* and *Aspergillus niger* are actually available in air; on the other hand, the sample surface starts to unevenly dehydrate and dry due to the evaporation of moisture in the desiccators storing the CPBs, which is unpleasant for moulds to live thus covering only part of the sample surface. However, in spite of its small quantities, the microbial biomass can live on with the carbon source stored in the sample, indicating that the cottonseed protein-derived bioplastics is biodegradable to a certain extent. Still, it is necessary to use a more standard test of biodegradability for the synthesized bioplastics—for example, the measurements in a nutrient agar culture medium, which contain a large number of microbial fungi (e.g. *B. subtilis, Staphylococcus aureus, Bacillus, Escherichia coli, Aspergillus flavus, A. oryzae* and *A. niger*) to degrade almost all organic matter under ideal conditions.

Figure 8b illustrates how the biodegradability of the synthesized bioplastics was measured in soil environment. Specifically, soil was firstly collected at the campus of Zhongkai University of Agriculture and Engineering, crushed, sieved and transferred to a wide-mouth bottle.

Secondly, the samples were carefully added in the bottle in the way that they were buried in parallel in the soil. Then, the bottle was kept in an incubator and thirdly the samples were taken out after a certain period of time, rinsed with 75% ethanol solution as well as deionized water, dried and weighed. The ability of soil to degrade organic matters is often quantified by the weight loss (%) of the sample after the soil-burial test, shown as

$$\text{Weight loss} = \frac{W_a - W_b}{W_b} \times 100\% \tag{1}$$

where W_b and W_a are the weight of the bioplastic sample before and after the soil-burial test, respectively. Background experiments for comparison, the same bioplastics, were stored in an empty wide-mouth bottle under the same condition, and their weight loss measured using Eq. (1) following exactly the same procedure as described above. **Figure 8c** shows the weight loss of a typical CPB bioplastic after the soil-burial measurement as a function of the recorded degrading time. It can be seen that the bioplastic degrades fast in the first 30 days, losing its weight up to 40%, followed by no obvious changes of its weight in the following month. The experimental data are fitted with multiple regression fitting, written as Weight loss = 0.1192

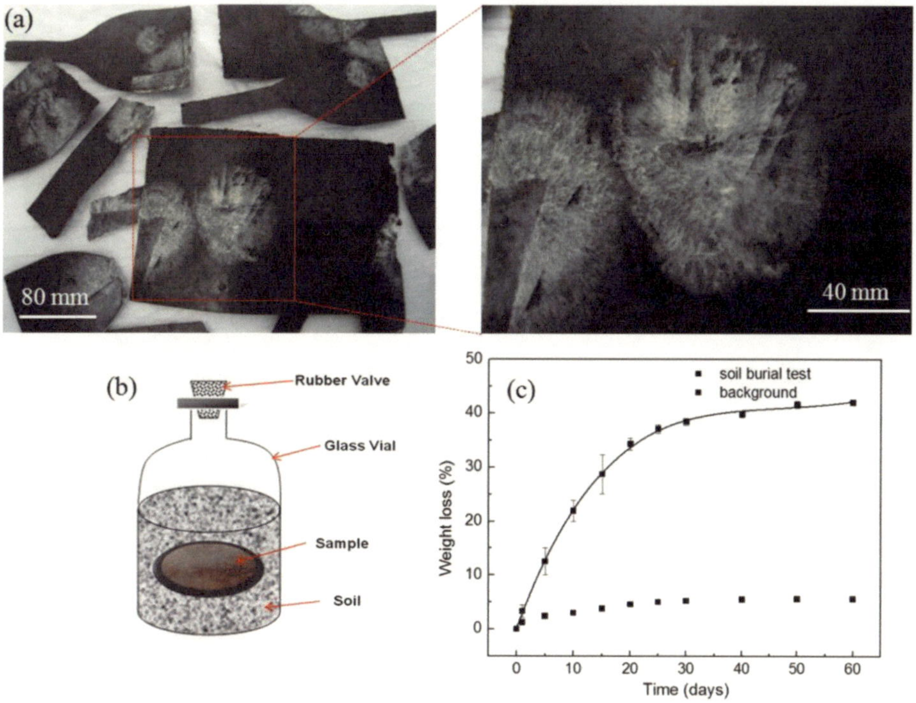

Figure 8. Biodegradability test of the CPB bioplastics. (a) Microbial fungi growth after 6 months under natural-storage condition (at room temperature and 40 RH%); (b) schematic of soil-burial test and (c) results of weight loss (%) of the bioplastics measured by soil-burial test referenced with a background.

$+ 2.8908t - 0.0772t^2 + 0.0001t^3$, where t is the number of days of degradation. The weight loss of the cross-linked (CP-GA) and non-cross-linked (CP-0CL) bioplastics, after 30 days of being buried in the soil, are 28 and 45%, respectively, indicating that the cross-linked treatment can effectively decrease the degree of biodegradation. It should be pointed out that the cottonseed protein reacts with the aldehyde under certain circumstances (Section 2.2.2), creating a high-density cross-linked network, in which the cross-linked/entangled macromolecules and their chains contribute to resisting the invasion of the microorganisms.

4. Thermal stability and thermomechanical relaxation

4.1. Thermogravimetry analysis of thermal stability

Thermal stability of glandless cottonseed protein bioplastics was evaluated by thermogravimetry analysis (TGA), which was carried out on a TG 209 under nitrogen atmosphere (protective gas flow was 15 ml min^{-1}) at a heating rate of 30°C min^{-1} from 25 to 500°C. Overall, the cross-linked bioplastics (CP-FA, CP-GX and CP-GA) have less mass loss compared with CP-0CL over the tested temperature range, implying an improvement to thermal stability. The formation of strong imine covalent bonds for the cross-linked samples after the hot press should account for the improved thermal stability, similar to the cross-linked soy protein bioplastics [16].

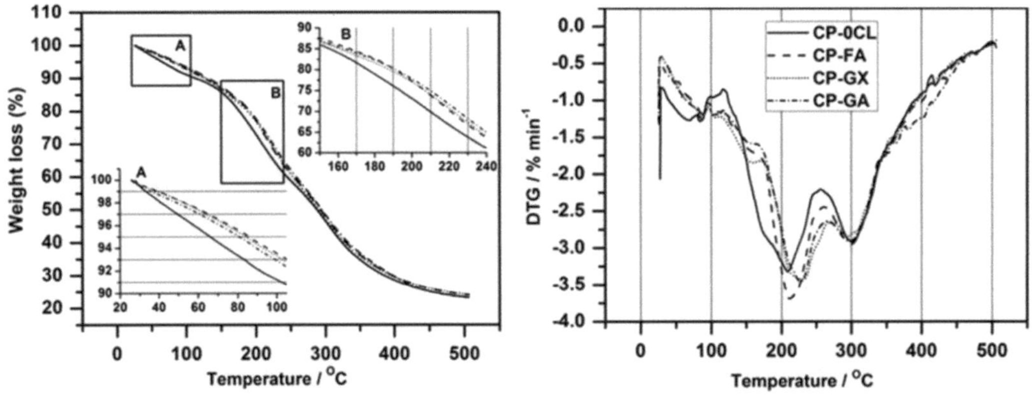

Figure 9. Weight loss and DTG curves of the CPBs as a function of temperature. Inset graphs denote the first stage (A) and second stage (B) of the CPB weight loss [15]. Reproduced with permission from The Royal Society of Chemistry (2012).

Specifically, three distinct stages of mass loss for the CPBs are observed from the TGA curves in **Figure 9**. In the first one (Inset graph A, **Figure 9**), less than 10 wt% of sample mass losses between room temperature and 100°C, mainly because of the evaporation of moisture previously absorbed by samples. In the next stage from 160 to 230°C (Inset graph B, **Figure 9**), the CPBs decomposed rapidly with a mass loss of 20–40 wt%, which is due to the decomposition of small molecules (glycerol and urea residues), as verified by Zhang et al. [17]. In the last one, decomposition of CP occurs at temperature of >260°C, in which the volatile molecules such as CO_2, CO and NH_3 are released as a consequence of degradation. Unsaturated compounds with carbonyl groups may also present in this stage, according to the study carried out by Schmidt et al. [18] using FTIR spectra.

It is also interesting to see that the CP-FA sample showed the least mass loss at temperature below 190°C, suggesting the best thermal stability among all the CPBs, while CP-GA was the best at temperature above 190°C. This might suggest that the interactions between CP and GA are greater than that between CP and FA with increasing temperature, probably due to the higher cross-linking efficiency of GA compared to FA at elevated temperatures [19].

4.2. Differential scanning calorimetry and dynamic mechanical analysis of thermal relaxation behaviours

To investigate the thermal relaxation behaviours of glandless cottonseed protein bioplastics, both differential scanning calorimetry (DSC) and dynamic mechanical analysis (DMA) were carried out; see the detailed experimental testing conditions in the published papers [15, 20]. **Figure 10a** shows a baseline increase from the minima at ~150°C, suggesting a complete denaturation of the pristine CP within the bioplastic matrix, in contrast to other proteins in particular soy protein, which exhibited two similar temperature characteristic of gossypin and congossypin globulin fractions [21]. In addition, all the modified CPBs regardless of the type of aldehyde cross-linking agent used showed such trend at similar denaturation temperature (T_d). Since protein macromolecules comprise a large number of amino acid species, multiple movements simultaneously occur during the CP denaturation including hydrogen bonding, dipole-dipole, charge-charge and hydrophobic interactions. As a consequence of these

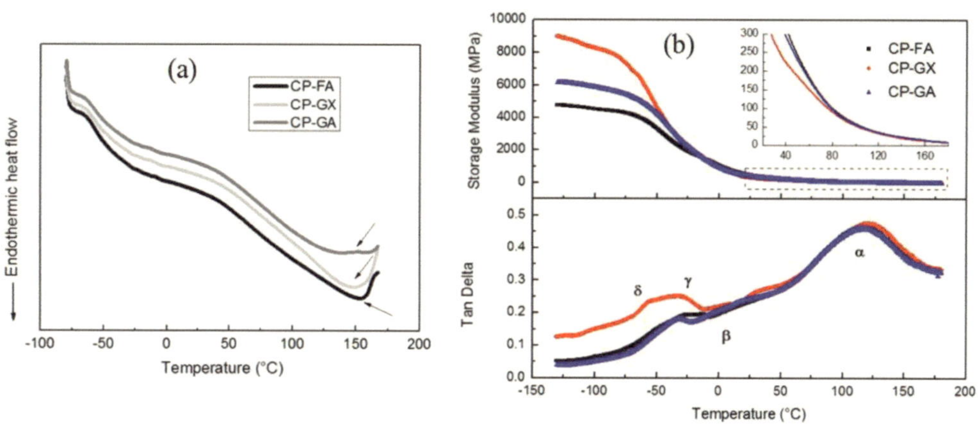

Figure 10. DSC (a) and DMA (b) thermograms of the aldehyde cross-linked CP-FA, CP-GX and CP-GA CPBs. The temperatures marked in DSC curves indicate the T_d. Inset is the enlarged plots marked by dashed rectangle [20]. Reproduced with permission from The Royal Society of Chemistry (2014).

interactions, insoluble protein aggregation is often formed, which is, however, accompanied by a low transitional energy [22], thus making it difficult to detect using DSC.

Dynamic mechanical analysis has better sensitivity to detect thermal events such as thermo-mechanical relaxation of macromolecule chains, similar to the sub-T_g transitions. Denaturation temperature of the cross-linked CPBs can be clearly identified from DMA curves (**Figure 10b**) at T_d about 120°C, corresponding to the α-transition temperature. In line with DSC results, DMA signals suggest that cross-linking leads to little change in T_d, meaning that the three aldehydes—formaldehyde, glyoxal and glutaraldehyde—cross-linked network have a similar density, which is nonetheless dependent on the type of plasticizer [23]. A small β-transition peak at ~0°C, shown in the Tan δ graph, **Figure 10b**, is probably associated with the absorption of moisture from air. A similar behaviour occurring at a relative humidity of >35% for soy protein-glycerol-water ternary systems was observed by Zhang's group [17].

The large decrease/increase in E' from DMA graphs usually suggests the occurrence of glass transitions of macromolecules. Storage modulus, E' profile shown in **Figure 10b**, indicates a broad glass transition irrespective of the type of cross-linking agent used, specifically showing two transitions below 0°C from the tan delta curves—γ and δ observed at approximately -25 and -55°C, respectively.

It is well acknowledged that protein-based bioplastics have more than one T_g [17, 24] due to its heterogeneous feature. A sub-T_g transitional behaviour is apparent for the CP-GX sample at the start of the E' decrement at approximately -100°C, but is less obvious in the other samples. Changes in storage modulus at low temperatures are more severe: the highest E' value (~8500 MPa) was found for CP-GX and the lowest for CP-FA (~4500 MPa) at -140°C. However, after the glass transition, a slightly lower value of E' for CP-GX may suggest a lower cross-linking density, implying longer molecular chain length between cross-links. This may lead to the increase of chain mobility favouring the formation of multiple intra- and intermolecular interactions such as hydrogen bonding, which would contribute to the mechanical reinforcement in the glassy state. Indeed, glyoxal is more easy to form hydrogen bonds with electronegative elements in the protein (O, S, N, etc.) than formaldehyde would, according to hydrogen-bonding theories [25].

5. Interaction between bioplastics and water

5.1. Water absorption and transportation kinetics

Water absorption of the CPB (CP-0CL, CP-FA, CP-GX and CP-GA) films was carried out according to ASTM D570-98 standards. Briefly, the pre-dried and weighed CPBs were firstly immersed in distilled water at room temperature, removed from the water at regular time intervals, dabbed with filter paper to remove excess water on the sample surface and the weight of the sample registered.

Water absorption (WA) is calculated using Eq. (2)

$$\mathrm{WA}(\%) = \frac{W_t - W_0}{W_0} \times 100 \tag{2}$$

where W_0 and W_t are the initial weight of the bioplastics and the weight of the sample after being immerged in water for t min, respectively. It is found that water absorption of all bioplastics increased markedly over the first 2 h of immersion, followed by a gradual decrease in absorption rate in the subsequent 8 h. After this stage, water absorption reaches an equilibrium state, ensuring no further mass increase. It is found that cross-linking helps reducing water absorption, as the bioplastics (CP-FA, CP-GX and CP-GA) absorbed less water than the control sample (CP-0CL) over the course of testing period. These bioplastics have a more compact and tightly bound network, which limits the distance water molecules can diffuse within, and hence lowers the total capacity of water that can be absorbed; so a lower amount of water absorption is obtained, compared with the control sample.

Water absorption is a big concern, in general, for practical applications of protein-based plastics due to the fact that most proteins contain a big number of carboxyl and hydroxyl groups that are typically characteristic of hydrophilicity. For example, soy protein-derived plastics increase in mass by 78.66% after being immersed in distilled water for 2 h at room temperature [26]. Strikingly, the mass increase of the cottonseed protein-derived plastics (CP-0CL, CP-FA, CP-GX and CP-GA CBPs) studied in this work, under the same experimental conditions, was much lower (19.39, 16.35, 14.15 and 13.51%, respectively), suggesting a significant improvement in water resistance properties.

The results of CPB water absorption test were further analysed using theories of Fickian diffusivity, Liquid transport and Liquid permeability, to evaluate the liquid transit properties of the polymer network [20]. As rate indicators between polymer chain relaxation and water diffusion, values of the kinetic exponent n and characteristic constant of water absorption k vary from different bioplastics, with the n value increasing, whereas the k value decreases after addition of the cross-linking agent. Interestingly, a high diffusion coefficient D value for the cross-linked bioplastics indicates that water diffuses easily in the cross-linked networks according to the theory of Liquid transport. Furthermore, the findings based on the theory of Liquid permeability suggest that the presence of cross-linked structure promotes the physical transport process, including water diffusion and permeability, while that in the absence of cross-linking, it is chemical interaction such as hydrogen bonding or van der Waals interactions that facilitate water transport within the protein.

5.2. Different water states

Differential scanning calorimetry measurements were performed on a TA Instruments Q200 DSC under nitrogen atmosphere, in order to find out possible water states within the CPBs after their water absorption. In a typical experiment, a specimen (weighed ~5–6 mg) was placed into an Al pan and a known amount of water added by a micro-syringe. The pan was then hermetically sealed by an Al lid and conditioned for 24 h at room temperature to enable the water absorption states to equilibrate. The conditioned samples were first equilibrated at

-80°C for 10 min, and then heated up to 50°C at a rate of 10°C min^{-1}, with the same programme repeated three times to verify reproducibility. All the hermetic Al pans were weighed after the measurements to confirm no loss of sample weight during the experiment.

Water content ω_{H_2O} of the bioplastics was calculated as

$$\omega_{H_2O}(\%) = \left(W_{H_2O}^{add} / W_{CPBs}\right) \times 100 \tag{3}$$

where $W_{H_2O}^{add}$ and W_{CPBs} stand for weight of added water and that of the CPBs tested, respectively. W_{CPBs} is the total mass of the sample, namely the sum of the dried sample and the water added. Free water contains both freezable bulk water and that weakly bound to the polymer, and whose weight percentage $\omega_{H_2O}^{free}$ is expressed as

$$\omega_{H_2O}^{free}(\%) = \left(W_{H_2O}^{free} / W_{H_2O}^{add}\right) \times 100 \tag{4}$$

$$W_{H_2O}^{free} = \left(\Delta H_{W_{CPBs}} / \Delta H_{pure\ H_2O}\right) \times W_{CPBs} \tag{5}$$

where $W_{H_2O}^{free}$ is the weight of the free water component within the bulk sample, obtained by multiplying the weight fraction of water (determined as $\Delta H_{W_{CPBs}}/\Delta H_{pure\ H_2O}$) with the total mass of the tested sample (W_{CPBs}). Here, $\Delta H_{W_{CPBs}}$ is calculated by integrating the endothermic ice-melting peak, related to the total mass of the tested sample (sum of the dried sample and water added). $\Delta H_{pure\ H_2O}$ is the melting enthalpy of pure water; it equals to 365 J g^{-1} using distilled water as a reference for all samples in this study. The weight percentage of non-free water $\omega_{H_2O}^{non\text{-}free}$ is estimated from the difference between the weight of water added and that of free water:

$$\omega_{H_2O}^{non\text{-}free}(\%) = \left(W_{H_2O}^{non\text{-}free} / W_{H_2O}^{add}\right) \times 100 \tag{6}$$

$$W_{H_2O}^{non\text{-}free} = W_{H_2O}^{add} - W_{H_2O}^{free} \tag{7}$$

If no endothermic peak can be detected by adding very small amount of water, it is considered to be strongly bound to the polymer and thus non-freezable.

Figure 11 shows the change in the DSC fusion of water within the CPBs as a function of water concentration. The heat of fusion changes significantly for each sample by increasing the water

http://dx.doi.org/10.5772/64045

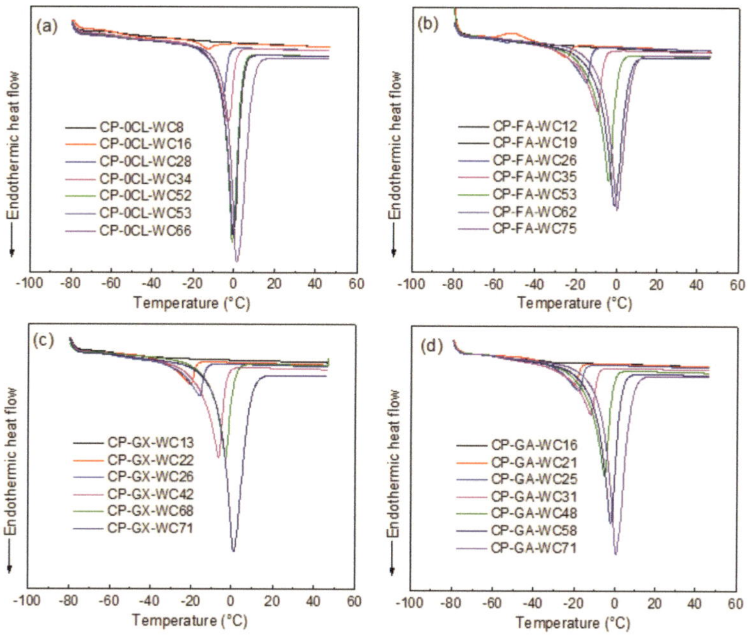

Figure 11. DSC thermograms showing the change in enthalpy and peak fusion temperature of the CPBs with respect to water content (WC, %). (a) CP-0CL, (b) CP-FA, (c) CP-GX and (d) CP-GA series [20]. Reproduced with permission from The Royal Society of Chemistry (2014).

content, from almost no endothermic signal at a water content below 15% to a strong response at water contents above 70%, causing a broad peak to appear centred around 0°C. Furthermore, increases in water content can bring about increases in the peak fusion temperature. For example, the heat fusion maximum temperature of the CP-FA sample changes by 25°C (from -24.9 to 0.1°C) as a result of the increase of the amount of water added, from 19 to 75%. We believe that the formation of water layers on/within the biomass surface largely depends on water content added into the bioplastics—being strongly bound to CPBs at a lower content, both strongly and weakly bound at a slightly higher concentration, and ultimately a ternary strongly to weakly bound to free system at an even higher water content (i.e. saturation).

The trend of the heat of fusion shown in **Figure 11** indicates that different states of water contained within the CPB structures exist, namely non-freezable water, free bulk-like water and freezable bound water, as reported for other hydrophilic polymers [27]. **Figure 12** schematically demonstrates the bonding ability of CPB polymer networks with the water molecules, correspondingly showing the presence of a fraction of strongly-bound-to-polymer water that could not freeze upon cooling, freezable weakly-bound-to-polymer water whose mobility is partially retarded and a certain amount of freezable bulk-like water.

With increasing water content within the CPB network, it is believed that water adopts at least three different states. At lower concentrations, water is present in strongly-bond-to-polymer state where it is strongly connected to protein polymer chains, and thus cannot freeze. When the CPB system contains a content of water above a certain threshold, it appears as weakly-bond-to-polymer water, the intermediate state, suggesting a boundary where water molecules whose mobility is partially retarded could not sufficiently interact with the polymer chains to prevent the state of fusion, yet are able to crystallize. Lastly, excess water or bulk-like water is free of interactions with the protein chains, and is a predominant fraction at higher water contents.

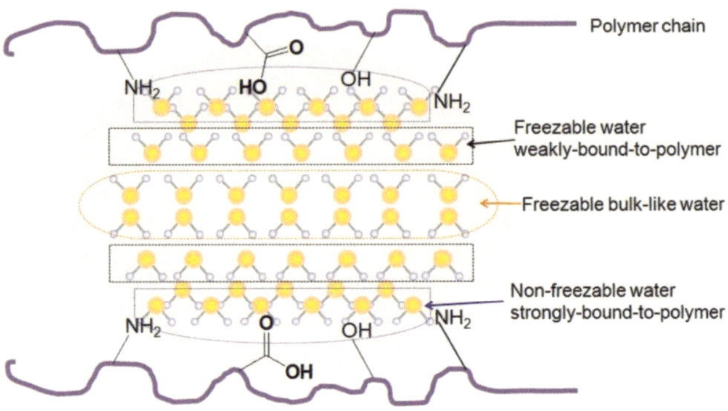

Figure 12. Schematic of CPB polymer chains affinity to water molecules, illustrating the presence of different states of water: freezable bulk-like water, freezable and non-freezable bound-to-polymer water [20]. Reproduced with permission from The Royal Society of Chemistry (2014).

6. Concluding remarks

Environmentally friendly bioplastics were successfully synthesized utilizing glandless cottonseed protein that was subjected to the processes of protein denaturation, plasticizing, cross-linking and hot compression; they are readily biodegradable, fairly thermal stable and resistive of water absorption while showing a fraction of the structural heterogeneity. The results presented in this chapter could be valuable for further development of protein-derived bioplastics with demanding properties as well as extending the value of cottonseed protein in non-feed industries. However, both the intrinsic heterogeneity feature and unsatisfied mechanical performance of protein-derived bioplastics (in general) impose large challenges to their large-scale industrial production. Future directions in this field may be taken as follows: (i) controllable design of protein-derived bioplastics with balanced properties—biodegradable, mechanical performance and the extension of service life—is needed; (ii) desired functions of the bioplastics are required to meet the needs in value-added applications where extreme environments, for example, high temperature and/or high moisture content, might be involved; and (iii) exploring new protein resources will play an important role in the development of biodegradable plastic industry. Genetically modified crops for instance can be used in the future to provide specific amino acid composition of protein as known building blocks for the resulting bioplastics, in order to optimize their structure and properties.

Acknowledgements

The authors are grateful to P. Shuttleworth, G. Ellis and J. P. Fernández-Blázquez for fruitful discussions, and to the National Natural Science Foundation of China (Grant no. 20776164; 33 21176269), Natural Science Foundation of Guangdong Province (Grant no. 9251022501000003), China Scholarship Council and China Postdoctoral Science Foundation for financial support of this work.

Author details

Hangbo Yue[1*], Guoqiang Yin[2*] and Yingde Cui[1,3]

*Address all correspondence to: yuehangbo@163.com and yingq007@163.com

1 School of Chemical Engineering and Light Industry, Guangdong University of Technology, Guangzhou, China

2 Institute of Green Chemical Engineering, Zhongkai University of Agriculture and Engineering, Guangzhou, China

3 Guangzhou Vocational College of Science and Technology, Guangzhou, China

References

[1] Gennadios A, Protein-Based Films and Coatings. Florida: CRC Press. 2002. pp. 1–42. DOI: 10.1201/9781420031980

[2] Song F, Tang D-L, Wang X-L, Wang Y-Z, Biodegradable soy protein isolate-based materials: a review. Biomacromolecules. 2011; 12: 3369–3380. DOI: 10.1021/bm200904x

[3] Zhang H, Mittal G, Biodegradable protein-based films from plant resources: a review. Environmental Progress & Sustainable Energy. 2010; 29: 203–220. DOI: 10.1002/ep.10463

[4] Mekonnen T, Mussone P, Khalil H, Bressler D, Progress in bio-based plastics and plasticizing modifications. Journal of Materials Chemistry A. 2013; 1: 13379–13398. DOI: 10.1039/c3ta12555f

[5] Mülhaupt R, Green polymer chemistry and bio-based plastics: dreams and reality. Macromolecular Chemistry and Physics. 2013; 214: 159–174. DOI: 10.1002/macp.201200439

[6] Santin M, Ambrosio L, Soybean-based biomaterials: preparation, properties and tissue regeneration potential. Expert Review of Medical Devices. 2008; 5: 349–358. DOI: 10.1586/17434440.5.3.349

[7] Zhang B, Cui Y, Yin G, Li X, Liao L, Cai X, Synthesis and swelling properties of protein-poly(acrylic acid-co-acrylamide) superabsorbent composite. Polymer Composites. 2011; 32: 683–691. DOI: 10.1002/pc.21077

[8] Scheller J, Conrad U, Plant-based material, protein and biodegradable plastic. Current Opinion in Plant Biology. 2005; 8: 188–196. DOI: 10.1016/j.pbi.2005.01.010

[9] Verbeek C, van den Berg L, Recent developments in thermo-mechanical processing of proteinous bioplastics. Recent Patents on Materials Science. 2009; 2: 171–189. DOI: 10.2174/1874464810902030171

[10] Marquie C, Guilbert S, Formation and properties of cottonseed protein films and coatines. In: Gennadios A, Ed. Protein-Based Films and Coatings. Florida: CRC Press. 2002. pp. 139–158. DOI: 10.1201/9781420031980.ch5

[11] Marquié C, Chemical reactions in cottonseed protein cross-linking by formaldehyde, glutaraldehyde, and glyoxal for the formation of protein films with enhanced mechanical properties. Journal of Agricultural and Food Chemistry. 2001; 49: 4676–4681. DOI: 10.1021/jf0101152

[12] Bennion BJ, Daggett V, The molecular basis for the chemical denaturation of proteins by urea. Proceedings of the National Academy of Sciences. 2003; 100: 5142–5147. DOI: 10.1073/pnas.0930122100

[13] Krimm S, Bandekar J, Vibrational spectroscopy and conformation of peptides, polypeptides, and proteins. In: Anfinsen CB, Edsall JT, and Richards FM, Eds. Advances in Protein Chemistry. Salt Lake City: Academic Press. 1986. pp. 181–364. DOI: 10.1016/S0065-3233(08)60528-8

[14] Kiernan JA, Formaldehyde, formalin, paraformaldehyde and glutaraldehyde: what they are and what they do. Microscopy Today. 2000; 1: 8–12.

[15] Yue HB, Cui YD, Shuttleworth PS, Clark JH, Preparation and characterisation of bioplastics made from cottonseed protein. Green Chemistry. 2012; 14: 2009–2016. DOI: 10.1039/C2GC35509D

[16] Chabba S, Matthews GF, Netravali AN, 'Green' composites using cross-linked soy flour and flax yarns. Green Chemistry. 2005; 7: 576–581. DOI: 10.1039/b410817e

[17] Chen P, Zhang L, Cao F, Effects of moisture on glass transition and microstructure of glycerol-plasticized soy protein. Macromolecular Bioscience. 2005; 5: 872–880. DOI: 10.1002/mabi.200500072

[18] Schmidt V, Giacomelli C, Soldi V, Thermal stability of films formed by soy protein isolate-sodium dodecyl sulfate. Polymer Degradation and Stability. 2005; 87: 25–31. DOI: 10.1016/j.polymdegradstab.2004.07.003

[19] Hopwood D, A comparison of the crosslinking abilities of glutaraldehyde, formaldehyde and α-hydroxyadipaldehyde with bovine serum albumin and casein. Histochemistry and Cell Biology. 1969; 17: 151–161. DOI: 10.1007/bf00277781

[20] Yue HB, Fernandez-Blazquez JP, Shuttleworth PS, Cui YD, Ellis G, Thermomechanical relaxation and different water states in cottonseed protein derived bioplastics. RSC Advances. 2014; 4: 32320–32326. DOI: 10.1039/c4ra01794c

[21] Mo X, Sun X, Thermal and mechanical properties of plastics molded from urea-modified soy protein isolates. Journal of the American Oil Chemists Society. 2001; 78: 867–872. DOI: 10.1007/s11746-001-0357-1

[22] Donovan JW, Ross KD, Increase in the stability of avidin produced by binding of biotin. Differential scanning calorimetric study of denaturation by heat. Biochemistry. 1973; 12: 512–517. DOI: 10.1021/bi00727a024

[23] Sears JK, Darby JR. Mechanism of plasticizer action. In: Sears JK and Darby JR, Eds. The Technology of Plasticizers. Chichester: Wiley. 1982. pp. 35–77.

[24] Chen P, Zhang L, New evidences of glass transitions and microstructures of soy protein plasticized with glycerol. Macromolecular Bioscience. 2005; 5: 237–245. DOI: 10.1002/mabi.200400179

[25] Emsley J, Very strong hydrogen bonding. Chemical Society Reviews. 1980; 9: 91–124. DOI: 10.1039/cs9800900091

[26] Mo X, Sun X, Plasticization of soy protein polymer by polyol-based plasticizers. Journal of the American Oil Chemists Society. 2002; 79: 197–202. DOI: 10.1007/s11746-002-0458-x

[27] Ping ZH, Nguyen QT, Chen SM, Zhou JQ, Ding YD, States of water in different hydrophilic polymers – DSC and FTIR studies. Polymer. 2001; 42: 8461–8467. DOI: 10.1016/s0032-3861(01)00358-5

Chapter 13

Synthesis of Nanometal Oxide–Coated Cotton Composites

Issa M. El Nahhal, Abdelraouf A. Elmanama and Nadia M. Amara

Additional information is available at the end of the chapter

http://dx.doi.org/10.5772/63505

Abstract

Several selected studies dealing with the development of novel antimicrobial metal oxide–coated cotton nanocomposites and their antimicrobial applications have been reviewed in this chapter. Synthesis of metal oxide nanoparticles (NPs) and its deposition onto cotton fibers were conducted using various methods. These include the high energy γ-radiation, thermal treatment-assisted impregnation, "pad-dry-cure" of the impregnated fabric in the colloid formulation of metal oxide soluble, and ultrasonic radiation methods. The coated metal oxide nanoparticles have shown an effective enhancement for antimicrobial activity. They reduce the chance of diseases originating from hospital infections. The antimicrobial properties of cotton fabrics finished with metal oxide NPs against a variety of bacterial strains commonly associated with nosocomial infections, caused by *Staphylococcus aureus* and *Escherichia coli*, have been investigated by four different methods. The morphology of the cotton-coated metal oxide nanoparticles and their chemical structure have been analyzed by UV-vis, Fourier transform infrared spectroscopy (FTIR), scanning electron microscopy (SEM), X-ray diffraction (XRD) and X-ray photoelectron spectra (XPS). SEM and XRD analyses revealed that the shape and size of the coated nanoparticles are dependent on the nature of the metal oxide and its preparation conditions.

Keywords: antimicrobial activity, metal oxide–coated cotton, coated cotton nanocomposites, CuO and ZnO nanoparticles, ultrasonic radiations

1. Introduction

Textile fabric, especially those made from natural fibers, provides an excellent environment for the growth of microorganisms because of their large surface area and the ability to retain moisture. A large number of chemicals have been used to impart antimicrobial activity to textile materials. The development of new clothing products based on the immobilization of nanophased materials on textile has recently received growing interest from both academic and industrial sectors [1]. Currently, a wide range of nanoparticles (NPs) with various structures can be immobilized onto the textile fibers in order to bring new properties to the textile product [1]. In this scene, the preparation and applications of nanoparticle coatings onto cotton fibers have received much attention due to its promising applications.

There are three general methods to impregnate metal oxide nanoparticles onto the cotton fibers: the first method is "pad-dry-cure process" while the second method is ultrasonic irradiation, which is an effective method for the deposition of nanoparticles onto the surface of cotton textile fibers and other substrates. The third method is a thermal chemical treatment [2–4]. Among these methods, ultrasonic irradiation represents a promising tool in nanosynthesis and deposition of NPs on/into the natural cotton fiber as it reduces the operation time, allows one-step preparation and deposition of nanomaterials on textile substrates, and enhances the quality of products [5]. In addition, the sonication method results in an appreciable quantity of coating, higher dispersion, and more diffusion of the particles onto the substrate compared to the other coating methods [6]. Moreover, sonication results in a smooth and homogeneous layer of coating, and it is capable of projecting nanoparticles toward the fabric surface at a very high speed, which causes nanoparticles to adhere strongly to fabric surfaces [7]. Abramov and his coworkers [8] have developed a method for introducing copper oxide NPs (CuO-NPs) into cotton fabrics using sonochemical reactor and their antimicrobial activity has been studied.

Gouda and his coworkers [4] have succeeded in the synthesis of some nanometal oxides via microwave irradiation technique and applied them onto cotton fabric to study their multifunctional properties. Antibacterial activity was evaluated quantitatively against Gram-positive bacteria such as *Staphylococcus aureus* and Gram-negative bacteria such as *Escherichia coli*. The antimicrobial activity of cotton fiber coated with zinc oxide (ZnO) and CuO-NPs was investigated against *E. coli* and *S. aureus* cultures by El-Nahhal and his coworkers [2, 3]. In this study, they have prepared crystalline ZnO of hexagonal and CuO of monoclinic phases with an average crystallite size of 12 and 50 nm, respectively. These nanoparticles were physically adsorbed onto the cotton fiber surface by ultrasonic irradiation. These results proved that the coated cotton samples have displayed a high activity with a great reduction in the bacterial growth [2, 3].

Shateri-Khalilabad and Yazdanshenas [9] have synthesized ZnO-NPs on the surface of cotton fabric via a simple wet chemical method to impart antimicrobial activity and ultraviolet (UV) protection. SEM images revealed that significant amounts of hierarchical ZnO-NPs were homogeneously formed on the fibers' surface; most of them were bundle-/flower-like particles having different sizes. It was stated that the ZnO-NP–coated cotton fabric has a good bacter-

http://dx.doi.org/10.5772/63505

iostatic activity against two representative bacteria, *Klebseilla pneumoniae* and *S. aureus*, which was demonstrated by the zone of inhibition. It was proved that the coated fibers have an excellent ability to block the UV radiation [9]. Several authors have examined and investigated the antimicrobial activity of metal oxide–coated cotton nanocomposites, and they have showed an effective reduction in the bacterial activities [10–16]. ZnO nanoparticle assembly for the multilayer film formation on the cotton fabrics was prepared by layer-by-layer deposition process [17]. Hongjum and others have successfully synthesized ZnO films deposited onto the surface of cotton fibers by a simple two-step process [18]. The growth of ZnO films was carried out in Zn $(CH_3COO)_2$ solution, with NaOH solution [18]. In this chapter, we discussed the synthesis, characterization, and antimicrobial activity of metal oxide nanoparticles with emphasis on CuO and ZnO.

2. Antibacterial agents

Antibacterial agents are classified into two types: organic and inorganic. The organic materials are often less stable than that of the inorganic antibacterial agents with respect to the high temperatures and pressures compared to inorganic antibacterial agents [19]. The inorganic materials such as metal and metal oxides are considered to be stable at harsh processing conditions. Among these materials are the metal oxides ZnO, CuO, and MgO. One of these inorganic materials is zinc oxide (ZnO). ZnO belongs to a group of metal oxides that are characterized by several properties [20]. ZnO is generally regarded as a safe material for human beings and animals, and it has been used extensively in the formulation of many personal care products [21, 22].

CuO-NPs are very efficient in imparting antibacterial effect to fabric [7, 1]. They have been investigated as antibacterial agent against Gram-negative and Gram-positive microorganism *E. coli*. These copper oxide-plated or impregnated synthetic fibers possess broad spectrum biocidal properties: they are antibacterial, antifungal, antiviral, and they kill dust mites. Moreover, animal studies demonstrated that these fibers do not possess skin-sensitization properties [23].

3. Deposition methods

Various methods have been developed for depositing metal oxide nanoparticles on the textiles. There are only a few methods in the literature that describe the coating of fabrics with metal oxide nanoparticles, for example, the "pad-dry-cure" method [24–26], radiation, and thermal chemical treatment [4, 27, 28]. These techniques have some disadvantages: first, they are rather complicated and involve several stages; second, a stabilizer agent is used in order to get small nanoparticles, resulting in the presence of impurities in the final products. A new simple method for coating fabric surfaces with metal oxides is via ultrasound irradiation. Sonochemical irradiation has been proven as an effective technique for the synthesis of nanophased materials [1, 24, 29, 30]. The deposition and insertion of nanoparticles on/into the mesoporous ceramic and polymer supports, fabrics, and glasses is also reported [31–33]. The process involves the formation of metal oxide nanoparticles and subsequent deposition on fabrics in a one-step reaction. This coating process is not only safe and cheap but also shows that even with a low coating concentration of metal oxides in the composite, excellent antibacterial activity is maintained. In other systems, cross-linkers or binder agents are used to increase the adherence of inorganic agents NPs onto cotton fiber [17, 34–36]. In our unpublished research, surfactants were used as catalysts, which increase the homogeneity and adsorption of inorganic NPs onto cotton substrate [37].

3.1. Ultrasonic irradiation method

In this method, metal salt (CuX_2 or ZnX_2) precursor was dissolved in aqueous ethanolic solution. The pH was adjusted to 8–9 by the addition of $NH_3 \cdot H_2O$ or NaOH. The reaction mixture was irradiated with a high-intensity ultrasonic radiation under a flow of Ar. The sonication flask was placed in water bath maintained at a constant temperature of 30°C. The coated fibers were washed thoroughly with water and dried under vacuum at 60°C. The CuO- or ZnO-NPs–coated cotton fiber was obtained by the deposition of the corresponding nanoparticles onto the cotton fibers via the ultrasound irradiation of metal hydroxide according to the reaction in a similar way as previously reported [1–3].

During the formation process, a blue fresh product of $Cu(OH)_2$ is formed immediately after the addition of OH^-, which turns into brown color of copper oxide, after a few minutes of sonication. The CuO nanoparticles produced by the reaction were probably physically adsorbed onto cotton fibers (**Figure 1**).

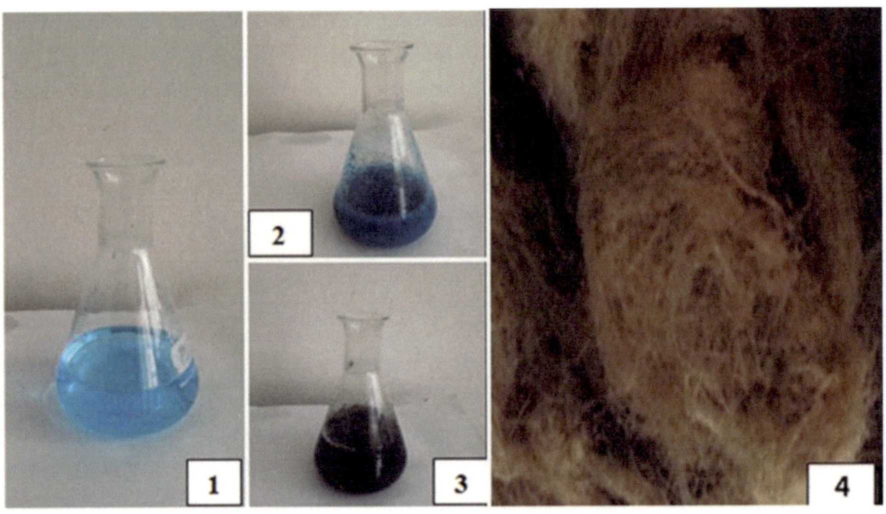

Figure 1. Coating steps of CuO-NPs onto cotton fibers: (1) aqueous solution of copper sulfate, (2) copper hydroxide "dark blue precipitate," (3) CuO-NPs, and (4) CuO-NP–coated cotton. M.Sc. thesis 2016, Islamic University Gaza.

3.2. Pad-dry-cure method

The metal oxide nanoparticles were treated with the fabric by pad-dry-cure method. Two percent of metal oxide nanoparticles were treated with 20% of wet pickup of cotton fabrics. Subsequently, these fabric samples were padded continuously for 15 min using two bowl-padding mangles. Then, the fabrics were cured at 120°C for 3 min. The excess of nanoparticles were removed by washing with sodium lauryl sulfate solution. The coated fabrics were completely washed with water and dried.

3.3. Microwave method

The thiol-modified cotton fabrics chelated with metal salt were prepared [4]. This was done by dipping the modified cotton fabrics into a conical flask containing 100 ml of metal ion solution. The flask was shaken overnight using Bench-top Shaker. Dipped fabric samples were squeezed at 100% wet pickup. Modified cotton fabrics containing metal salt were then placed in the microwave oven (MARS6, CEM microwave systems CEM GmbH, Germany) operating at a power of 1800 W and a frequency of 2455 MHz and subjected to microwave irradiation at 100°C for 5 min. Upon microwave irradiation, the cotton fabric samples gained a color corresponding to the metal oxide nanoparticles. The fabric samples containing metal oxide nanoparticles obtained were washed with double distilled water and then dried in an oven at 70°C for 1 h.

4. Influence of surfactants

Several surfactants include sodium dodecyl sulfate (SDS), cetyl trimethylammonium bromide (CTAB), Triton-X (TX)-100%, and HY were used for coating process to form metal oxide (ZnO and CuO)–coated cotton nanocomposites [37]. Surfactants were used as stabilizing agents for the metal oxide controlling their shape and size as encapsulated species within which were interacted with cellulose chain and metal oxide nanoparticles [38] (**Figure 2**).

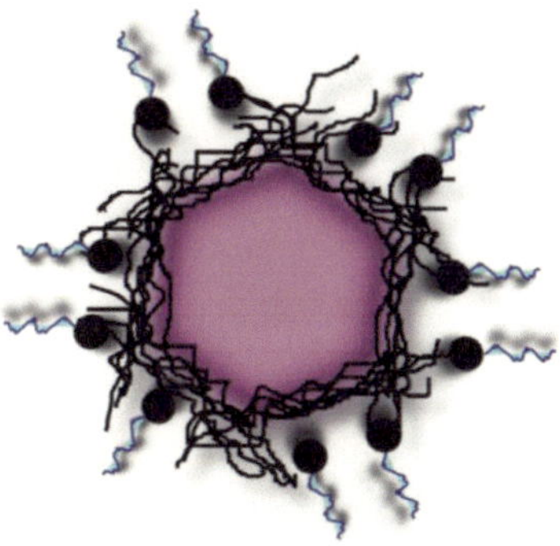

Figure 2. Interaction of ZnO with surfactant and cellulose, Manufacturing Nanostructures, chapter 4 (2014) 109-127.

5. Proposed antibacterial activity mechanism

Several studies have reported the mechanism responsible for the antibacterial action of the coated materials. The results showed that hydrogen peroxide and/or radical species are formed by the metal oxide-modified hybrid polymer, which probably contributes to the antibacterial activity. The generation of highly reactive species such as OH-H_2O_2 and O_2 is explained as follows, since both UV and UV light can activate MO with defects, electron hole pairs can be created. The holes split H_2O molecules into OH^-, H^+ and then they react with hydrogen ions to produce molecules of H_2O_2. The generated H_2O_2 can penetrate the cell membrane and kill the bacteria [39].

6. Wash durability of coated cotton materials

Wash durability test carried out on coated cotton fabrics showed that the different washing cycles resulted in significant release of MO-NPs out of the cotton substrate [37].

The results showed that CuO-NPs are adhered well onto the surface of the cotton fibers compared with ZnO-NPs (**Figure 3**).

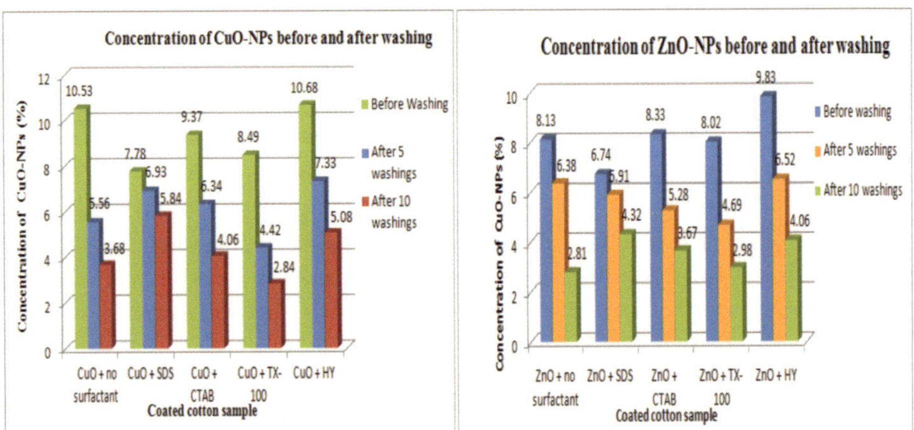

Figure 3. Concentration of CuO and ZnO-NPs before and after washing, M.Sc. thesis 2016, Islamic University Gaza.

7. Characterization methods

7.1. FTIR analysis

The infrared spectra of blank sample showed characteristic absorption peak at 3329 cm^{-1}, which is attributed to OH-stretching vibration; the band at 2887 $cm^{-1}$is assigned to the C-H-stretching vibration peak, and the band at 1427 cm^{-1} is ascribed to C-H bending vibration peak [18]. The strongest absorption peak of pristine cotton samples appears at 1037 cm^{-1}, which is characteristic of the OH-stretching vibration peak. The absorption peak at 1159 cm^{-1} is observed for all samples, which may refer to C-O-C asymmetric-stretching vibrations. The peak at 1643 cm^{-1} indicates the presence of water. FTIR spectra were recorded at room temperature for pristine- and ZnO-coated cotton fibers, respectively (**Figure 4**). Both spectra are characterized by two intense and broad bands in the range of 3300–3500 cm^{-1} and 1400–1500 cm^{-1}, assigned to the existence of hydroxyl groups on the surface [18]. It indicates that both of them show the characteristic bands of cellulose. An additional peak at 464 cm^{-1} is observed for ZnO-coated cotton fibers, which is attributed to the Zn-O vibration band [40].

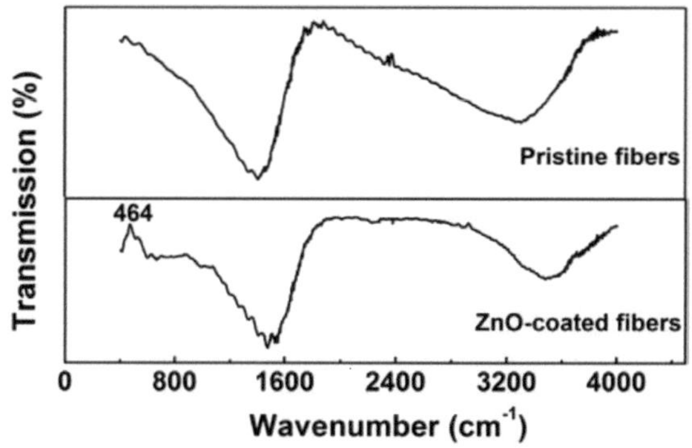

Figure 4. FTIR spectra of pristine fibers and ZnO-coated fibers, Materials Letters 65 (2011) 1316–1318.

7.2. UV/vis spectra

UV visible spectrum of ZnO nanoparticle synthesized with 0.5% soluble starch (**Figure 5**) shows an absorption peak at 361 nm. By using effective mass approximation, the size (diameter) was calculated to be 40 nm [38].

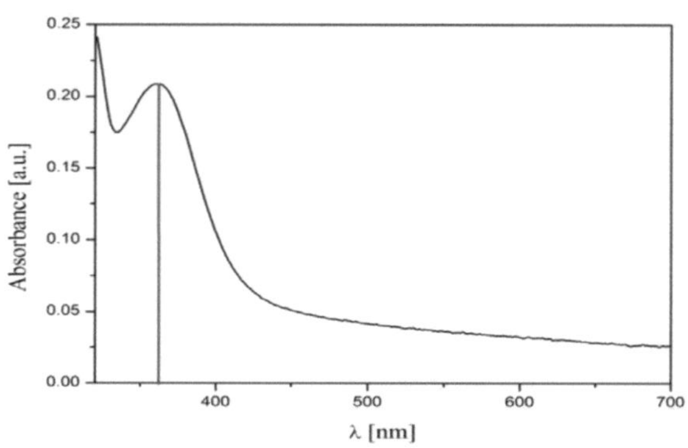

Figure 5. Absorption spectra of ZnO-NPs in ethanol. Manufacturing Nanostructures, chapter 4 (2014) 109-127.

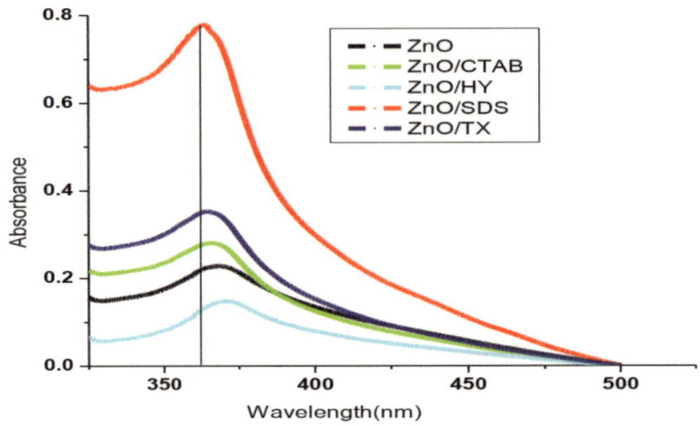

Figure 6. UV-spectra of ZnO-NPs in different surfactants, M.Sc. thesis (2015), Islamic University Gaza.

Figure 6 displays the absorption spectra of ZnO-NPs prepared in different surfactants (CTAB, HY, SDS, and TX-100). There was a blue shift of the peak maximum from 371 for ZnO/HY to 362 nm for ZnO/SDS [37]. It is also shown that the highest peak intensity was obtained when SDS was used whereas the lowest intensity resulted when HY was used. This is in consistence with the fact that smaller particles "in case of using SDS" were bound strongly to the fiber surface compared with the larger particles "in case of using HY" which were not strongly adhered to the surface. This explains why the addition of SDS shows the least leaching of CuO- and ZnO-NPs compared with HY (**Figure 3**).

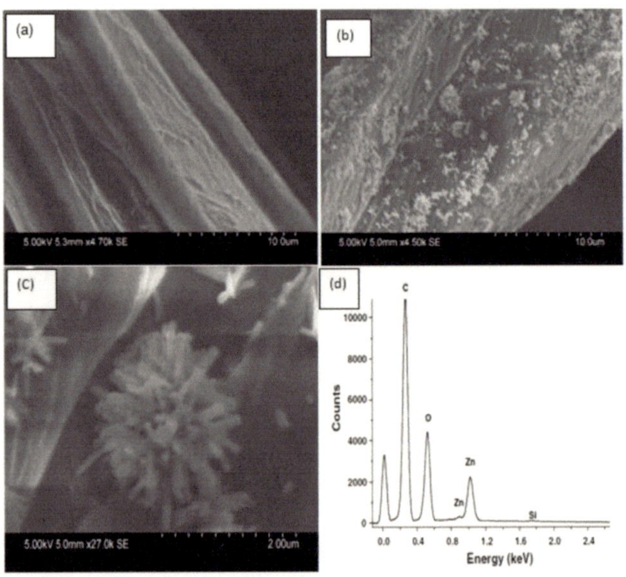

Figure 7. SEM images: (a) blank cotton, (b) ZnO-coated cotton, (c) ZnO nanorods onto cotton fiber (high magnified), and (d) EDX spectra of coated ZnO. J Mater Sci:Mater Electron 24 (2013).

7.3. SEM results

The morphology of the fiber surface before and after coating with ZnO nanoparticles was reported [3]. **Figure 7a** shows the SEM image of the original cotton fiber before coating where grooves and fibrils could be easily seen on the surface of the fiber. **Figure 7b** presents the SEM image of ZnO-NP–coated fibers, where ZnO nanoparticles can be easily observed. Under these conditions, it is found that nanorod crystals of various sizes as well as assemblies of well-defined flower of nanorods of ZnO are observed (**Figure 7c**). That is in agreement with previously reported results [41]. The chemical composition of the ZnO-coated cotton samples is presented in **Figure 7d**. EDX spectrum of the ZnO-coated cotton composite showed C, Zn, and O components.

Surfactants can play an important role in synthesizing nanomaterials of different interesting morphologies. It has found that surfactants can be used to control the size, shape, and agglomeration among the particles [37].

7.4. XRD results

The crystalline nature of the commercial ZnO and CuO was analyzed by XRD (**Figure 10a** and **b**), respectively. According to the results, the ZnO pattern is assigned to the hexagonal phase of zincite and the CuO pattern corresponds to the monoclinic tenorite phase [1–3, 16].

X-ray diffraction analysis revealed the presence of the crystalline zinc oxide on the cotton fibers (**Figure 8a**). The pattern corresponds to the hexagonal phase of ZnO. The pattern can be indexed for diffractions from the (10 0), (0 0 2), (1 0 1), (1 0 2), (1 1 0), (1 0 3), and (112) planes of wurtzite crystals. The average crystallite size of zinc oxide nanoparticles estimated by XRD data was around 12 nm, which is very close to the reported values of similar ZnO-coated cotton materials, which provides evidence that a sphere crystallite shape of ZnO is more probable.

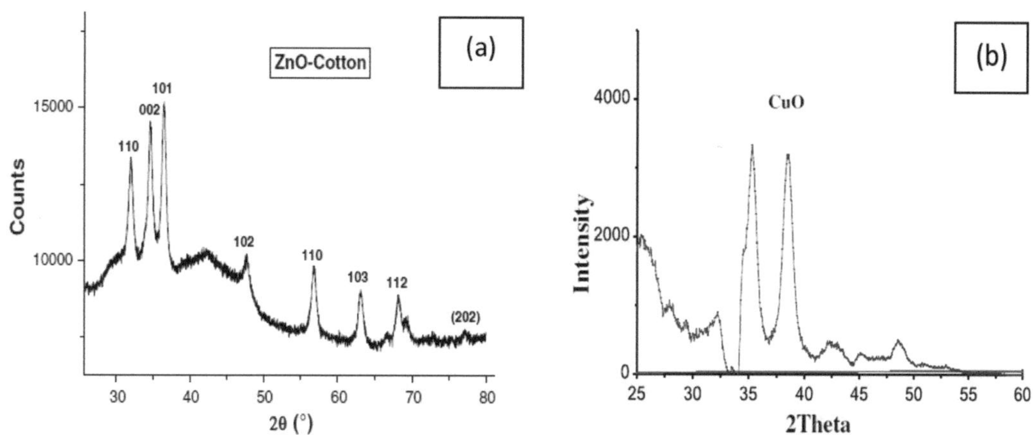

Figure 8. XRD analysis for (a) ZnO, J Mater Sci:Mater Electron 24(2013) and (b) CuO-NP–coated cotton substrate, Intern. Nano Lett. 2, 62 (2012).

The XRD pattern of the coated cotton (**Figure 8b**) reveals that copper oxide is present onto the cotton fibers. The pattern corresponds to the monoclinic phase of CuO; the diffraction peaks match very well with the PDF file 80–1916. The peaks at $2\theta = 35.53$ and 38.37 are assigned to the (−111) and (111) reflection lines of monoclinic CuO particles. Scherer's equation was used to estimate the mean size of nanoparticles.

7.5. XPS results

X-ray photoelectron spectroscopy was used to examine ZnO nanoparticle film coated onto the cotton fabrics. The survey scan XPS spectrum of cationized cotton fabric showed distinctive peaks at 283.95, 399.6, and 530.11 eV, which indicate the presence of carbon, nitrogen, and oxygen, respectively (**Figure 9a**). **Figure 9b** showed a survey scan XPS spectrum of 16 multi-layer ZnO nanoparticle film deposited on cationized cotton fabrics. Distinctive peaks at 283.95, 530.11, and 1033.7 eV indicate the presence of carbon, oxygen, and zinc, respectively.

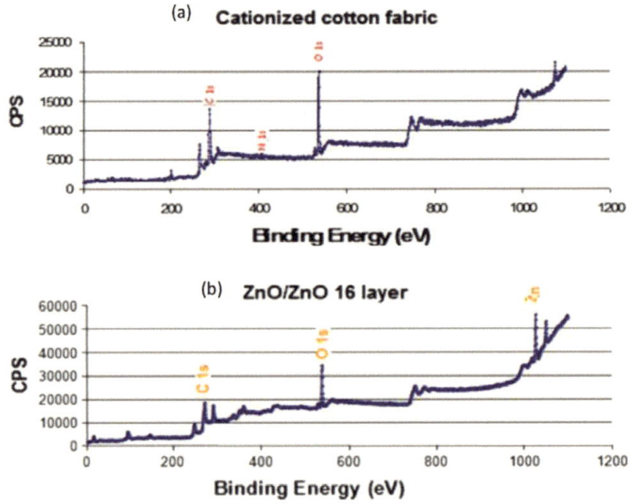

Figure 9. XPS survey for (a) cationized cotton and (b) ZnO/cotton composite, Nanoscale Res Lett 5 (2010) 1204–1210.

8. Antimicrobial activity

8.1. Antibacterial tests

Two different types of cell wall in bacteria, called Gram-positive and Gram-negative, are well known. The Gram-positive bacteria have a thick cell wall and bear many layers of peptido-glycan and teichoic acids, whereas the Gram-negative bacteria are characterized by a relatively thin cell wall with a few layers of peptides surrounded by a second lipid membrane containing lipopolysaccharides and lipoproteins.

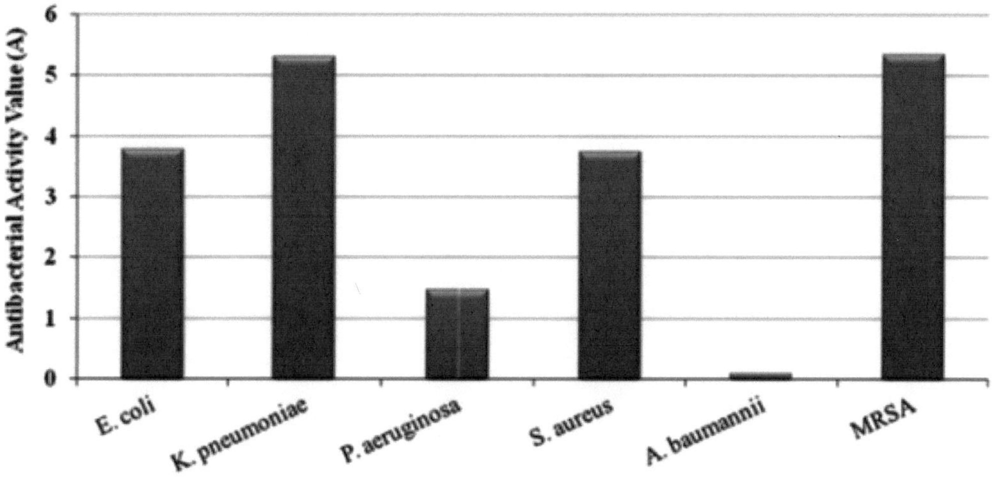

Figure 10. Antimicrobial activity of cotton coated with CuO-NPs, Applied Material Interface, 2 (2010) 1999-2004.

Coated cotton with antimicrobial activity materials (metal oxides) showed good antibacterial activity against *E. coli, K. pneumoniae, S. aureus,* and methicillin-resistant *Staphylococcus aureus* (MRSA). Less antibacterial activity was also observed against *Pseudomonas aeruginosa* and no activity was observed against *Acinetobacter baumannii* [8]. The antibacterial activity of the CuO-NP–coated fabrics was assessed using the absorption method from BS EN ISO20743:2007. The results of the analysis are shown in **Figure 10**.

The antimicrobial activity of cotton coated with ZnO-NPs and CuO-NPs was tested against *E. coli* and *S. aureus* cultures by El-Nahhal and his coworkers [3]. Their results have reported that coated cotton samples displayed high activity with a great reduction in the bacteria population. The antibacterial activity of ZnO-NPs coated onto cotton against *E. coli* is shown in **Figure 11**. No growth was observed in the tubes containing the ZnO-coated cotton as evident by the clear appearance of the tubes and the absence of growth from the subcultured samples. Similar results were observed against *S. aureus*.

Shateri-Khalilabad and Yazdanshenas [9] have confirmed that the ZnO-NP–coated cotton fabric have a good bacteriostatic activity against two representative bacteria, *K. pneumoniae* and *S. aureus,* which was demonstrated by the zone of inhibition and it was proved that the coated fibers have an excellent ability to block the UV radiation.

Singhand and his coworkers [10] have characterized the antimicrobial properties of cotton fabrics finished with ZnO-NPs against a variety of bacterial strains commonly associated with nosocomial infections, *S. aureus* and *E. coli*. In their work, they have investigated the antibacterial properties by four different tests including semi-quantitative testing: agar diffusion method, shake-flask method, quantitatively by the shake-flask method (saline), and the absorption method. The results showed a very high antimicrobial activity of ZnO-coated material against both types of bacteria, with a slightly higher activity for *S. aureus* than for *E. coli* [10].

The antibacterial activity of ZnO nanoparticles was assessed using four different methods in order to investigate the efficacy under different conditions. The ability of the antibacterial agent to inhibit bacterial growth was first tested using a disk diffusion method. Cotton disks (10 mm) with or without the ZnO nanoparticle coating were examined. **Figure 12** shows a clear zone of inhibition around ZnO-treated fabric disk, with higher inhibition zone against *S. aureus as compared with E. coli.*

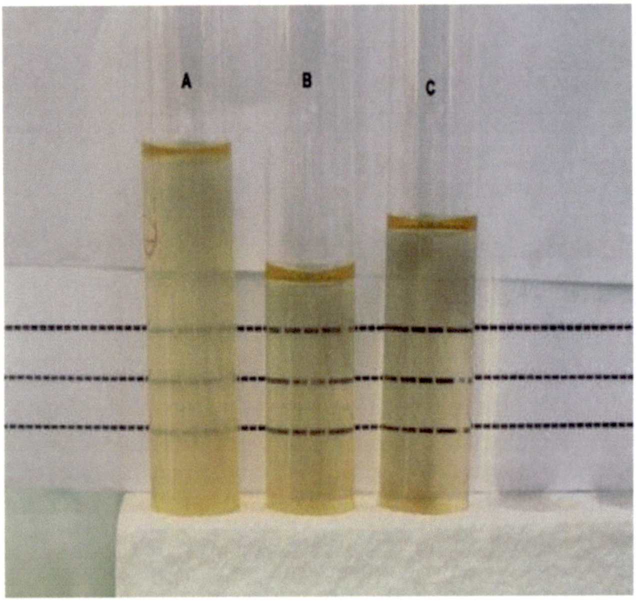

Figure 11. Photos of antimicrobial activity of ZnO-NPs/cotton, J Mater Sci:Mater Electron 24 (2013) 3970–3975, (middle sample; right negative control).

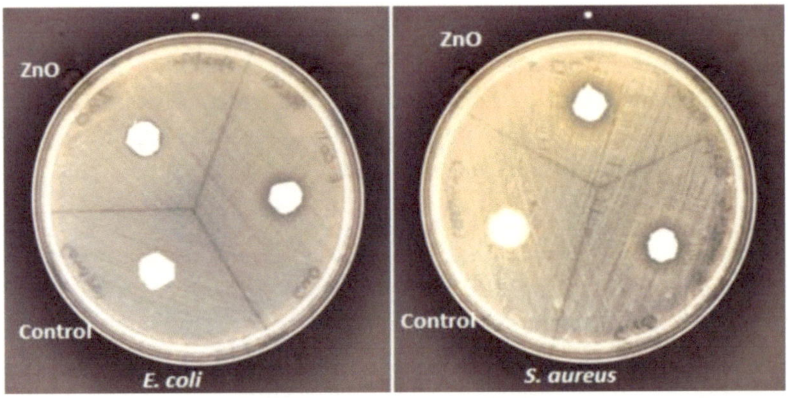

Figure 12. Antibacterial activity of ZnO-NP-treated fabrics by a disk diffusion method, J Microbial Biotechnol Food Sci 2(2012) 106-120.

The antibacterial activity of ZnO-coated cotton was determined using two shake-flask methods, with nutrient broth, and saline as media. The bacterial growth was monitored by measuring the optical density of the medium versus time. **Figure 13** shows the change in absorbance over time. A very high antimicrobial activity was seen against both bacteria.

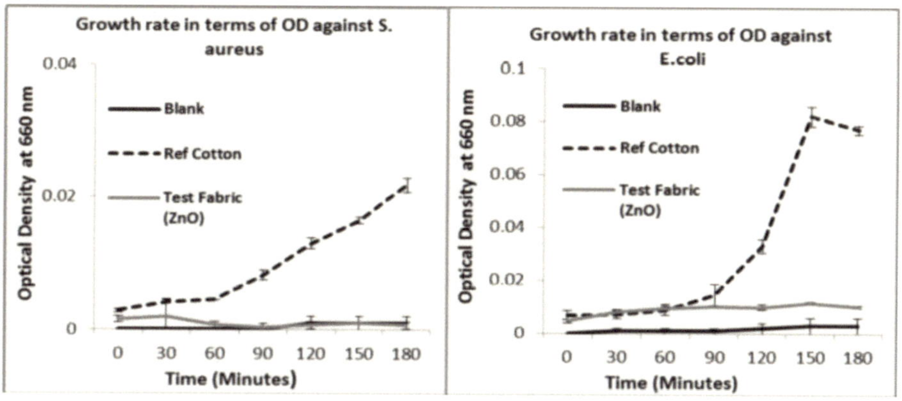

Figure 13. Graphs showing change in absorbance over time (3 h) for nutrient broth shake and flask tests, J Microbiol Biotechnol Food Sci 2(2012) 106-120.

The antibacterial activity of the finished fabrics was assessed against *S. aureus* and *E. coli*, qualitatively by agar diffusion, parallel streak method, and quantitatively by percentage reduction test. The results demonstrated that ZnO-NP–coated cotton fabrics showed higher antimicrobial activity against *S. aureus* in both qualitative and quantitative tests [11]. The results of the qualitative antibacterial assessment by agar diffusion show that the fabric sample treated with ZnO-NPs showed a maximum inhibitory effect against *S. aureus*. It is observed that the ZnO-NP-treated fabric showed higher antibacterial activity when compared with ZnO bulk-treated fabrics, whereas the untreated fabrics showed no antibacterial activity (**Figure 14a–c**).

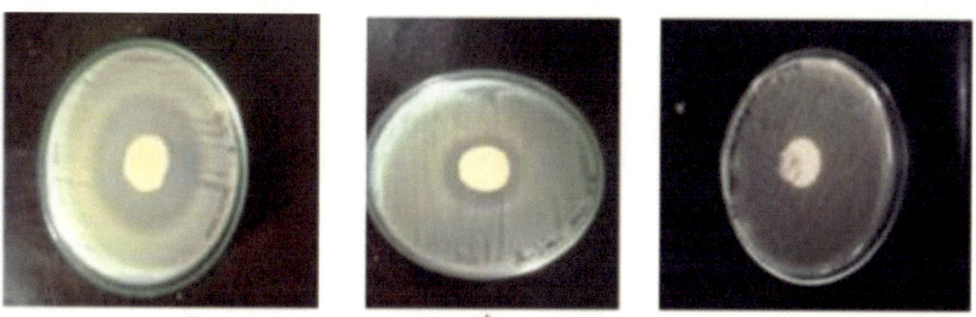

Figure 14. Antibacterial activity of (a) ZnO-NP-treated fabric, (b) ZnO bulk-treated fabric, and (c) untreated fabric (control) by disk diffusion method, International Journal of Engineering, Science.

Perelshtein and his colleagues [42] have prepared CuO-NP–coated cotton bandages and tested their antimicrobial activity against *E. coli* and *S. aureus*. The viable bacteria were monitored by counting the number of colony-forming units from the appropriate dilution on nutrient agar plates. As shown in **Figure 15**, treatment for 1 h with the coated cotton leads to the complete inhibition of *E. coli* and *S. aureus* growth [42].

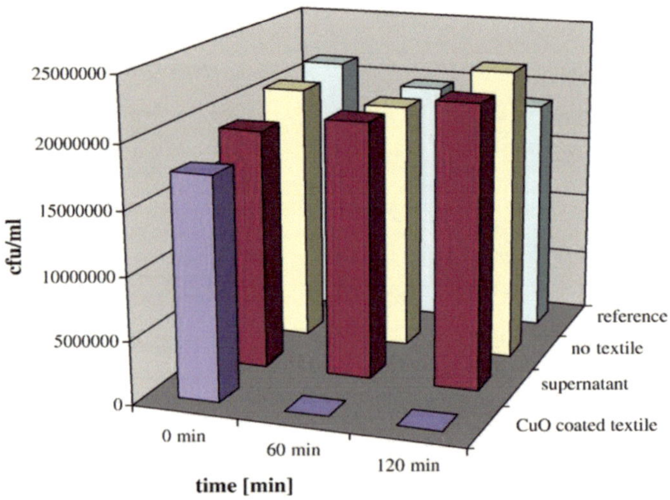

Figure 15. Antimicrobial activity of the CuO-coated bandages against *E. coli* and *S. aureus*, Surf Coat Technol204, 1-2, (2009) 54-57.

Vigneshwaran and his team [12] have prepared ZnO-soluble starch nanocomposites using water as a solvent and soluble starch as a stabilizer. The synthesized ZnO-NPs of 38 ± 3 nm were then impregnated onto cotton fabrics and its antibacterial and UV protection functions of ZnO-NP–coated cotton fabrics were studied. It was reported that the ZnO-NP–coated cotton fabrics showed an excellent antibacterial activity against two representative bacteria, *S. aureus* and *K. pneumoniae*. In addition, nano-ZnO impregnation enhanced the protection of cotton fabrics against UV radiation in comparison with the untreated cotton fabrics [12].

The antibacterial properties of nanometal oxides (ZnO, CuO) are based on the formation of reactive oxygen species (ROS). This work reveals that the antibacterial properties of these nanometal oxides are strongly dependent on their crystalline structure. The sonochemically prepared nanometal oxides are better antimicrobials than commercially available metal oxides with the same particle size range [16].

8.2. Antifungal test

The ZnO and CuO NP–coated cotton composites were assessed and investigated for antifungal activity against *Candida albicans* and *Microsporum canis* [37]. The results showed that both CuO-NP- and ZnO-NP–coated cotton showed greater antifungal activity against *C. albicans* compared with *M. canis* and that CuO-NP–coated cotton has greater activity against both fungal species (*C. albicans* and *M. canis)* compared with ZnO-NP–coated cotton (**Figure 16**). It was also shown that NP-coated cotton fabric was able to retain the antifungal activity against both fungal species even after 10 washes. However, this activity (expressed as % reduction) was reduced as the number of washes increased.

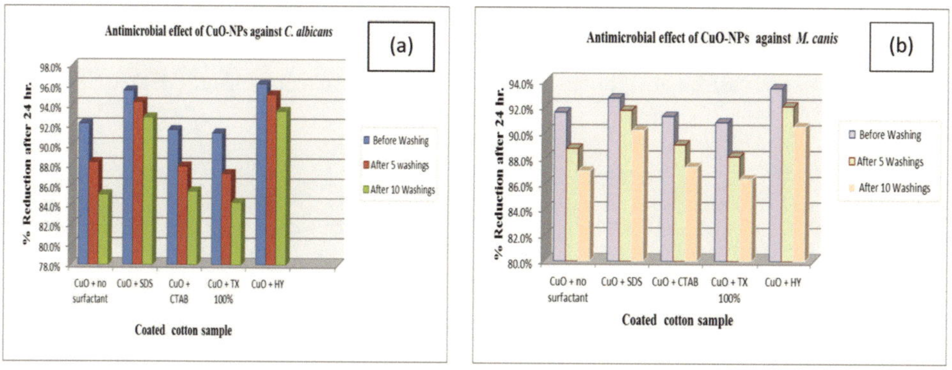

Figure 16. Antifungal activity of CuO-NPs against (a) *Candida albicans* and (b) *Microsporum canis*, M.Sc. thesis 2016, Islamic University Gaza.

9. Conclusion

In this chapter, selected studies dealing with the development of antimicrobial metal oxide–coated cotton nanocomposites and their antimicrobial applications have been reviewed with respect to the synthesis of metal oxide NP–coated cotton composites and their application for antimicrobial activities. The deposition onto cotton fibers was conducted in various methods: high-energy γ-radiation, thermal treatment-assisted impregnation, and "pad-dry-cure" of the impregnated fabric in the colloid formulation of metal oxide nanocomposites; these methods are mostly based on long-duration multistage procedures and require some binding agents for the anchoring of the nanoparticles onto the substrate. A third effective method was used for the synthesis and deposition of nanoparticles onto the substrate in a one-step process without using any type of binding agents. This method was based on using ultrasonic radiations. It has been demonstrated that the use of surfactants increased the durability of the NPs and its activity in the coated fabric. The results showed that there was subsequent decrease in the concentration of the adsorbed NPs accompanied with reduction in the antibacterial efficiency as the number of washes increased. SDS was the most effective surfactant in minimizing the leaching of both MO-NPs and it helped in getting the smallest size for CuO and metal oxides. The physical and chemical characteristics of the cotton-coated material prepared in the presence of surfactants were markedly different from those prepared in the absence of surfactants. It is also shown that the size of the MO-NPs, which were obtained when surfactants were used, is smaller than that obtained in the absence of surfactants.

The coated metal oxide nanoparticles have shown an effective enhancement for protection against UV radiation and antimicrobial activity, and they reduce the chance of disease originating from hospital infections. In this work, the antibacterial and antifungal activities were examined by several different methods. The results showed a very high antimicrobial activity of metal oxide–coated material against both types of bacteria, with a slightly higher activity for *S. aureus* than for *E. coli*. The morphology of the cotton-coated metal oxide nanoparticles and their chemical structure. Several methods have been employed for their chemical and structural characterization, and these include UV-vis spectrophotometer, FTIR, SEM, XRD, and XPS.

Author details

Issa M. El Nahhal[1*], Abdelraouf A. Elmanama[2] and Nadia M. Amara[2]

*Address all correspondence to: issanahhal@hotmail.com

1 Al-Azhar University of Gaza, Gaza, Palestine

2 Islamic University of Gaza, Gaza, Palestine

References

[1] Perelshtein I, Applerot G, Perkas N, Wehrchuetz-Sigl E, Hasmann A, Guebitz G M, Gedanken A, Sonochemical co-deposition of antibacterial nanoparticles and dyes on textiles. Surf Coat Technol. 2009;204:54–57. DOI:10.1016/j.surfcoat.2009.06.028

[2] El Nahhal I M, Zourab S M, Kodeh F, Selman M, Genoid I, Babonneau F, Nanostructured copper oxide–cotton fibers: synthesis, characterization and applications. Intern Nano Lett. 2012;2:14:1–5. DOI:10.1186/2228-5326-2-14

[3] El Nahhal I M, Zourab S M, Kodeh F S, Elmanama A, Selman M, Genois I, Babonneau F, Nano-structured zinc oxide–cotton fibers: synthesis, characterization and applications. J Mater Sci: Mater Electron. 2013;24:3970–3975. DOI:10.1007/s10854-013-1349-1

[4] Gouda M, Aljaafari A, Al-Fayz W E, Preparation and characterization of some nanometal oxides using microwave technique and their application to cotton fabrics. J Nanomater. 2015; 2015:1–9. DOI:10.1155/2015/586904

[5] Harifi T, Montazer M, A review on textile sonoprocessing: a special focus on sonosynthesis of nanomaterials on textile substrates. Ultrason Sonochem. 2015;23:1–10. DOI: 10.1016/j.ultsonch.2014.08.022

[6] Firdhouse M J, Lalitha P, Fabrication of antimicrobial perspiration pads and cotton cloth using amaranthusdubius mediated silver nanoparticles, J Chem. 2013;2013:1–5. DOI:org/10.1155/2013/741743

[7] Abramov OV, Gedanken A, Koltypin Y, Perkas N, Perelshtein I, Joyce E, Mason T. Pilot scale sonochemical coating of nanoparticles onto textiles to produce biocidal fabrics. J Surf Coat Technol. 2009;204:718–722. DOI:10.1016/j.surfcoat.2009.09.030

[8] Abramov A, Gedanken A, Popov V, Ooi E-H, Mason T J, Joyce E, M, Beddow J, Perelshtein I, Bayazitov V, A sonochemical technology for coating of textiles with antibacterial nanoparticles and equipment for its implementation. Mater Lett. 2013;96:121–124. DOI:10.1016/j.matlet.2013.01.041

[9] Shateri-Khalilabad M, Yazdanshenas M E, Bifunctionalization of cotton textiles by ZnO nanostructures: antimicrobial activity and ultraviolet protection. Text Res J. 2013;83:993–1004. DOI:10.1177/0040517512468812

[10] Singh G, Joyce E M, Beddow J, Mason T J, Evaluation of antibacterial activity of ZnO nanoparticles. J Microbiol Biotechnol Food Sci. 2012;2:106–120. DOI:org/10.1039/C2JM31054F

[11] Rajendran R, Balakumar C, Ahammed H A M, Jayakumar S, Vaideki K Rajesh E, Use of zinc oxide nano particles for production of antimicrobial textiles. Int J Eng Sci Technol. 2010;2:202–208.

[12] Vigneshwaran N, Kumar S, Kathe A, Varadarajan P, Prasad V, Functional finishing of cotton fabrics using zinc oxide-soluble starch nanocomposites. Nanotechnology. 2006;17:5087.http://dx.doi.org/10.1088/0957-4484/17/20/008

[13] Perelshtein I, Applerot G, Perkas N, Grinblat J, Hulla E, Wehrschuetz-Sigl E, Hasmann A, Guebitz G, Gedanken A, Ultrasound radiation as a "throwing stones" technique for the production of antibacterial nanocomposite textiles. Appl Mater Interf. 2010;2:1999–2004. DOI:10.1021/am100291w

[14] Sedighi A, Montazer M, Samadi N, Synthesis of nano Cu2O on cotton:morphological, physical, biological and optical sensing characterizations. Carbohydr Polym. 2014;110:489–498. DOI:10.1016/j.carbpol.2014.04.030

[15] Manna A C, Synthesis, characterization, and antimicrobial activity of zinc oxide nanoparticles. Nano-Antimicrobials. 2012; 151–180. DOI:10.1007/978-3-642-24428-5_5

[16] Perelshtein I, Lipovsky A, Perkas N, Gedanken A, Moschini E, Mantecca P, The influence of the crystalline nature of nano-metal oxides on their antibacterial and toxicity properties. Nano Research. 2015;8:695–707. DOI:10.1007/s12274-014-0553-5.

[17] Ugˇur S S, Sarıısık M, Aktas A H, Ucar M C¸ Erden E, Modifying of cotton fabric surface with nano-ZnO multilayer films by layer-by-layer deposition method. Nanoscale Res Lett. 2010;5:1204–1210. DOI:10.1007/s11671-010-9627-9

[18] Hongjun W, AnvarZakirov S U, Yuldashev J L, Dejun Fu T K, ZnO films grown on cotton fibers surface at low temperature by a simple two-step process. Mater Lett. 2011;65:1316–1318. DOI:10.1016/j.matlet.2011.01.072

[19] Sawai J, Quantitative evaluation of antibacterial activities of metallic oxide powders (ZnO, MgO and CaO) by conductimetricassay. J Microbiol Methods. 2003;54:177–182. DOI:10.1016/S0167-7012(03)00037-X

[20] Coyle S, Wu Y, Lau K T, De Rossi D, Wallace G, Smart nanotextiles:a review of materials and applications. MRS Bull. 2007;32:434–442. DOI:http://dx.DOI:.org/10.1557/mrs2007.67

[21] Stoimenov P K, Klinger R L, Marchin G L, Klabunde K, Metal oxide nanoparticles as bactericidal agents. J Langmuir. 2002;18:6679–6686. DOI:10.1021/la0202374

[22] Axtell H C; Hartley S M; Sallavanti R A. U.S. Patent 5,026,778, 2005.

[23] Borkow G, Gabbay J. Putting copper into action: copper-impregnated products with potent biocidal activities. FASEB J. 2004;18:1728–1730. DOI:10.1096/fj.04-2029fje

[24] Vigneshwaran N, Kumar S, Kathe A A, Varadarajan P V, Functional finishing of cotton fabrics using zinc oxide–soluble starch nanocomposites. Nanotechnology. 2006;17:5087–5095. DOI:http://dx.doi.org/10.1088/0957-4484/17/20/008

[25] Anita S, Ramachandran T, Rajendran R, Koushik C, Mahalakshmi M, A study of the antimicrobial property of encapsulated copper oxide nanoparticles on cotton fabric. Text Res J. 2011;81:1081–1088. DOI:10.1177/0040517510397577

[26] Xu B, Cai Z, Fabrication of a superhydrophobicZnOnanorod array film on cotton fabrics via a wet chemical route and hydrophobic modification. Appl Surf Sci. 2008;254:5899–5904. DOI:10.1016/j.apsusc.2008.03.160

[27] Borkow G, Gabbay Copper, An ancient remedy returning to fight microbial, fungal and viral infections. J Curr Chem Biol. 2009;3:272–278. DOI:10.2174/187231309789054887

[28] El-Naggar A M, Zohdy M H, Hassan M S, Khalil, E M, Antimicrobial protection of cotton and cotton/polyester fabrics by radiation and thermal treatments. I. Effect of ZnO formulation on the mechanical and dyeing properties. J Appl Polym Sci. 2003;88:1129–1137. DOI:10.1002/app.11722

[29] Gedanken A, Using sonochemistry for the fabrication of nanomaterials. Ultrason Sonochem. 2004;11:47–55. DOI:10.1016/j.ultsonch.2004.01.037

[30] Perkas N, Amirian G, Dubinsky S, Gazit S, Gedanken A, Ultrasound-assisted coating of nylon 6,6 with silver nanoparticles and its antibacterial activity. J Appl Polym Sci. 2007;104:1423–1430.DOI:10.1002/app.24728

[31] Kotlyar A, Perkas N, Amiryan G, Meyer M, Zimmermann W, Gedanken A, Coating silver nanoparticles on poly(methyl methacrylate) chips and spheres via ultrasound

irradiation. J Appl Polym Sci. 2007;104:2868–2876. DOI:10.1002/app.25893Key:citeulike:5687740

[32] Pol V G, Srivastava D N, Palchik O, Palchik V, Slifkin M A, Weiss A M, Gedanken A, Sonochemical deposition of silver nanoparticles on silica spheres A. Langmuir. 2002;18:3352–3357. DOI:10.1021/la0155552

[33] Pol V G, Wildermuth G, Felsche J, Gedanken A, Calderon-Moreno J,Antimicrobial protection of cotton and cotton/polyester fabrics by radiation and thermal treatments. Effect of ZnO formulation on the mechanical and dyeing properties. J Nanosci Nanotechnol. 2005;5:975–979. DOI:10.1002/app.11722

[34] Xu ZJ, Tian YL, Liu HL, Du ZQ, A situ hydrothermal synthesis of $SrTiO_3/TiO_2$ heterostructurenanosheets with exposed (0 0 1) facets for enhancing photocatalytic degradation activity. Appl Surf Sci, 2015;324:68–75.DOI:10.1016/j.apsusc.2014.07.100

[35] Galkina O L, Sycheva A, Blagodatskiy A, Kaptay G, Katanaev V L, Seisenbaeva G V, Kessler V G, Agafonov A V, The sol–gel synthesis of cotton/TiO_2 composites and their antibacterial properties. Surf Coat Technol. 2014;253:171–179. DOI:10.1016/j.surfcoat.2014.05.033

[36] Kalimuthan R, MahalingamS, Grafting of cellulose fabric using PVP with MgO nanoparticles for improve performance of bacterial and fungal pathogens. World J Pharm Pharm Sci. 2014;13:1989–2004.

[37] Amara N M, Antibacterial and antifungal activity of metal oxides nanoparticles coated onto cotton fibers [MSc thesis]. Islamic University, Gaza; 2016.

[38] Marta Fiedot, Olga Ra, PatrycjaSuchorska Woźniak, IwonaKarbownik, Helena Teterycz.Polymer-surfactant interactions and their influence on zinc oxide nanoparticles morphology. In: Waqar Ahmed and Nasar Ali, editors, Manufacturing nanostructures; 2014, pp. 108–127. ISBN (eBook):9781910086070.

[39] Blake D M, Maness P-C, Huang Z, Wolfrum E J, Jacoby W A, Huang application of the photocatalytic chemistry of titanium dioxide to disinfection and the killing of cancer cells. J Sep Purif Methods. 1999;28:1–50. DOI:10.1080/03602549909351643

[40] Bagreev S, Bashkova DC, Locke TJ, Bandos, Sewage sludge-derived materials as efficient adsorbents for removal of hydrogen sulfide. Environ Sci Tech. 2001;35:1537–1543. DOI:10.1021/es001678h

[41] Cullity BD, Elements of x-ray diffraction, 2nd edition. Addison-Wesley, Reading. ISBN 10:0201011743 ISBN 13:9780201011746

[42] Perelshtein I, Applerot G, Perkas N, Wehrschetz-Sigl E, Hasmann A, Guebitz G, Gedanken A, Antibacterial properties of an in situ generated and simultaneously deposited nanocrystallineZnO on fabrics. ACS Appl Mater Interf. 2008;1:361–366.DOI:10.1021/am8000743